Diagnostic and Interventional Radiology in Gynecological and Obstetric Diseases

Raffaella Niola • Antonio Pinto
Francesco Giurazza
Editors

Diagnostic and Interventional Radiology in Gynecological and Obstetric Diseases

Springer

Editors
Raffaella Niola
Vascular and Interventional Radiology Department
Ospedale Antonio Cardarelli
Naples, Italy

Antonio Pinto
Radiology Department
Azienda Ospedaliera Dei Colli-CTO
Naples, Italy

Francesco Giurazza
Vascular and Interventional Radiology Department
Ospedale Antonio Cardarelli
Naples, Italy

ISBN 978-3-031-11909-5 ISBN 978-3-031-11910-1 (eBook)
https://doi.org/10.1007/978-3-031-11910-1

This Springer imprint is published by the registered company Springer Nature Switzerland AG
The registered company address is: Gewerbestrasse 11, 6330 Cham, Switzerland

Foreword

Most people think of Radiology as a diagnostic specialty. Of course, it plays an essential role in diagnosis in obstetrics and gynecology. But it is also used successfully to guide minimally invasive interventions and so effective treatment. Interventional Radiology has grown out of the diagnostic imaging specialty and has come a long way since it was first conceived by Charles Dotter. Its increasingly successful application is due not only to technological advances in equipment but also to the imagination of its proponents who have applied their skills across all specialties and lobbied for its inclusion in modern medicine.

This has led to profound changes in the way many conditions are now managed from trauma, peripheral vascular disease, cancer, and prostate disease to fibroids and massive obstetric hemorrhage. The application of interventional radiology in obstetrics and gynecology is particularly important to this predominantly young, well informed and otherwise healthy group of women. It is a tragedy when a young mother loses her life or womb because placenta percreta has not been diagnosed before delivery and the chance missed to plan her management including interventional radiology to help control hemorrhage.

For Interventional Radiology to be successfully applied in O&G, we not only need a cohort of skilled interventional radiologists willing to fully participate in the clinical management of these women but also obstetricians and gynecologists with open minds and a willingness to understand how these new techniques and their colleagues in Interventional Radiology are integral to their service.

Collaboration and combining the skills of obstetricians, gynecologists, and interventional radiologists broadens treatment options, leads to new therapeutic methods, and improves outcomes for women. This book and its contributors show the way.

Anna Maria Belli

Radiology Department
St George's Hospital and Medical School
London, UK

Preface

First time we (my coworkers and I) approached the role of Interventional Radiology in Obstetrics and Gynecology, many years ago, were not thought to walk so fast ahead.

When one looks at the place that uterine embolization has in the current management in Obstetrics and Gynecology, it seems a long way from the genesis of the procedure.

Especially about the predelivery embolization in preventing PPH.

Personally, my "primum movens" for going ahead in the way of uterine arteries embolization in PPH was the silhouette I met, of a child, orphan, whose mother died due to PPH; he looked so alone, sad, serious, shy. He was living with his two sad grandparents in a big, dark, old house.

What's happened to me? I felt something telling me to study, to try to help in avoiding women suffering from hemorrhage during the childbirth.

PPH is still the first cause of mother mortality in the world.

Interventional Radiology treatment, by using embolization of uterine arteries, seems to make a great deal in avoiding/decreasing hemorrhage, and anyway reduces the number of transfused blood units.

Applying this concept to the other O&G diseases, we realize the infinity of possibilities Interventional Radiology has, not only for PPH, but for ectopic pregnancy, AVM, fibroid, cancer, before surgery, and bail-out.

All these aspects and more will be described in details in this book, that collects our intentions to give to Interventional Radiologists and trainees especially, suggestions about this interesting field.

I am pleased to introduce this text to you; hopefully, it will help providers caring for patients undergoing these procedures to understand techniques and related clinical managements.

Many thanks to the colleagues who helped us in this adventure.

Special thanks to Professor Anna Maria Belli, a great woman and Interventional Radiologist, who accepted to write the preface for this book.

Naples, Italy Raffaella Niola

Introduction

Nowadays, the multidisciplinary approach is the key factor for the success of any medical challenge.

In obstetric and gynecological diseases, the gynecologist is supported by multiple medical figures including anesthesiologists, neonatologists, and radiologists [1]; the strict cooperation between gynecologists and radiologists allows to improve the diagnostic process and the quality of the medical care. In order to be part of the decisional process, radiologists need to learn clinical skills from colleagues involved in women health.

This book focuses mainly on interventional radiology (IR); however, fine diagnostic radiology is of paramount importance for any procedure the interventionalists perform: it represents the basis for the primary diagnosis, but also for procedural planning and treatment outcome evaluation. No interventional radiologist can approach properly a procedure without having clearly performed the diagnostic radiological process.

Both obstetric and gynecological diseases are analyzed with first level (Ultrasound) and second level radiological examinations (Computed Tomography and Magnetic Resonance). In the first section of this book, the main aspects of diagnostic radiology in these fields are reviewed.

Section II is dedicated to the general aspects that an interventional radiologist should be aware of before starting any procedure: materials, radioprotection, pharmacology, and safety are part of the basilar background.

The materials development, sustained by industries, requires a continuous update of the operators; the technological progress allows to expand the boundaries of the percutaneous procedures and the global number of interventions performed is growing year by year.

The radioprotection is a hot topic in IR community; in Europe, the recent directive 2013/59/EURATOM [2] has included the dosimetric information into all radiological reports. The new radiological apparels allow to reduce the radiations emission in both CT scans and angiographic procedures; however, especially in young women, radioprotection is a crucial aspect to consider.

The pharmacology is another aspect to analyze carefully in any procedure, considering also drugs assumed before the intervention and prescribed thereafter.

The last chapter of Section II focuses on ethics and safety; all radiologists, both diagnostic and interventional, act in the boundaries of these principles.

Section III focuses on IR in gynecological diseases; endovascular, percutaneous and extracorporeal techniques will be described. In 1995, Ravina introduced embolization for uterine myomas [3], today the most applied IR procedure in women health; interestingly, he was a gynecologist and already understood the potential of cooperation with IR. Today, myomas can be treated also by percutaneous ablation and even extracorporeal high intensity focused ultrasound. Furthermore, the number of diseases treated with mini-invasive methods has grown, apart from myomas; the range of pathologies managed with IR includes many other conditions, from infertility due to Fallopian tube occlusion, to pelvic congestion syndrome, arteriovenous malformations and malignancies.

On the other hand, Section IV analyzes the role of IR in the obstetrics scenario; here, IR includes both elective and emergent procedures. The goal of elective interventions is to occlude definitively or temporarily the uterine arteries to minimize the risk of a possible bleeding; instead, in emergency embolization must interrupt an already existing hemorrhage. Thanks to the progress of diagnostic radiology, more and more patients receive an antenatal diagnosis of placental anomalies; these patients, at high risk for uterine hemorrhage, should be referred to trained centers where proper endovascular preventive strategies could be applied to avoid dramatic life-threatening bleedings.

In this book, the main aspects of all these arguments are discussed; the table of content has been designed to provide an overview of all the modern IR procedures applicable in these fields. Certainly, readers will not perform all of the mentioned techniques in their daily practice; however, the authors have provided all efforts to transmit to students, residents, and trainees the basilar concepts to understand the relevance of diagnostic and interventional radiology in these scenarios; already trained radiologists will find a quick refresher of their knowledge and may receive the adequate stimulus to expand their interests in modern interventional procedures in gynecological and obstetric diseases.

References

1. Weston M, Soyer P, Barral M, et al. Role of interventional procedures in obstetrics and gynecology. Radiol Clin North Am. 2020;58(2):445–62.
2. European Society of Radiology (ESR). Summary of the European Directive 2013/59/Euratom: essentials for health professionals in radiology. Insights Imaging 2015;6(4):411–7.
3. Ravina J H, Herbreteau D, Ciraru-Vigneron N, et al. Arterial embolisation to treat uterine myomata. Lancet 1995;346:671–72.

Radiology Department, Azienda Ospedaliera dei Colli—CTO Napoli
Naples, Italy
Raffaella Niola
Francesco Giurazza

UOC Radiologia Vascolare e Interventistica
AORN Cardarelli di Napoli
Naples, Italy
Antonio Pinto

Contents

Part I

Imaging

Imaging in Gynecology

1

Francesca Iacobellis, Marco Di Serafino, and Luigia Romano

1.1 Introduction

Several imaging techniques can be adopted to image the female genital tract. The choice of the most suitable imaging approach and the related imaging protocols varies depending on the clinical indications and patient's conditions. In this chapter, the role of each imaging method in the gynaecological setting will be briefly reviewed, as well as the most common pathologies, particularly considering those of interventional radiology interest.

1.2 Imaging Methods

1.2.1 Ultrasound

Pelvic ultrasound (US) is considered the ideal investigative tool to adopt as first-line examination for suspected gynaecological disorders in patients of all ages. It has the advantages of being widely available, inexpensive, and free from ionising radiation, but on the other hand, the examination may be variably limited by patient habitus, presence of pelvic cutaneous medication, and bowel overdistension. Transabdominal sonography (TAS) and transvaginal sonography (TVS) are complementary techniques [1]; saline infusion sonohysterography (SIS) is another technique that is sometimes used for further specific evaluation (Table 1.1) [1].

F. Iacobellis · M. Di Serafino · L. Romano (✉)
Department of General and Emergency Radiology, Ospedale Antonio Cardarelli, Naples, Italy

R. Niola et al. (eds.), *Diagnostic and Interventional Radiology in Gynecological and Obstetric Diseases*, https://doi.org/10.1007/978-3-031-11910-1_1

Table 1.1 Sonographic methods, protocol, utility, and limits for examining the female pelvis

Sonographic methods	Probe	Protocol	Utility	Limits
Transabdominal sonography (TAS)	Lowfrequency probe (convex probe 3–5 MHz)	The standard protocol for examining the female pelvis involves an initial TAS with the urinary bladder completely full, so it can act as an acoustic window. Following bladder emptying, the patient assumes a lithotomy position, and TVS is performed. The two imaging techniques are complementary and often provide different diagnostic information	TAS offers a wider field of view than TVS and allows better visualisation of the superficial and distal structures of the vagina by bringing the probe closer to the target organs	• Empty bladder • Obese patients • Retroverse uterus where the fundus is located beyond the focal zone of the transducer • Less effective for characterisation of adnexal masses
Transvaginal sonography (TVS)	High-frequency probe (endocavitary probe >7 MHz)	The protocol often also calls for the execution of Doppler, power Doppler, and pulsed wave Doppler flowmetry depending on the clinical situation and pathology that emerge from grayscale imaging. The use of 3D ultrasound has also become standard, and it is particularly useful for assessing the correct positioning of the IUD and submucosal leiomyomas, as well as the contour of the bottom of the uterus and foetal morphology in the case of suspected congenital anomalies	TVS approach requires a greater penetration depth to avoid the attenuating soft tissues that cover the pelvic organs. Therefore, it requires the use of a higher frequency probe, which, in turn, provides greater resolution of the anatomical details of the uterus, ovary, and adnexal structures	• Limited field of view • Should not be performed on patients who are unable or unwilling to consent to the procedure, as well as on most virgin patients and for those in which the insertion of the probe produces marked discomfort • It is contraindicated in pregnant patients
Sonohysterography with solution infusion (SIS)		SIS involves the instillation of sterile saline into the endometrial cavity under ultrasound guidance The SIS examination should be scheduled close to the fourth to seventh day of the menstrual cycle, this scheduling avoids the possibility of performing the examination on a pregnant patient and reduce the possibility of false positive results in the study of the endometrium. In the study of endometrial cavity, false positives may be due to normal irregularities and increased thickness of the endometrium in the secretory phase of the cycle. This examination may allow also the evaluation of Fallopian tube patency	SIS is a simple, low-cost, minimally invasive exam with a high level of diagnostic accuracy. SIS is more sensitive than TVS for the detection of focal endometrial anomalies and is equivalent to hysteroscopy in the identification and characterisation of focal lesions. Echogenic contrast media such as air bubbles can be used, particularly when evaluating the patency of the fallopian tubes	

Sonographic methods	Probe	Protocol	Utility	Limits
Alternative approaches: Transperineal, translabial, and transrectal ultrasound	High-frequency (7–10 MHz) linear probe often alternating with low-frequency (3–5 MHz) convex probe (transperineal or translabial)	Patient evaluation does not require specific preparation except for transrectal examination, where cleansing of the rectum with enemas is recommended	Useful in evaluating the postmenopausal uterus, cervix, and lower urinary tract	• Specific local contraindications or patient refusing the transrectal access
	High-frequency (>7 MHz) endocavitary probe (transrectal)			

1.2.2 X-Ray

In gynaecological setting, X-rays are used to perform hysterosalpingography. This method has a very specific indication, where the aim is to assess the patency and the morphology of the fallopian tubes and the endometrial cavity in the diagnostic work-up of infertility [2].

1.2.3 Magnetic Resonance Imaging

Magnetic resonance imaging (MRI) is increasingly used as second-level examination to evaluate gynaecological pathologies due to its panoramicity, excellent soft-tissue contrast, its ability to provide good tissue characterisation, multiplanar imaging capabilities, and the absence of ionising radiation, that is particularly relevant in women in childbearing age. The examination can be integrated by the injection of Gadolinium-based intravenous (iv) contrast media (cm) to evaluate the vessels and tissues enhancement. The main contraindications are represented by the presence of non-MR compatible devices and by patient claustrophobia.

The imaging protocol may slightly vary depending on the clinical indication, and this is basically described in Table 1.2.

Table 1.2 MRI protocol for the study of the pelvis

Magnet	Sequences	Aim
≥1.5 T	T2-weighted (W)	Acquired in at least two orthogonal planes, oriented on the uterine axis to adequately evaluate uterine diseases or secondary uterine and parametrial involvement. Imaging in a third orthogonal plane can be performed to clarify and confirm the findings
	T1-W	Useful to compare the signal variations among them characterising oedema, blood, and fat components
	T1-W and T2-W fat suppressed (FS)	
	DWI/ADC	Increasingly used to detect high cellularity areas suspected of malignancy. With some limitations, these sequences associated with T2-W may solve diagnostic doubts, avoiding the administration of iv cm
	Dynamic three-dimensional unenhanced and contrast-enhanced T1-W FS sequences	Used when it is necessary to study vessels opacification (MR angiography) and tissue enhancement. Sequences are oriented depending on the main indication, that is sagittal, when it is mainly needed to study the uterine wall, or axial and coronal planes when a more panoramic view of the pelvis is needed

1.2.4 Computed Tomography

In the presence of an acute abdomen associated with suspected haemoperitoneum or severe vaginal bleeding, imaging is necessary for a prompt and accurate diagnosis [3].

Although US is generally the first-line abdominal and pelvic investigative modality, Multidetector Computed Tomography (CT) can provide the diagnosis of acute gynaecologic disorders when US is inconclusive or partially conclusive, or genital abnormalities extend beyond the sonographic field of view [3–6].

An exhaustive CT protocol is recommended (Table 1.3). Comparing the base-line scan with the following contrast-enhanced multiphase scans, it is possible to detect early arterial or late active bleeding and differentiate any pre-existing hyperattenuation due to calcifications, clots, or other causes, from contrast medium extravasation (Fig. 1.1) [7]. In case of intermittent haemorrhage, venous source of bleeding, or decreased perfusion related to vasospasm and hypotension, active bleeding may appear on portal or even late venous phase images (Fig. 1.2) [8].

Table 1.3 CT protocol

Scanner	Phases	Aim
MDCT	Precontrast scan	Detect pre-existing hyperattenuation due to calcifications, clots, or to other causes and differentiate them from contrast medium extravasation
	Arterial phase (acquired at 30 s after the start of iv cm injection or, better, timed with bolus tracking)	To evaluate the opacification of the arterial vessels and to detect arterial active bleeding
	Portal venous phase (acquired at 60–70 s after the start of iv cm injection)	To evaluate the opacification of the venous vessels and of the parenchymal organs, to evaluate the entity of an arterial active bleeding, and to detect a venous bleeding
	Delayed excretory venous phase (acquired at 120–160 s after the start of iv cm injection)	To detect slight minor active bleeding, to evaluate the involvement of the urinary system

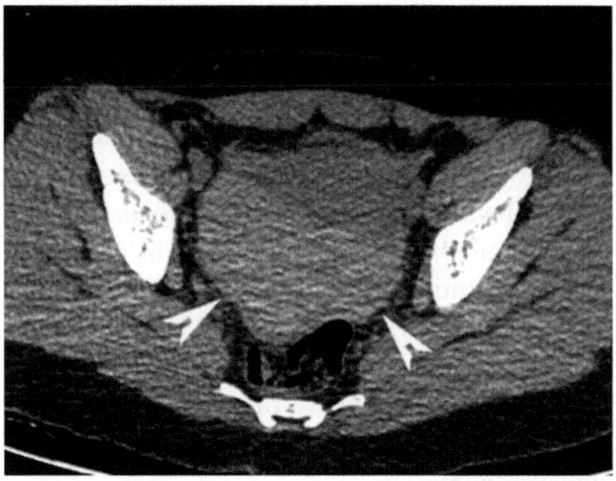

Fig. 1.1 Axial baseline CT image evidences hyperdense blood in pelvic peritoneal cavity (arrows)

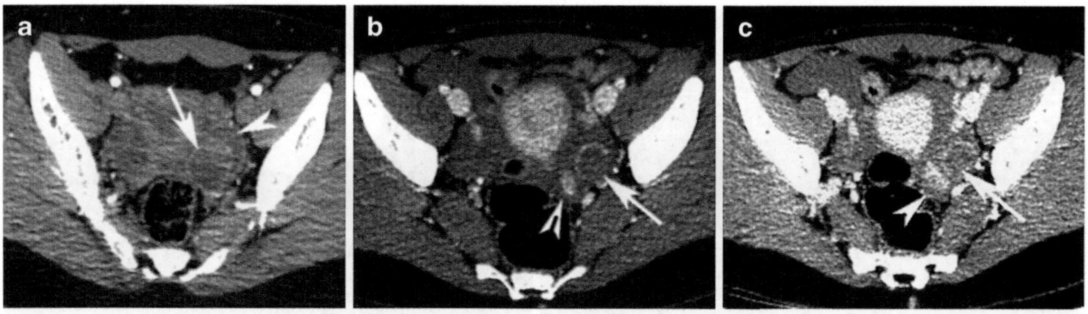

Fig. 1.2 Axial post-contrast arterial CT (**a**) phase depicts an adnexal cyst surrounded by an enhancing rim due to vascularity within the wall (**a**, arrow). There is haemoperitoneum (**a**, arrowhead) without active extravasation of contrast medium in this phase. Post-contrast portal CT phase (**b**) depicts the rupture of the cystic wall (**b**, arrow) with pooling of contrast medium in the cul-de-sac (**b**, arrowhead). Post-contrast excretory CT phase (**c**) demonstrates an enlargement of contrast medium pooling outside the haemorrhagic cyst (**c**, arrowhead)

1.3 Gynaecologic Haemorrhages

Haemorrhage associated with gynaecologic disorders is an important cause of morbidity and even mortality. The recognition and characterisation of these conditions is fundamental in order to allow timely diagnosis and appropriate treatment, frequently consisting in endovascular procedures when acute bleeding is detected [9].

1.3.1 Gynaecologic Causes of Haemoperitoneum

1.3.1.1 Haemorrhagic Ovarian Cyst

Internal haemorrhage may occur following the rupture of different kinds of adnexal cyst (Fig. 1.3), the most common type being the corpus luteum cyst (Fig. 1.4) [10–13]. In this setting, CT's role is to promptly diagnose and characterise the presence of active bleeding to orient the treatment.

Corpus Luteum Cyst

The CT characteristic of a corpus luteum is a well-circumscribed, adnexal unilocular cystic structure, surrounded by an enhancing rim due to vascularity within a thickened wall. When a corpus luteum doesn't regress, a luteal cyst develops and could be filled with blood, forming a haemorrhagic corpus luteum. Bleeding is caused by the hypervascularisation and fragile vessels of the granulosa layer within the wall of the cyst. Increased vascularity of the ovary during the luteal phase may determine the risk of rupture of the cyst wall and bleeding inside the peritoneal cavity. The rupture may often involve the right ovary because the left ovary is protected by the sigmoid colon.

At CT, non-haemorrhagic follicular and corpus luteum cysts appear as unilocular lesions, usually measuring less than 50 mm, with thin walls and homogeneous fluid with water-like attenuation. The presence of blood determines an increased attenuation (>40 Hounsfield Units, HU) within the cyst at the pre-contrast CT phase. After iv cm administration, the wall of the luteal cyst appears thicker than those of follicular cysts and highly vascularised (Fig. 1.4) [10]. The ruptured luteal cyst is seen as a discontinuity of the thickened wall, often surrounded by hyperattenuating sentinel clot sign. Occasionally, active bleeding may be detected as contrast extravasation near the cyst (Fig. 1.5) [14]. Haemoperitoneum appears as hyperdense (>40 HU) peritoneal-free fluid, with higher attenuation of the peritoneal cul-de-sac, due to clots (Fig. 1.6). In every circumstance clots may be useful in identifying the bleeding source since they generally develop close to the organ from which the haemorrhage originates ('sentinel clot' sign) [4]. After a few days, a fluid-fluid level inside the peritoneal cul-de-sac can develop. This appearance corresponds to the CT

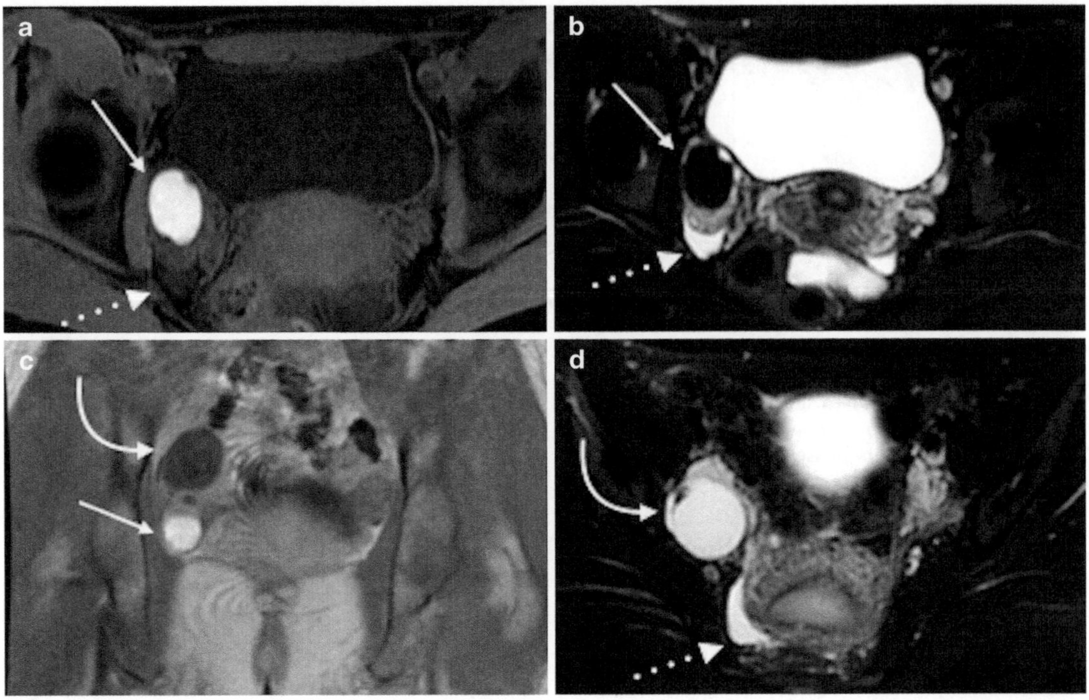

Fig. 1.3 Twenty-two-year-old patient with right iliac fossa pain: (**a**) T1-W FS axial, (**b**) T2-W FS axial, (**c**) T1-W coronal, and (**d**) T2-W FS axial sequences showing a right ovarian cyst with hyperintense content in the T1-W and T1-W FS sequences and hypointense content in T2-W FS sequences (**a–c** straight arrows) related with an early subacute intracystic bleeding. On the same ovary there is also a simple follicular cyst with hypointense content in the T1-W sequence (**c**, curved arrow) and hyperintense content in T2-W FS sequence (**d**, curved arrow). A small volume of free fluid is present in the pelvis (**a, b, d** dashed arrows)

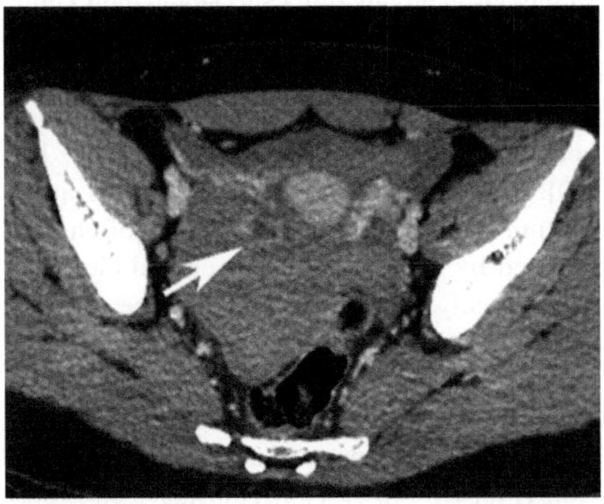

Fig. 1.4 Axial post-contrast CT phase depicts a luteinic cyst with vascularised wall (arrow)

'haematocrit effect', due to sedimented erythrocytes producing a layer of high attenuation [11].

At US, when ruptured, the corpus luteum presents as a small cystic lesion (typically less than 3 cm) with a crenate wall and is characterised by a homogeneous hypoechoic appearance, with mild internal echoes [13, 15]. In most cases, there is a peripheral margin characterised by an increase in vascularity, typically in a 'ring of fire' shape, detectable at Doppler examination. Generally, haemorrhagic ovarian cysts contain areas of solid appearance due to clots and have concave or straight edges without a detectable flow inside [13, 15]. At US it is possible to detect the corpus luteum (Fig. 1.7) but not the active bleeding eventually present.

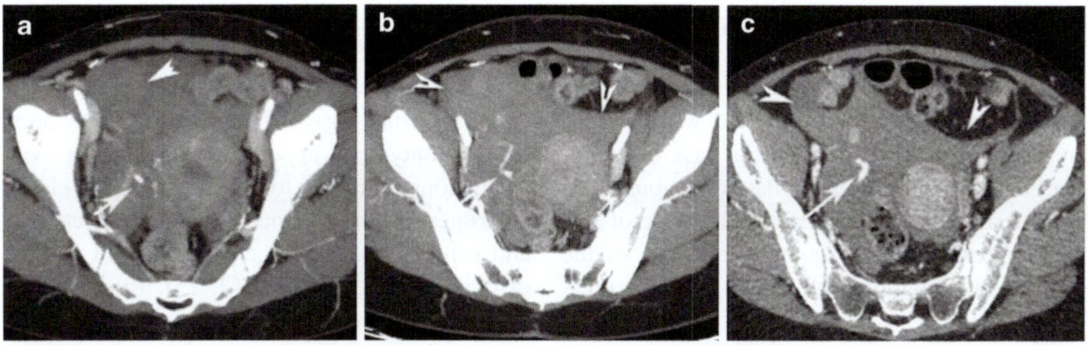

Fig. 1.5 Axial post-contrast arterial CT phase (**a**) depicts an adnexial vascularised cyst with pooling of contrast medium within the wall (**a**, arrow). There is haemoperitoneum (**a**, arrowhead). Post-contrast portal CT phase (**b**) depicts a jet of contrast medium (**b**, arrow) inside the blood peritoneal collection (**b**, arrowheads). Post-contrast excretory CT phase (**c**) demonstrates an enlargement of contrast medium pooling (**c**, arrow)

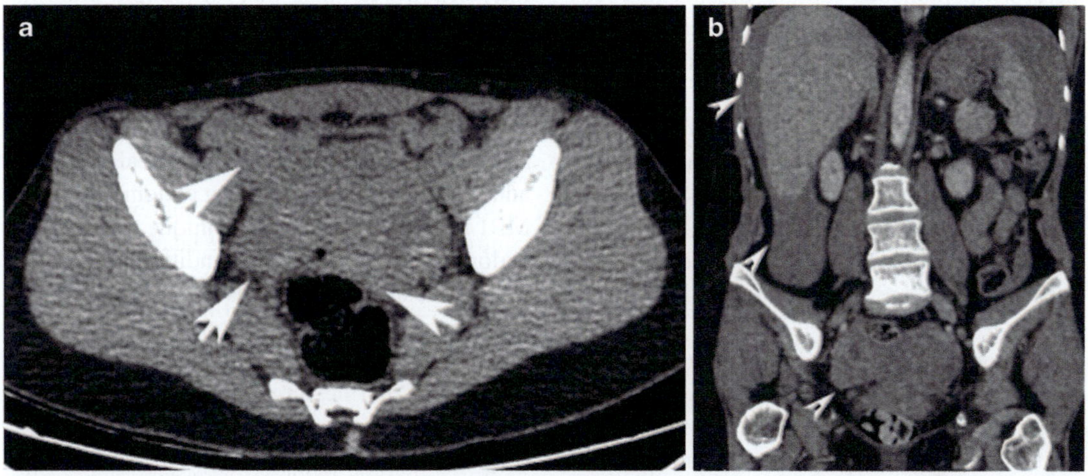

Fig. 1.6 Haemoperitoneum in pelvic cavity in axial CT view (**a**, arrows). Coronal abdominal CT (**b**) evidences large haemoperitoneum occupying abdominal and pelvic recesses (**b**, arrowheads)

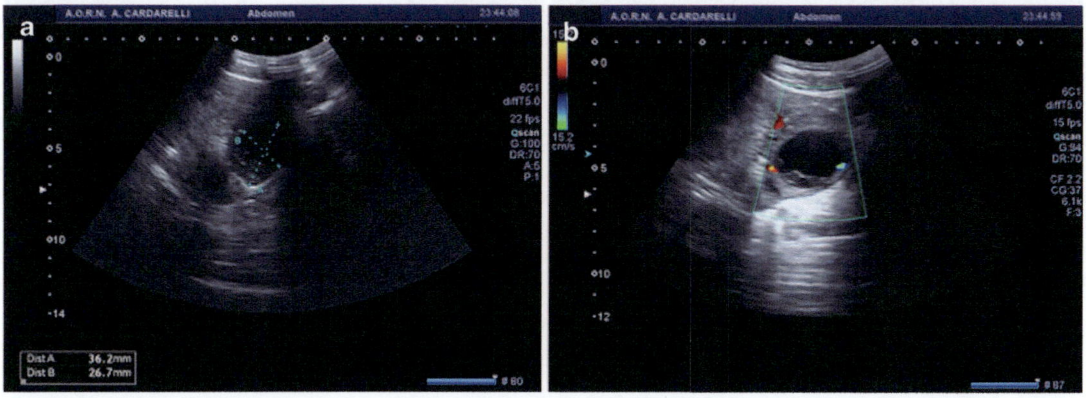

Fig. 1.7 Transabdominal sonography of left adnexa shows a haemorrhagic corpus luteum with blood deposits (**a**). Circumferential blood flow is also showed on colour-Doppler imaging (**b**) [16]

At MRI the corpus luteum appears as small-sized, unilocular fluid-containing structure, with typical homogenous T1-hypointense signal and T2-hyperintense signal, thickened walls with a crenulated enhancing rim. In the case of bleeding, the content becomes heterogeneous. The hemoperitoneum may show a wide range of signals depending on the quantity and age of the blood; sedimentation with level(s) may be present [17, 18].

Endometriotic Cysts

Endometriomas have highly variable, often heterogeneous CT appearance, and often mimic mixed solid/cystic or predominantly solid masses. Spontaneous rupture of an endometriotic cyst is a rare complication that causes a severe acute abdominal pain due to chemical peritonitis from the leakage of old blood (Fig. 1.8). Rupture commonly occurs at menstruation due to an increase in internal pressure. The CT findings of ruptured endometriotic cyst are a cystic mass with a slightly high-attenuation content and loculated ascites around the mass. These findings are not specific and similar to ovarian torsion [12].

US findings of endometriomas may coincide considerably with other adnexal masses [1]. Endometriomas appear as uni- or multiloculated cysts containing diffuse, low-level homogenous echoes, which is also known as a 'ground glass' appearance [13, 15]. However, this typical appearance is only present in 85–90% of surgically confirmed cases. The remaining cases present a nontypical appearance, with cyst wall projections (thought to represent blood clots), heterogeneous appearance of the internal echoes, and solid appearances seen (possibly in chronic ovarian endometriomas) [13, 15]. Rupture may be suspected by the presence of free fluid, but US cannot detect the active bleeding eventually present.

At MRI typical findings of endometriosis are represented by adnexal mass with high signal intensity on T1-weighted MR images and signal intensity lower than that of simple fluid on T2-weighted images, and furthermore, depending on the age of the blood, hemosiderine deposits may be present (Fig. 1.9) [19]. However, at MRI also other related findings may be detected, such as small superficial peritoneal implants, adhesion, and deep infiltrating endometriosis. So MRI is the best imaging technique for mapping endometriosis in elective condition, but not to look for acute complications as active bleeding in emergency setting [20]. Rarely, implantation of endometrial cells may occur at the surgical site at the time of uterine surgery and then, under hormone changes, scar endometrioma may occur (Fig. 1.10).

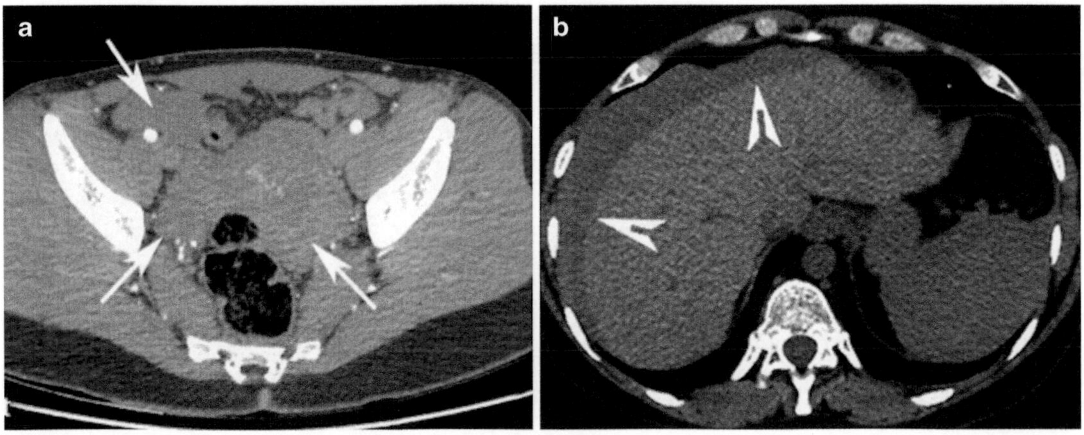

Fig. 1.8 Post-contrast portal CT phase depicts an endometriotic cyst rupture with haemoperitoneum (**a**, arrows) (**b**) spread up to perihepatic space (arrowheads)

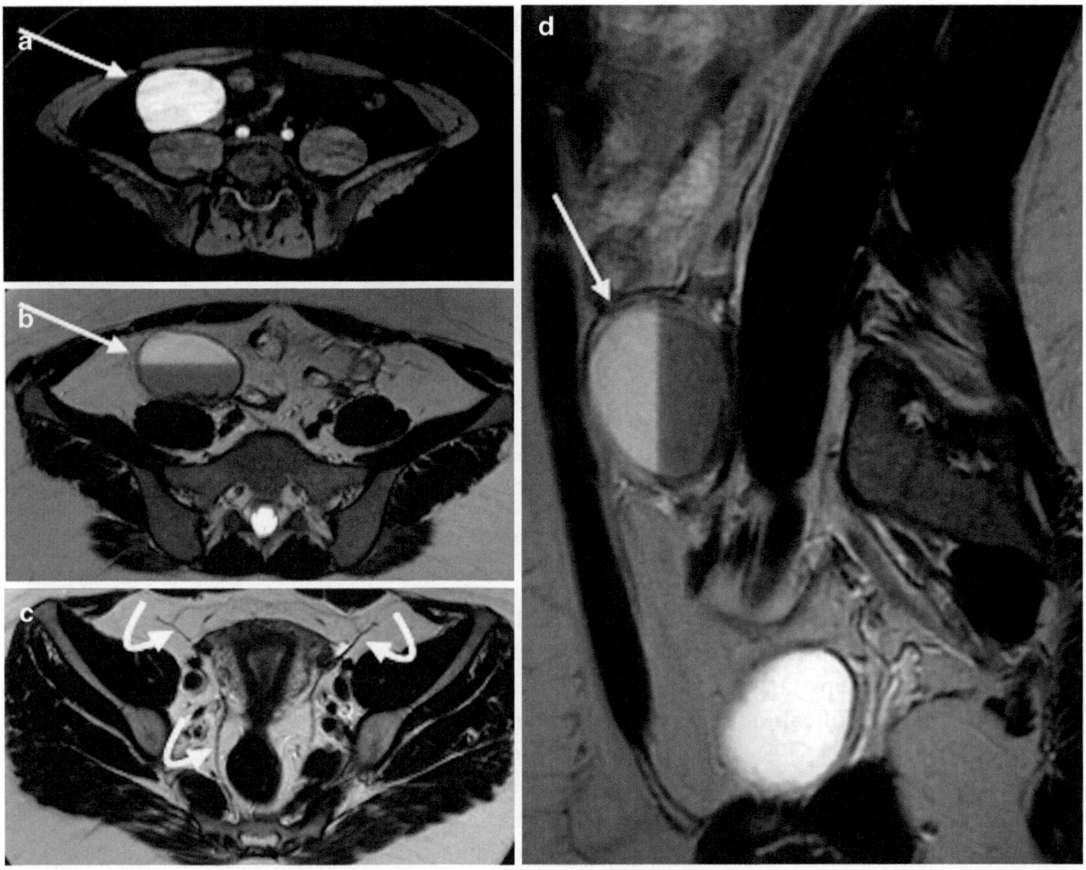

Fig. 1.9 Twenty-two-year-old patient with right iliac fossa pain: (**a**) T1-W FS axial, (**b, c**) T2-W axial, and (**d**) T2-W sagittal sequences showing a right ovarian endometrioma with high T1 signal on T1 FS sequence (arrow), (important for differentiating it from mature cystic teratoma of the ovary) and the typical 'shading sign' in T2-W sequences (**b, d** straight arrows), consisting in low signal in the declive portions of the cyst, due to the high concentration of protein and iron within the endometrioma from recurrent haemorrhage. There is also thickening of the supporting uterine ligament (**c**, curved arrows), related with endometriosis [16]

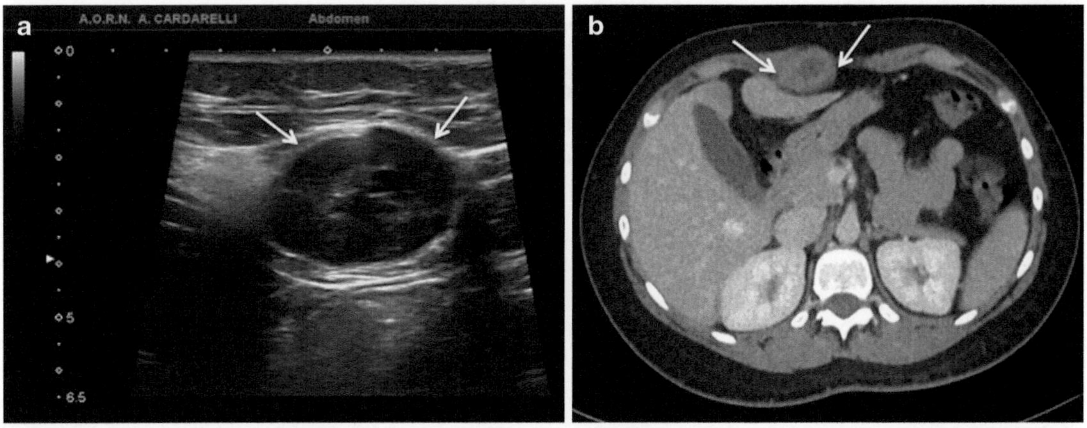

Fig. 1.10 Transabdominal sonography (**a**) of the abdominal wall shows a 35 mm abdominal wall endometriosis nodule with hypoechoic content and well-defined margins (**a**, arrows). The nodule is enclosed in the muscular fascia along the right rectal abdomen. Contrast-enhanced axial CT image shows heterogeneous enhanced mass in the right rectus sheath. The mass was subsequently proved to be abdominal endometriosis [16]

1.3.1.2 Ectopic Pregnancy

The second most frequent gynaecologic cause of haemoperitoneum is ruptured ectopic pregnancy [21]. About 2% of pregnancies are ectopic, with most implantations occurring in the fallopian tubes (95%). More rarely (3–4%) ectopic pregnancies occur in the uterine cornua, uterine cervix, broad ligaments, peritoneal cavity, and myometral scars of previous caesarean delivery; these may cause both hemoperitoneum and vaginal bleeding [22]. Frequently, patients with ectopic pregnancy undergo CT evaluation for the clinical diagnosis of severe acute abdomen associated with vaginal bleeding, without prior US. US has a high specificity (near 100%) but a very low sensitivity (about 15%) [22].

The characteristic CT findings include an adnexal cystic mass corresponding to the gestational sac, with mixed density blood clots and peripheral post-contrast enhancement, that is separate from an ipsilateral normal ovary (Fig. 1.11). The identification of bloody effusion (measuring 30–45 HU) in the Morrison pouch and in the cul-de-sac should raise concern for a ruptured ectopic pregnancy. The risk of rupture increases with the enlargement of the ectopic pregnancy. On contrast-CT enhanced images, active bleeding may be detected, especially in the case of a massive rupture [22]. The differential diagnosis includes haemorrhagic corpus luteum, cyst, and spontaneous abortion; however, the association of haemorrhagic fluid without an intrauterine pregnancy should raise suspicion for ectopic pregnancy [23].

MRI is occasionally used to initially detect an ectopic pregnancy as it is usually diagnosed, in elective conditions, on the basis of a combination of clinical, laboratory, and ultrasonographic findings [24].

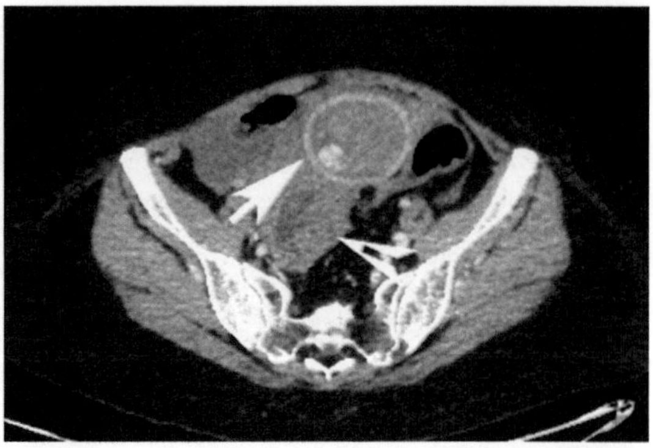

Fig. 1.11 Post-contrast portal CT phase shows an adnexal cystic mass corresponding to the gestational sac (arrow), with mixed density blood clots and peripheral post-contrast enhancement, that is due to ectopic ruptured pregnancy (arrowhead) with bloody effusion in the cul-de-sac

1.3.1.3 Caesarean Scar Pregnancy

Caesarean scar pregnancies (CSPs) are extremely rare [25]. The pathogenesis is unclear; however, theories suggest that the blastocyst enters a microscopic tract in the uterine scar and implants in the myometrium. The pregnancy may extend outside the uterus, attaching to adjacent pelvic structures. Scar ectopic pregnancies are associated with significant rates of uterine rupture, haemorrhage (Fig. 1.12), and haemoperitoneum [26], so these patients deserve a prompt diagnosis with enhanced CT and treatment usually consisting in embolisation, eventually followed by surgery (Fig. 1.12).

In elective conditions, US is the first-line imaging modality for the evaluation of a potential CSP, with the majority of CSPs diagnosed on the basis of TVUS. MRI is indicated when TVUS findings are equivocal, or when additional information is needed in preparation for surgery [27].

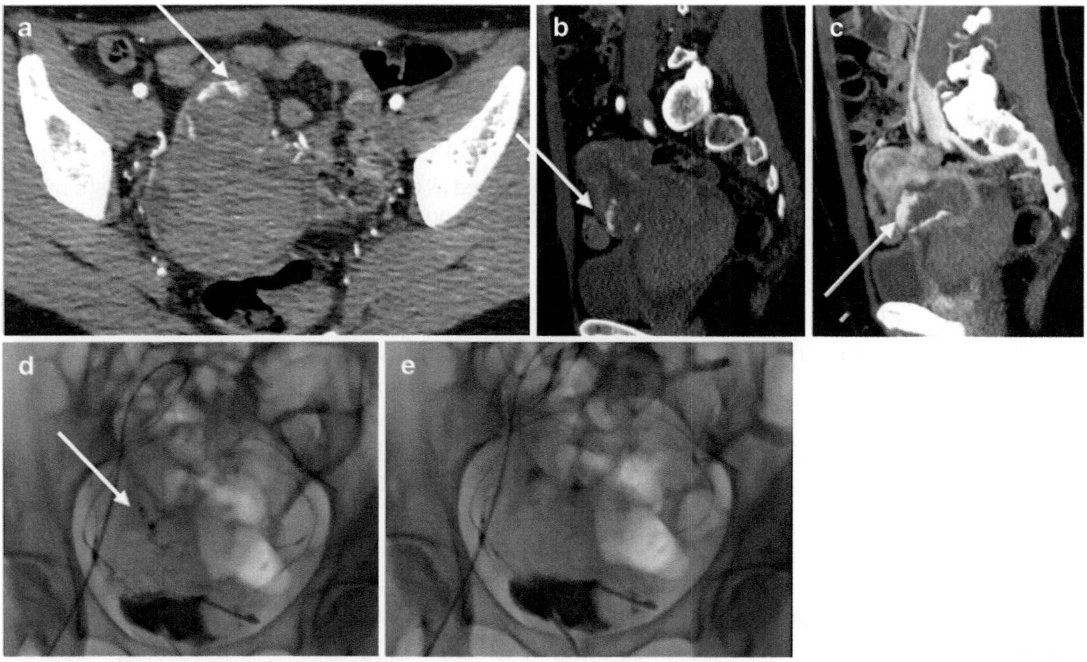

Fig. 1.12 Thirty-four-year-old patient with metrorrhagia. Axial (**a**) and sagittal (**b**) post-contrast arterial CT phase depict a pooling of active bleeding (**a**, **b**, arrows) due to pregnancy implant in the site of previous caesarean scar. The bleeding increases in the following portal phase (**c**, arrow). Patient was promptly and successfully treated with angioembolisation (**d**, active bleeding, arrow; **e**, control after embolisation) followed by hysterosuction of the scar pregnancy

1.3.2 Gynaecological Causes of Vaginal Haemorrhage

1.3.2.1 Uterine Artero-Venous Malformations

Uterine artero-venous malformations (AVMs) are rare congenital or acquired vascular lesions that consist of direct communications between arteries and veins, without intervening capillaries [28–34].

CT demonstrates a hypertrophic arterial/venous mass in the myometrium; the arteriovenous communications appear as intensely vascular multidirectional network of tortuous vessels (Fig. 1.13) [35].

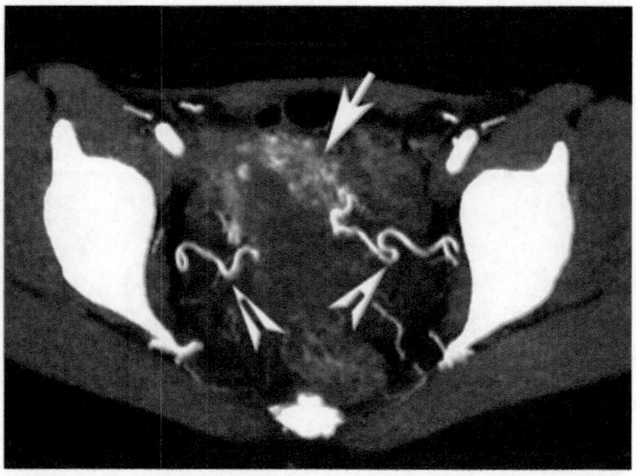

Fig. 1.13 Axial post-contrast arterial CT phase depicts a large 'nidus' of small artero-venous communication (straight arrow) between the branches of the uterine artery (arrowheads) and the myometrial venous plexus

US and Doppler, performed in elective conditions, may give extremely characteristic findings. Serpiginous cystic areas and blood vessel tangles can be observed in the scan with marked fillings from colour or power Doppler. Spectral Doppler enables visualisation of waveforms at high speed and low resistance (increased end-diastolic speed) in the supply artery and pulsatile flow at high speed in the drainage vein [1, 36, 37]. Pseudoaneurysms are also reported in the literature as another possible complication from intra-uterine procedures. These can be easily distinguished from AVMs by spectral Doppler. A pseudoaneurysm appears as an anechoic cystic structure with a turbulent blood flow with a 'yin-yang' waveform at colour Doppler analysis. Under spectral Doppler analysis, an undulatory waveform is detected at the neck of the pseudoaneurysm, with the flow heading towards the pseudoaneurysm during systole and away during diastole [1, 36, 37].

MRI gives its diagnostic contribution mainly due to its panoramicity. In this setting, enhanced-MRI sequences are particularly useful to study the vessel involvement and to correctly plan the following embolisation treatment (Fig. 1.14).

1.3.2.2 Post-Partum Haemorrhage

The World Health Organization estimates that severe bleeding complicates 10% of all live births and accounts for 24% of all maternal deaths annually [35, 38]. Post-Partum Haemorrage (PPH) is defined as blood loss of more than 500 cc after vaginal or 1000 cc after caesarean delivery [38, 39].

CT findings are represented by uterine active bleeding foci (Fig. 1.15) or pseudoaneurysms with extravasation of contrast medium associated with pelvic hypertrophied vessels or pelvic arteries vasospasm [40].

Retained products of conception refers to tissue that remains in uterus after delivery. The tissue is usually from the placenta. Contrast

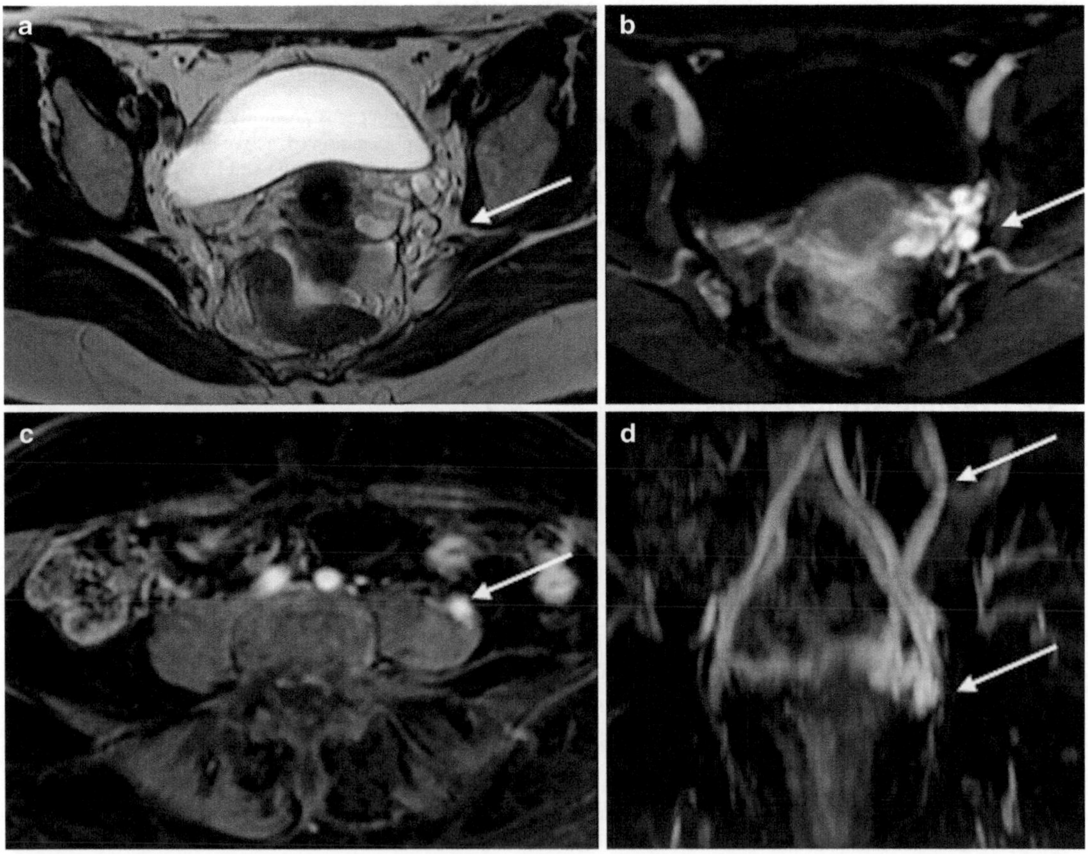

Fig. 1.14 Forty-three-year-old patient with chronic pelvic pain. (**a**) T2-W axial and (**b, c**) T1-W FS axial sequences after iv cm administration in arterial phase. (**d**) T1-W FS coronal sequence after iv cm administration in late phase. There is a pelvic varicocele on the left side (**a**, arrow), with early opacification, in arterial phase, of the left ovarian vein and arterialisation of the plexus consisting with AVM

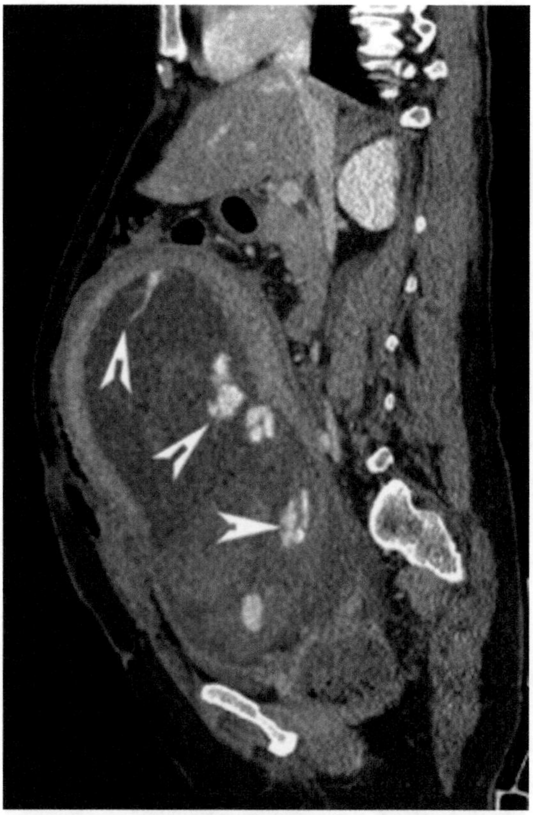

Fig. 1.15 Sagittal post-contrast CT image shows intrauterine active bleeding multiple foci (arrows) associated with haematometra in large post-partum uterus

enhanced CT shows in these cases an intensely enhanced mass in the uterine cavity during the early phase that can mimic a uterine AVM [41].

1.3.2.3 Cervical Pregnancy

Cervical pregnancy is one of the rarest ectopic pregnancies that may arise when the blastocyst passes through the uterine cavity and implants into the mucosa of the endocervical canal. It is potentially lethal for severe vaginal haemorrhage [42, 43].

At CT cervical pregnancy may appear as a haemorrhagic mass located below the internal cervical os, associated with active vaginal bleeding (Fig. 1.16) [44, 45].

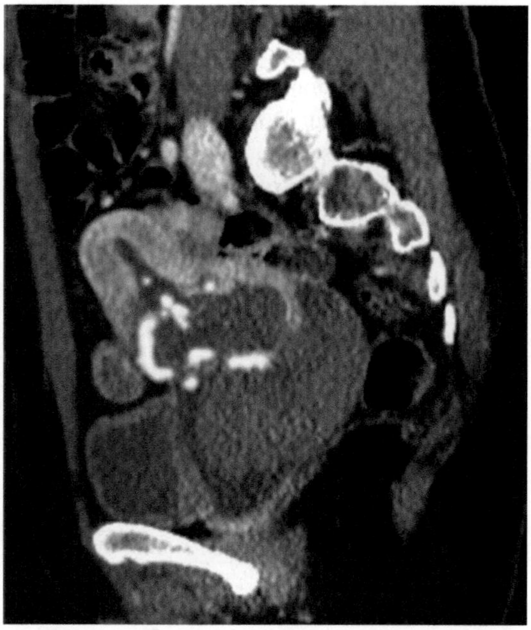

Fig. 1.16 Sagittal post-contrast CT image shows cervical pregnancy located below the internal cervical os, associated with active vaginal bleeding

1.4 Uterine Disorders

1.4.1 Adenomyosis

Adenomyosis is a common condition occurring more commonly in middle-aged, multiparous women who have pelvic pain, dysmenorrhoea, and menorrhagia [46–49]. It involves the migration of stroma and endometrial glands from the basal layer into the myometrium that is surrounded by reactive smooth muscle hyperplasia, which interdigitates with the ectopic endometrial tissue [46]. Adenomyosis can occur in diffuse (more common) and nodular forms.

US shows uterus with increased volume and a globular appearance, with hypoechoic areas a few millimetres in size distributed throughout the myometrium. Myometrial cysts and nodular or linear echogenic extension of the endometrium into the underlying myometrium can be detected during the second half of the menstrual cycle, as well as linear echogenic streaks or nodules that extend from the endometrium into the underlying myometrium. Colour Doppler aids in differentiating adenomyosis from leiomyomas [46–49]. Areas of adenomyosis often show diffuse intralesional hypervascularisation, while leiomyomas display peripheral rather than internal blood flow under colour Doppler. Focal adenomyosis or adenomyoma presents with a more atypical appearance, such as a focal mass with poorly defined margins, in contrast to leiomyomas which have clear margins (Table 1.4) [46–49].

MRI allows to better evaluate the extension of adenomyosis (Fig. 1.17) and diagnose the possible association with extrauterine endometriotic

Table 1.4 Ultrasound differential diagnosis between adenomyosis and intramural myoma

	Adenomyosis	Intramural myoma
Uterine morphology	Diffuse uterine enlargement	Distortion of external uterine contour
Echostructure	Inhomogeneous	Mixed, partly hyperechogenic and partly hypoechogenic
Posterior cone of shadow	Absent	Present
Morphology	Indistinct edges	Ovoid, round
Hypoechogenic lacunas	Present	Rare
Pseudocapsule	Absent	Present
Doppler	Few scattered vessels in the myometrium	Peripheral flow in the pseudocapsule, rarely inside the myoma

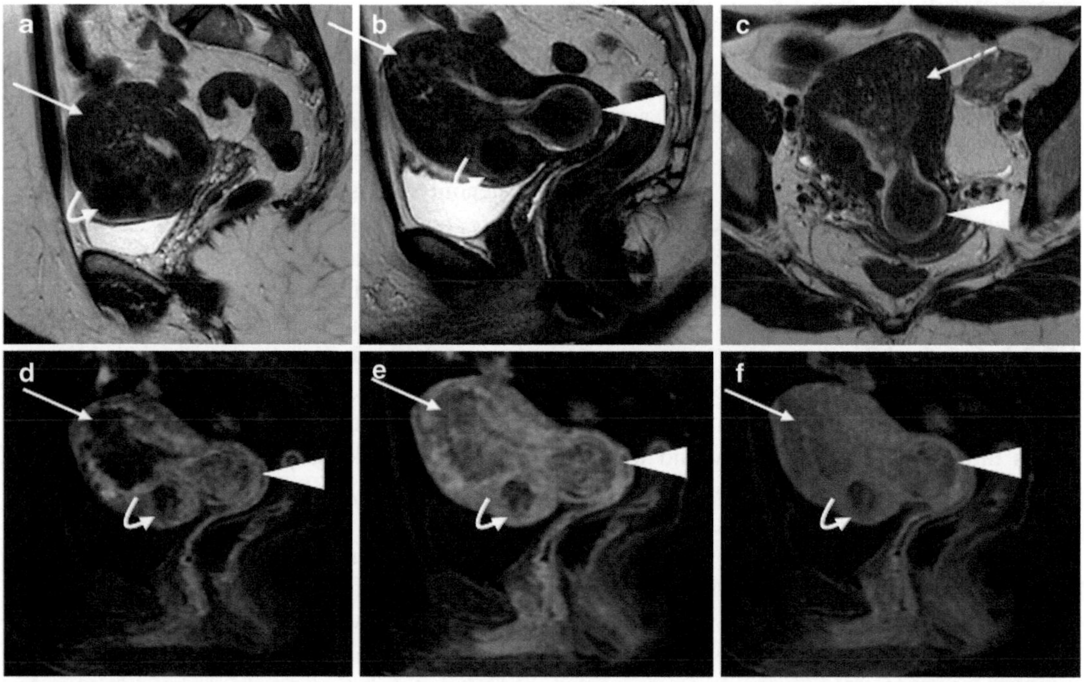

Fig. 1.17 Forty-year-old patient with pelvic pain and metrorrhagia. MRI T2-W sequences in sagittal (**a, b**) and coronal (**c**) planes and T1-W Fat Sat sequence in sagittal plane after iv cm injection in arterial (**d**), portal, (**e**) and late phases (**f**) show the presence of an extensive area of adenomyosis (**a–f**, straight arrows), multiple myometrial leyomiomas with typical hypointense T2-W signal (**a–f**, curved arrow), and a pedunculated leiomyoma (**b–e**, arrowhead) protruding into the cervical canal

foci [50]. At T2W sequences diffuse adenomyosis appears as ill-defined low-signal-intensity area in the myometrium containing multiple small high-signal-intensity areas, that are ectopic endometrial tissue and small cysts (Fig. 1.17). At T1W sequences, some of the high-signal-intensity spots can be seen, corresponding to some of the small high-signal-intensity areas seen on the T2-weighted image, representing haemorrhage within the ectopic endometrial tissue [51].

1.4.2 Leiomyoma

Leiomyomas (fibroids or myomas) are benign neoplasms comprised of smooth muscle and varying amounts of fibrous tissue. They are the most common uterine neoplasms. They can originate anywhere in the uterus and can occur singularly or in multiples, with sizes ranging from a few millimetres to several centimetres [48, 52, 53].

At US, leiomyomas are usually readily recognised, often with variable appearances. Most leiomyomas are readily identified as focal and sharply defined myometrial masses (Fig. 1.18), while an enlarged and diffusely heterogeneous uterus is more likely to indicate adenomyosis (Table 1.2) [48, 52, 53]. Leiomyomas can be hypoechoic, isoechoic, or echogenic compared to the myometrium; however, hypoechoic is most common. The surrounding myometrium can be compressed to form a pseudocapsule and is easily identifiable by US. Occasionally, the vascular or lymphatic channels may create a thin hypoechoic crown around the intramural leiomyoma. The blood vessels in myomas usually exist peripherally and parallel to the pseudocapsule. Small leiomyomas are usually homogeneous; however, those with a diameter greater than 3 cm tend to be heterogeneous. As leiomyomas increase in size, they tend to outgrow their vascular supply. This can cause degeneration, which can be hyaline, myxoid, cystic, or haemorrhagic [48, 52, 53]. When this occurs, the leiomyoma may present a more atypical appearance at US. Degeneration can lead to oedema, which in turn can lead to the presence of cystic spaces, echogenic haemorrhagic areas, and dystrophic calcification. The latter occurs predominantly in postmenopausal patients. Calcifications can be curvilinear, peripheral, or aggregate and may

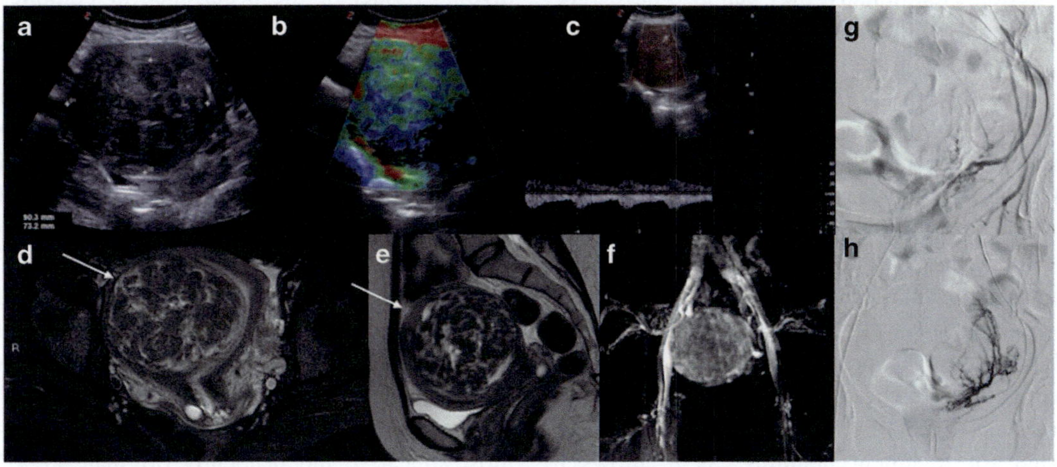

Fig. 1.18 Forty-five year-old patient with large uterine leiomyoma. US B-mode image in traverse plane depicting the myoma (**a**), note the inhomogeneous structure, with fibrous areas at the elastosonography evaluation (**b**) and high vascularity at the Doppler evaluation (**c**). MRI better depict the extension of the leiomyoma. T2W Fat Sat sequence (**d**, axial plane, arrow) and T2W sequence (**e**, sagittal plane, arrow) underline the lesion margin, the inhomogeneity and the oedematous component, slightly hyperintense. In (**f**), GRE T1W Fat Sat VR 3D contrast enhanced angiography, is showed the vascular supply and drainage. In (**g**) and (**h**) are shown images of the angiography performed to embolize the leiomyoma, demonstrating the high vascularity

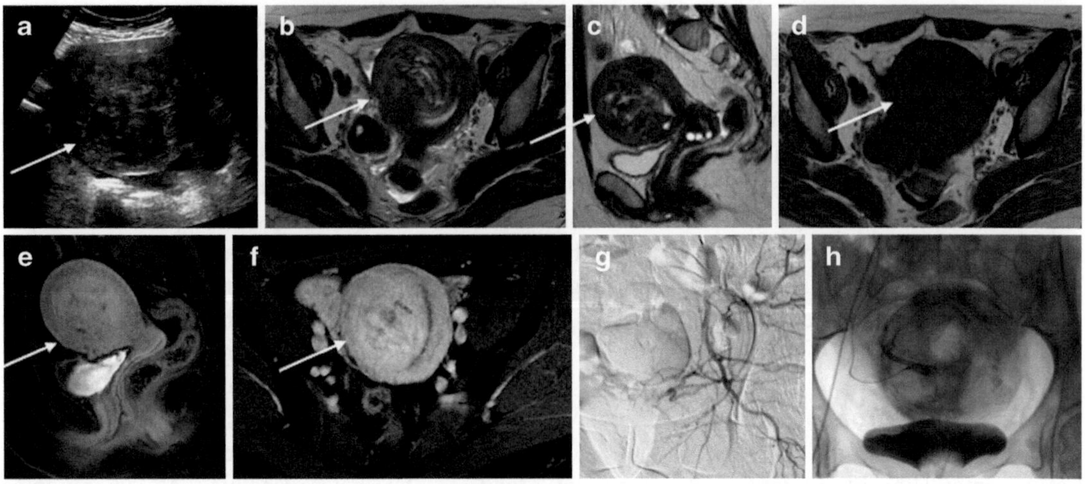

Fig. 1.19 Forty-year-old patient. US (**a**) and MRI T2-W sequences in axial (**b**) and sagittal (**c**) planes, T1-W sequence in axial plane (**d**), T1-W FS sequences after iv cm injection in sagittal (**e**) and axial (**f**) planes, and endovascular embolisation (**g, h**) in patient with a large uterine leiomyoma (**a–f**, arrows), with inhomogeneous structure due to the presence of fluid colliquative content [16]

show dense posterior shading [48, 52, 53]. However, many leiomyomas have characteristic areas of acoustic attenuation that are not always attributable to the presence of calcifications. Submucosal leiomyomas can present with symptoms of menorrhagia, menometrorrhagia, and anaemia and require definitive treatment with resection. Additionally, they can also have varying degrees of intracavitary extension, which can distort the cavity itself (Fig. 1.18) [48, 52, 53].

MRI findings are related with the described variability of the lesions, usually hypointense to the myometrium in the T2W sequences (Fig. 1.17), with variable presence of cystic or haemorrhagic degeneration (Fig. 1.19) and calcifications (these last best seen at CT). The contrast enhancement at the arterial phase is higher in the periphery, as well as at the venous phase (Fig. 1.19). The peak enhancement is usually seen in the late phase, at 3 min, but may be present even earlier [51]. MRI is particularly indicated for treatment planning, as it allows to evaluate the patient eligibility for the procedure and the post-treatment outcome (Fig. 1.19). For interventional endovascular treatment, it is important to describe the number of leiomyomas, the location and size, the stalk diameter if pedunculated (because of the risk of separation from the uterus) (Fig. 1.17), their vascular intake and percentage of enhancement, and the presence of adenomyosis (Fig. 1.17). These details give significant prognostic information about the potential success of the procedure. MRI is useful also in the follow-up after the endovascular treatment to evaluate the success of the procedure or the need of reembolisation of residual viable leiomyoma tissue, or the occurrence of complications as hematomas, unwanted tissue necrosis, and infections [54, 55].

CT isn't indicated for the diagnosis and characterisation due to the poor contrast resolution but may detect multiple large nodules and their complications (acute necrosis, torsion, and bleeding) in examination performed for differential diagnosis of acute pelvic pain (Fig. 1.20).

Although leiomyomas are mostly benign, leiomyosarcomas can occur, the cause of which remains uncertain. Although it has been hypothesised that a leiomyosarcoma may develop following degeneration of a pre-existing leiomyoma, most appear to independently originate [1, 52, 53, 56]. Imaging findings that suggest tumour presence include size variation, indistinct or infiltrative margins, unusually complex pattern, and internal vascularisation, particularly with uneven vessel distribution. However, these findings are not specific, and as such, there may not be a substantial imaging difference between a rapidly

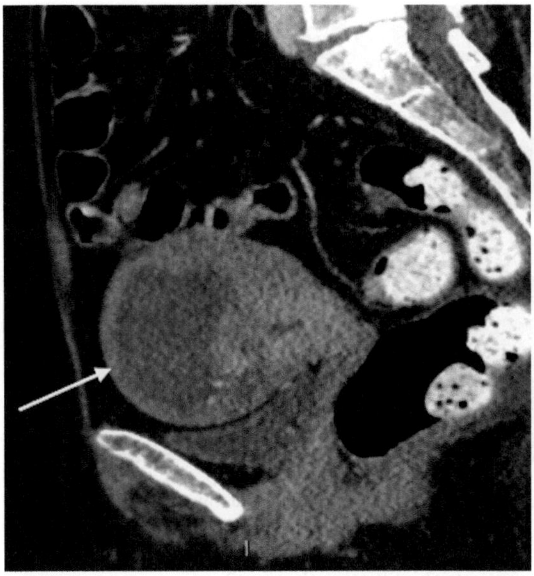

Fig. 1.20 Enhanced CT in sagittal view of a 45-year-old patient with a large necrotic uterine fibroid causing pelvic pain (arrow)

growing or degenerative myoma and a sarcoma. It may be useful to perform an MRI to confirm the contrast enhancement of the solid component [1, 52, 53, 56]. Other signs of malignant degeneration include local invasion and distant metastasis, which are both more easily detected with MRI or CT compared with US. However, even at MRI the differentiation with degenerative benign leiomyomas is not always possible due to the considerable variability of imaging appearance of these lesions [51].

1.4.3 Endometrial Polyps

Endometrial polyps are hyperplastic growths that consist of dense fibrous tissue or smooth muscle cells with disordered endometrial glands. Endometrial polyps can be sessile or pedunculated, unique or multiple. Polyps have been found to range in size from 1 mm to a few centimetres [36, 57].

US, preferably performed early after menstrual cycle, shows a diffuse or focal echogenic thickening of the endometrial echo pattern. The endometrium-myometrium interface is usually intact, and the polyp forms an acute angle with the endometrium. Colour Doppler can be useful as it shows the vascular pedicle present in almost half of polyps [1, 36, 57].

At MRI, small endometrial polyps (<1 cm) may be difficult to detect because of their signal intensity identical to that of normal endometrium on T1 and identical or slightly less intense than endometrium on T2 [58]. Larger polyps can be diagnosed at MRI on the basis of a fibrous core, intratumoural cysts, and focal enhancement within the endometrial cavity and with a regular interface with the junctional zone [59].

1.4.4 Endocervical Polyps

The exact cause of endocervical polyps is not known, but chronic inflammation and high oestrogen levels have been found to be predisposing factors. Patients may experience vaginal bleeding; however, many present as asymptomatic.

US can identify an endoluminal cervical mass. The presence of vascularisation or a vascular bundle distinguishes endocervical polyps from debris, blood clots, or mucous plugs. Large endocervical polyps can obstruct the endocervical canal and cause a prolapse to form in the vagina.

At MRI endocervical polyps are slightly hypointense than the endometrium and cervical mucosa in the T2-W sequences; an enhanced-MRI may show an increased arterial enhancement and the vascular pedicle [60].

1.4.5 Endometrial and Cervical Cancer

Endometrial cancer is defined as cancer that occurs above the level of the internal orifice of the cervix and affects the upper two-thirds of the uterus. It is the most common gynaecological cancer [1, 36, 61].

US shows diffuse endometrial thickening or an endometrial mass, which is often difficult to distinguish from endometrial hyperplasia or polyps. The thickened endometrial echo pattern is often hyperechoic but may have areas of reduced echogenicity. If myometrial invasion has not

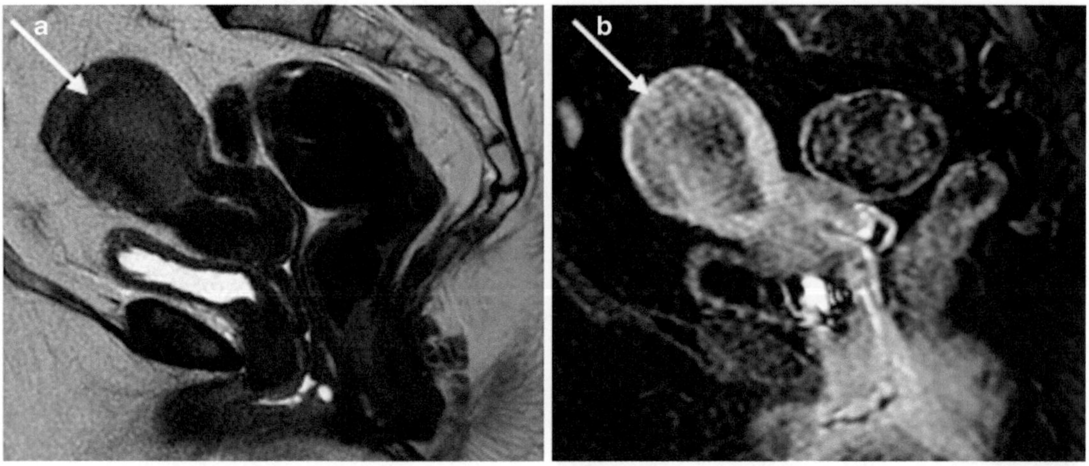

Fig. 1.21 Sixty-year-old patient with endometrial cancer (arrows); sagittal T2W sequence (**a**) and T1-W FS post iv cm injection (**b**). Note the typical T2 W signal (**a**) more intense than the adjacent myometrium and less intense than the normal endometrium (arrows). After iv cm injection (**b**) the pathological tissue enhances slowly than the myometrium, and furthermore it is better depicted the myometrial infiltration (**b**, arrow)

occurred, the myometrial interface can be well-defined with an intact subendometrial halo (inner layer of the myometrium). However, the focal or diffuse interruption of the subendometrial halo or the extension of the echogenic endometrial lesion in the underlying hypoechoic myometrium is worrying for myometrial invasion [1, 36, 61]. The Doppler assessment is not useful. TVS is the best and most widely used diagnostic imaging modality for the detection of endometrial cancer [1, 36, 61].

MRI is the modality of choice for the local staging of the tumour. For this purpose it is particularly important to acquire sequence on the three planes oriented on the main axis of the uterus, to correctly evaluate the infiltration of the junctional line and of the myometrium. The tumour is isointense to the adjacent myometrium in the T1W sequence, whereas it is hyperintense to the adjacent myometrium, in the majority of cases, in the T2W sequences (Fig. 1.21). After the administration of iv cm, endometrial cancer enhances earlier than normal endometrium but later than adjacent myometrium (Fig. 1.21). DWI sequences may be very useful and when fused with T2-W images seem to be better than enhanced-MRI for assessing the depth of myometrial invasion; in atrophic uterus, enhanced-MRI is more helpful to assess the myometrial invasion [58].

Carcinoma of the cervix is the third most common gynaecological malignancy after endometrial and ovarian cancer [36, 62].

At US, cervical cancer appears as a mass with variable echogenicity. Although the tumours can be well-defined and clearly delimited, especially if small or in the initial developmental stage, cervical cancers infiltrate and disrupt the normal zonal anatomy of the cervix by distorting the endocervical canal where they originate [36]. Ultrasound does not play a decisive role in the screening, diagnosis, or stage definition of cervical cancer. Screening and diagnosis are performed more effectively with the Papanicolaou (Pap) test, with cervical biopsy, and subsequent interventions performed clinically according to the FIGO (Fédération internationale de gynécologie et d'obstétrique) staging system [63, 64]. If further investigation is required, an MRI is typically performed in order to assess the extent of the local pathology and lymph node involvement, while a CT scan can be performed to determine lymphadenopathy and distant metastases [1, 36, 62].

At MRI cervical cancer is best viewed on T2-W sequences, with an intermediate signal between the cervical stroma and the adipose tissue, and the extension may be well visualised on DWI, so enhanced sequences are optional and may be adopted in particular cases [65].

In both endometrial and cervical cancer, CT has a role in whole body tumour staging and in the diagnosis of complications as acute bleeding, fluid and necrotic collections deserving percutaneous drainage, bowel involvement with infiltration, and consequent obstruction [66].

1.5 Adnexal Masses

Most ovarian masses are benign, and the majority show sufficiently typical US features that can be reliably characterised. Usually, malignant tumours of the ovary can also be recognised and diagnosed based on typical US characteristics [13, 15]. The American College of Radiologists (ACR) O-RADS US has a reliable diagnostic performance in differentiating between malignant and benign adnexal lesions [67].

A small minority of ovarian masses have indeterminate ultrasound findings, and therefore typically need to be further evaluated by follow-up ultrasound, MRI scanning, or surgical evaluation (Figs. 1.22 and 1.23). MRI is helpful due to its panoramicity and the possibility to directly characterise the lesions based on

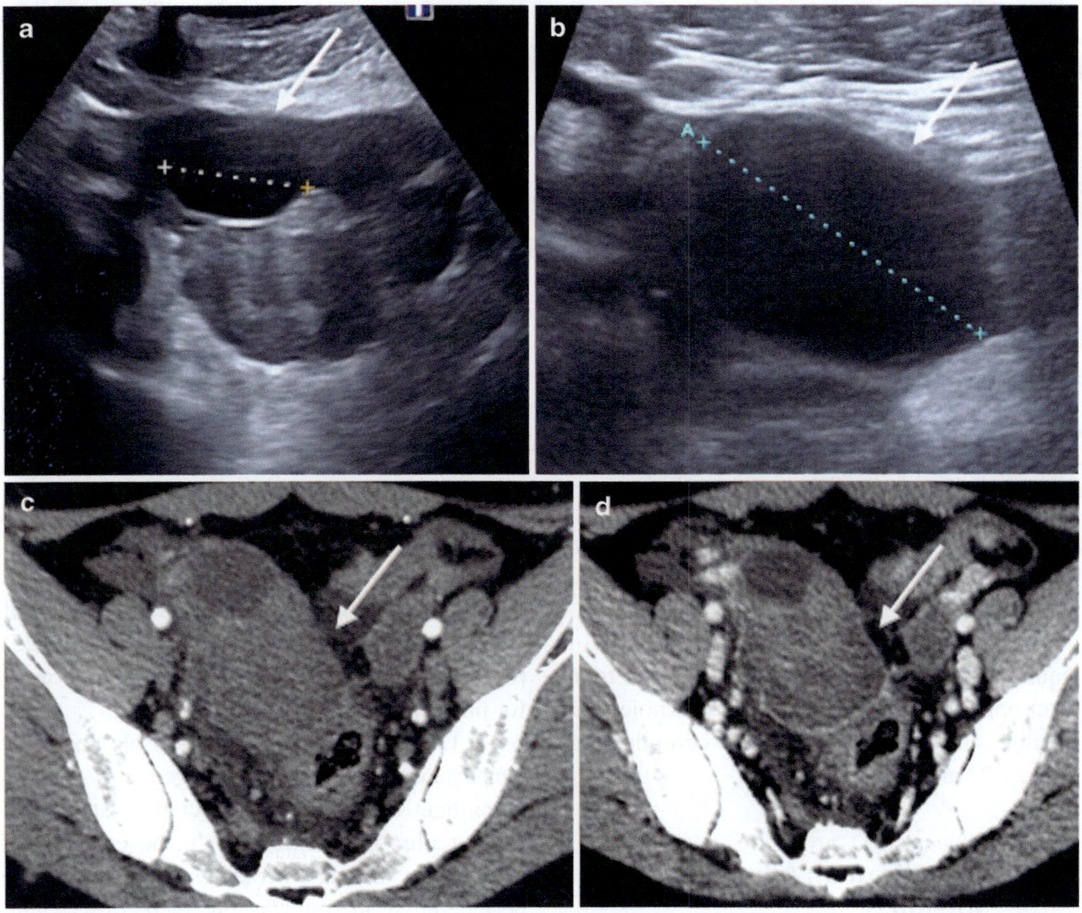

Fig. 1.22 Twenty-six-year-old patient complaining for right iliac fossa pain. (**a, b**) US scans, (**c, d**) CT scans, and axial views. There is a simple cyst at the right ovary (**a**, straight arrow) with smooth and regular margin and anechoic content. In the right adnexal area there is a further larger mass (**b**, arrow), 'cyst like' with hypoechoic content and blurred margin deserving further diagnostic test. CT shows a right adnexal inhomogeneous mass (**c, d** arrows) indissociable from the right ovary and suspected of malignancy. Presented in: Iacobellis F, Di Serafino M, Danzi R, Ponticiello G, Schillirò ML, Barbuto L, Nicola R, Scaglione M, Romano L. Gynecological and obstetric causes of acute right iliac fossa pain: imaging approach and related imaging findings. EPOS ECR 2021 doi: 10.26044/ecr2021/C-12876

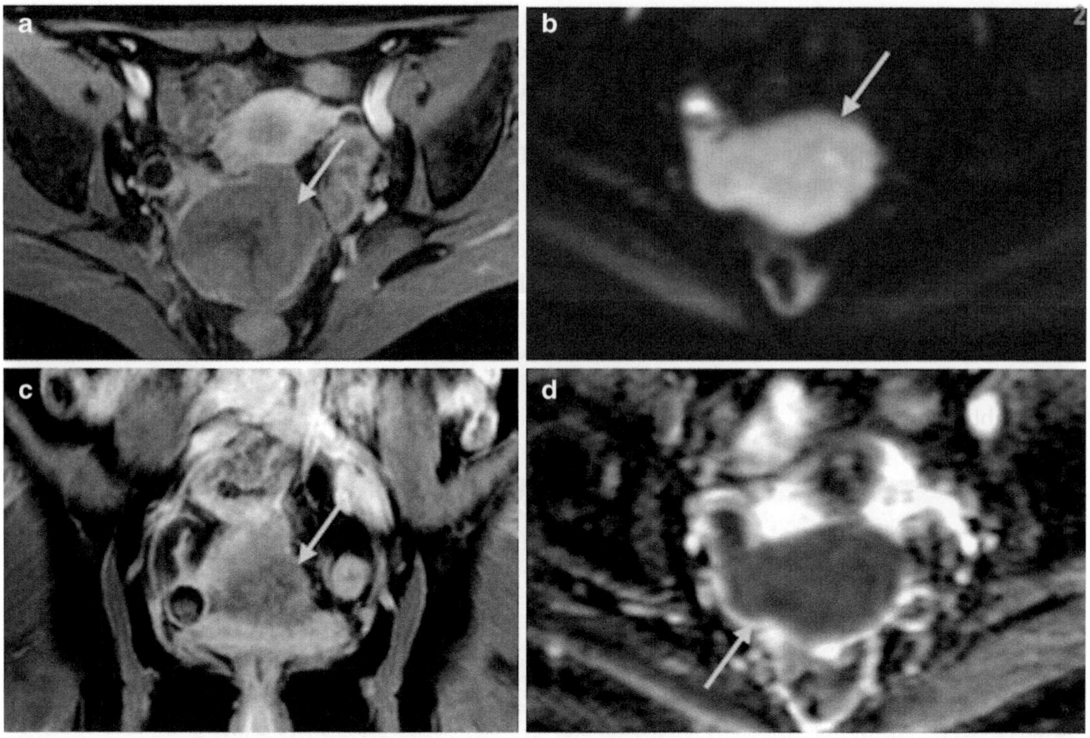

Fig. 1.23 Same patient of Fig. 1.21. (**a**) MRI T1-W fat sat axial sequence after iv cm administration, (**b**) coronal T1-W FS fat sat sequence after iv cm administration, (**c**) axial DWI, and (**d**) ADC map. There is an inhomogeneous vascularised mass in the right salpinx (**a–d** straight arrow) causing upstream luminal obstruction with tortuous appearance (**b**, curved arrow). The mass has restricted diffusion (**c, d**) due to high cellularity. At pathological examination the mass resulted in a tubal leiomyosarcoma. Presented in: Iacobellis F, Di Serafino M, Danzi R, Ponticiello G, Schillirò ML, Barbuto L, Nicola R, Scaglione M, Romano L. Gynecological and obstetric causes of acute right iliac fossa pain: imaging approach and related imaging findings. EPOS ECR 2021 doi: 10.26044/ecr2021/C-12876

the presence of fluid, fat, or blood components within them.

When malignant masses are detected, MRI is required for the local staging, to establish treatment opportunities. CT has a role in whole body staging and in detection of complications (Figs. 1.22 and 1.24).

1.5.1 Complication: Adnexal Torsion

It may be solicited by the presence of an adnexal mass, usually larger than 5 cm, but can occur also in absence. Adnexal torsion consists in a partial or complete rotation of the adnexal structures around the vascular peduncle, with occlusion of venous outflow and arterial inflow (Fig. 1.25) [68, 69]. Timely diagnosis and surgery are crucial for preserving the ovaries [68, 69].

At US, the most common grayscale finding is the presence of a one-sided enlarged ovary, usually larger than 4 cm, with or without associated mass. Further ultrasound findings are the presence of multiple small ovarian follicles positioned at the peripheral level on the enlarged ovary with hypoechoic formation (i.e. the 'pearl necklace' appearance) [1, 70]. Over time, the ovarian stroma may become more heterogeneous in ultrasound images due to haemorrhagic foci or necrosis [1,

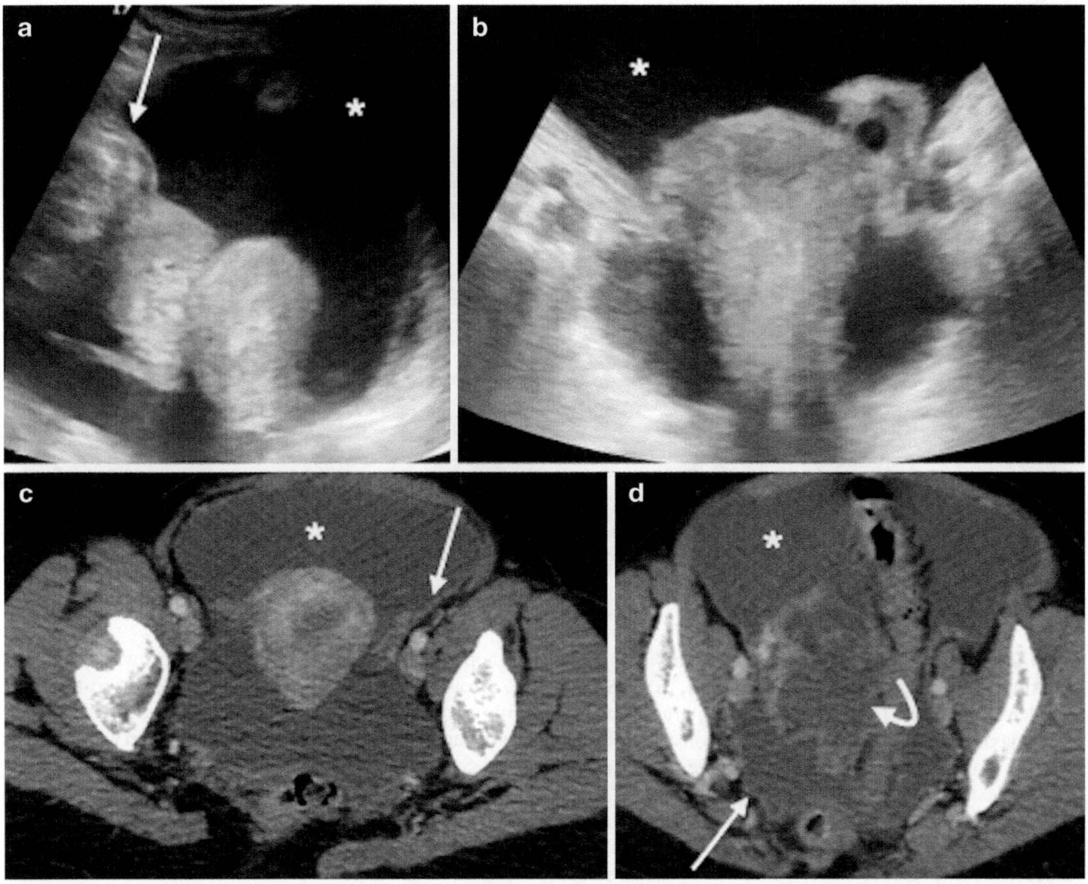

Fig. 1.24 Fifty-seven-year-old patient with persistent pelvic pain. (**a, b**) US scans, (**c, d**) enhanced CT scans in portal venous phase showing large amount of ascitic fluid (**a–d**, asterisks) with thickened peritoneum (**a, c, d**, arrows). This is related with peritoneal carcinosis due to an advanced ovarian cancer (**d**, curved arrow). Presented in: Iacobellis F, Di Serafino M, Danzi R, Ponticiello G, Schillirò ML, Barbuto L, Nicola R, Scaglione M, Romano L. Gynecological and obstetric causes of acute right iliac fossa pain: imaging approach and related imaging findings. EPOS ECR 2021 doi: 10.26044/ecr2021/C-12876

70]. Comparison with the asymptomatic ovary can help in detecting such changes. Abnormal positioning of the ovary, such as in the midline of the uterus, or higher or lower in the Douglas cavity, or a dislocation in the contralateral area of the pelvis are important observations. When subjected to twisting and congestion, the vascular peduncle may appear as an indistinct adnexal mass adjacent to the ovary. In addition to the grayscale findings, colour and spectral Doppler assessment are important for the assessment of adnexal torsion [1, 70, 71]. As with grayscale imaging, Doppler findings vary according to the degree of torsion, the time elapsed since the onset of the disease, and the degree of vascular compromise. The absence of detectable blood flow in the affected ovary allows a confident diagnosis, with a positive predictive value (PPV) of 94%. However, numerous reports have shown that the detection of flow within an ovary alone, using echocolour Doppler and spectral Doppler, cannot rule out the presence of torsion. The double arterial flow that supplies the ovary can aid in arterial flow maintenance, even with initial loss of venous flow. This means that

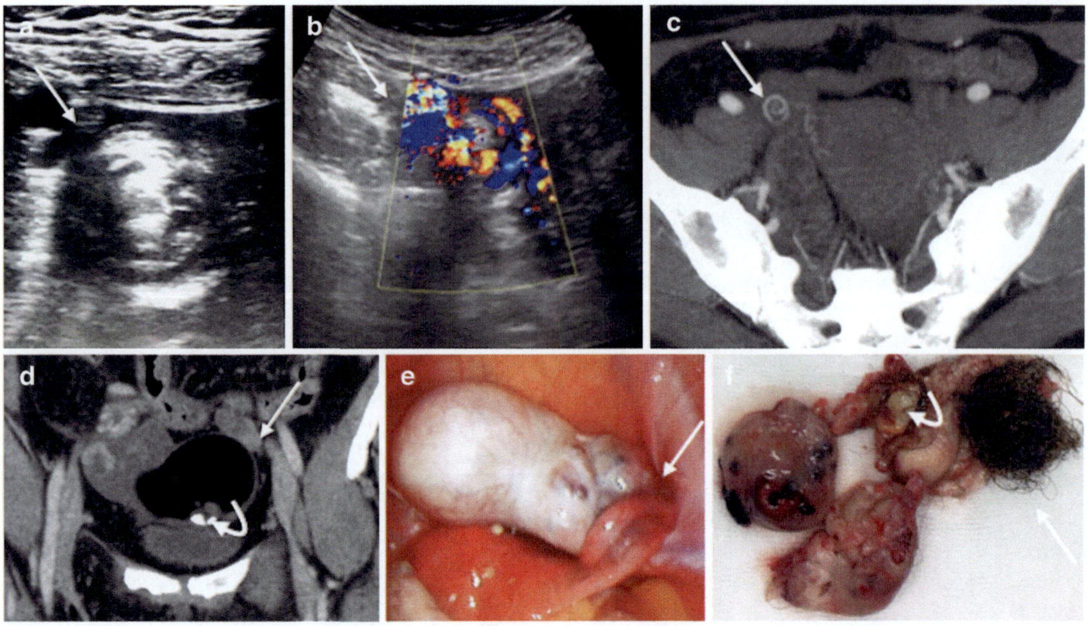

Fig. 1.25 Thirty-four-year-old patient complaining for remitting acute right iliac fossa pain. (**a, b**) US and Doppler scans; (**c**) CT scan in axial view, arterial phase, MIP (maximum intensity projection) reconstruction; (**d**) CT scan in coronal view; (**e**) intraoperative view; and (**f**) resected lesion. At the most painful site there is a 'whirl sign' (**a, b**, arrows), better seen with a Doppler evaluation (**b**, arrow) and confirmed at enhanced CT (**c**, arrow), related with the presence of a large mature cystic teratoma (**d**, straight arrow; contained teeth, curved arrow). At the intraoperative evaluation, ovarian torsion was confirmed (**e**, arrow), and the right ovary with the cystic teratoma with its mixed content (**f**, hairs, straight arrow and teeth, curved arrow) was resected. Presented in part in: Iacobellis F, Di Serafino M, Danzi R, Ponticiello G, Schillirò ML, Barbuto L, Nicola R, Scaglione M, Romano L. Gynecological and obstetric causes of acute right iliac fossa pain: imaging approach and related imaging findings. EPOS ECR 2021 doi: 10.26044/ecr2021/C-12876

whether the torsion is early, intermittent, or partial, both venous and arterial flow can be preserved [1, 70, 71]. The analysis of spectral Doppler waveforms can increase the sensitivity of torsion diagnosis. An arterial waveform with reversal of diastolic flow, which indicates high resistance, can suggest the presence of torsion, thus helping its diagnosis. However, overall, the grayscale findings and the clinical picture are considered to be more reliable than Doppler in diagnosing adnexal torsion. A twisted vascular pedicle or vortex sign is a useful finding in both grayscale and Doppler for diagnosing adnexal torsion (Fig. 1.25). On colour Doppler, coiled vessels in the pedicle appear as a spiral or vortex [1, 70, 71]. This spiral or vortex is best detected when the probe is moved back and forth in the transverse plane along the central axis of the twisted peduncle.

Although ultrasound is the primary method for assessing a suspected ovarian torsion at a clinical level, CT may be the first analysis performed in the emergency room for differential diagnosis of acute pelvic pain.

MRI is a second-level examination that can be very helpful in case of inconclusive US. MRI helps in identifying the organ of origin for adnexal masses, in masses characterisation, and in detecting alternative causes of acute pelvic pain. Furthermore, when ovarian torsion is detected, the MRI appearance guides the treatment suggesting if the ovary can be saved or is in a stage of advanced ischemia (Fig. 1.26) [72].

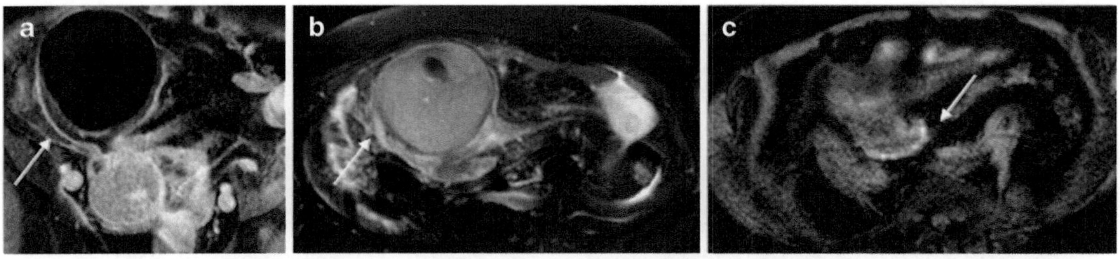

Fig. 1.26 Forty-year-old patient complaining of persistent lower abdominal pain. (**a**) T1-W Fat Sat, (**b**) T2-W Fat Sat, and (**c**) T1-W Fat Sat sequences show a cystic teratoma at the right ovary (**a, b** arrows), with proteinaceous components at the twisted pedicle (**c**, arrow), with increased signal in T1-W sequences due to haemorrhagic necrosis. This is an inveterate ovarian torsion. Presented in: Iacobellis F, Di Serafino M, Danzi R, Ponticiello G, Schillirò ML, Barbuto L, Nicola R, Scaglione M, Romano L. Gynecological and obstetric causes of acute right iliac fossa pain: imaging approach and related imaging findings. EPOS ECR 2021 doi: 10.26044/ecr2021/C-12876

1.6 Pelvic Pain

Pelvic pain often presents a diagnostic challenge, as there are a variety of potential causes, including both gynaecological and other disorders characterised by overlapping clinical symptoms. Pelvic ultrasound is the primary imaging method used, but MRI, when available, is increasingly used [68].

1.6.1 Pelvic Inflammatory Disease

Pelvic inflammatory disease (PID) refers to a spectrum of diseases that occur when microorganisms ascend from the lower genital tract to the uterus, fallopian tubes, and ovaries, and is a common cause of referral to the emergency department and hospitalisation for acute gynaecological disorders [73, 74]. The continuum of infection begins with cervicitis and progresses to endometritis, salpingitis, pyosalpinx, tubo-ovarian complex, and tubo-ovarian abscess.

Endometritis may be suspected in an appropriate clinical setting when the endometrium is thick and/or irregular, and the cavity may or may not contain fluid with or without echogenic particles. The filling of the endometrial cavity with pus is known as pyometra (Fig. 1.27) [75]. These findings may be firstly suspected at US and confirmed at second-level imaging tests.

Although salpingitis may not always be recognisable on US, infected fallopian tubes can show thickening of the walls and hyperaemia (Fig. 1.28). An occlusion of the ovarian fimbria of the fallopian tubes due to inflammation will result in a dilated tuba containing pus or in a pyosalpinx. A pyosalpinx appears as a dilated tubular structure with echogenic intraluminal fluid and sediment, sometimes with layered echoes indicating the presence of liquid and sediments (Fig. 1.28). The presence of thick, hypervascularised walls is indicative of acute disease (Fig. 1.28) [73, 74]. Left untreated, PID worsens, causing a tubo-ovarian complex as the inflammation spreads to the adjacent ovary. This ovary subsequently becomes enlarged, with indistinguishable margins and increased vascularity, although it remains distinguishable as a separate structure. The inflamed fallopian tube is often adjacent or adherent to the ovary. The final phase is the formation of a tubo-ovarian abscess (TOA), in which the ovary is no longer delineated, and an inflammatory mass covers both the ovary and the fallopian tube. Rupture of a TOA can result in septic shock (Fig. 1.29) [1, 73, 74].

CT is performed in acute setting for differential diagnosis of acute pain, whereas MRI is preferable as second-level imaging examination when the clinical indication is mainly oriented on gynaecological disease and in the follow-up.

1.6.2 Pelvic Congestion Syndrome

Pelvic congestive syndrome (PCS) can be a cause of chronic pelvic pain and is caused by defective

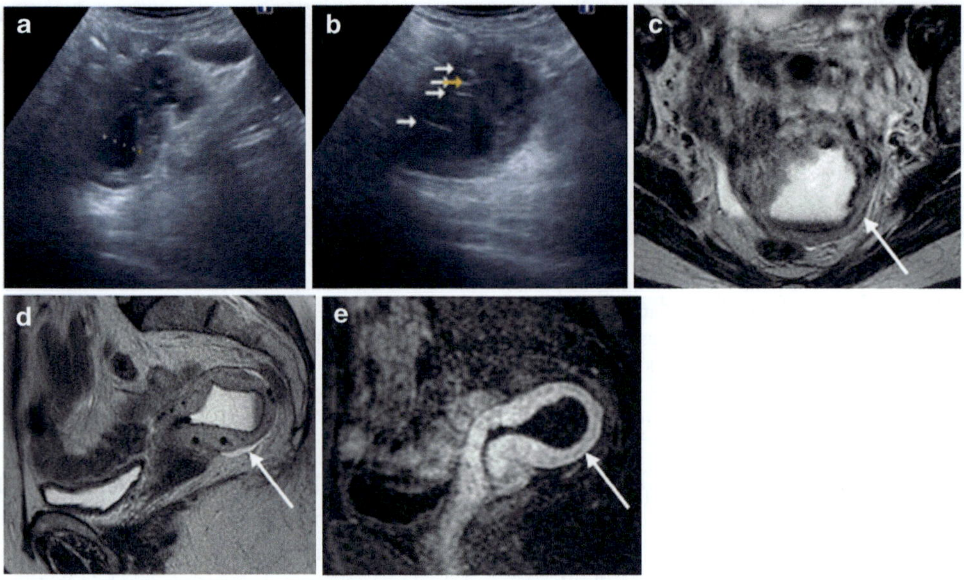

Fig. 1.27 Fifty-nine-year-old patient with right iliac fossa and pelvic pain and fever. At US there is a distended hypoechoic endometrial cavity (**a**, dashed line), with some hyper echoic spots inside (**b**, arrows). MRI was performed (**c**, sagittal T2-W and **d**, sagittal T1-W fat sat with iv cm) confirming the endometrial cavity distention with increased myometrial enhancement due to pyometra [16]. Presented in: Iacobellis F, Di Serafino M, Danzi R, Ponticiello G, Schillirò ML, Barbuto L, Nicola R, Scaglione M, Romano L. Gynecological and obstetric causes of acute right iliac fossa pain: imaging approach and related imaging findings. EPOS ECR 2021 doi: 10.26044/ecr2021/C-12876

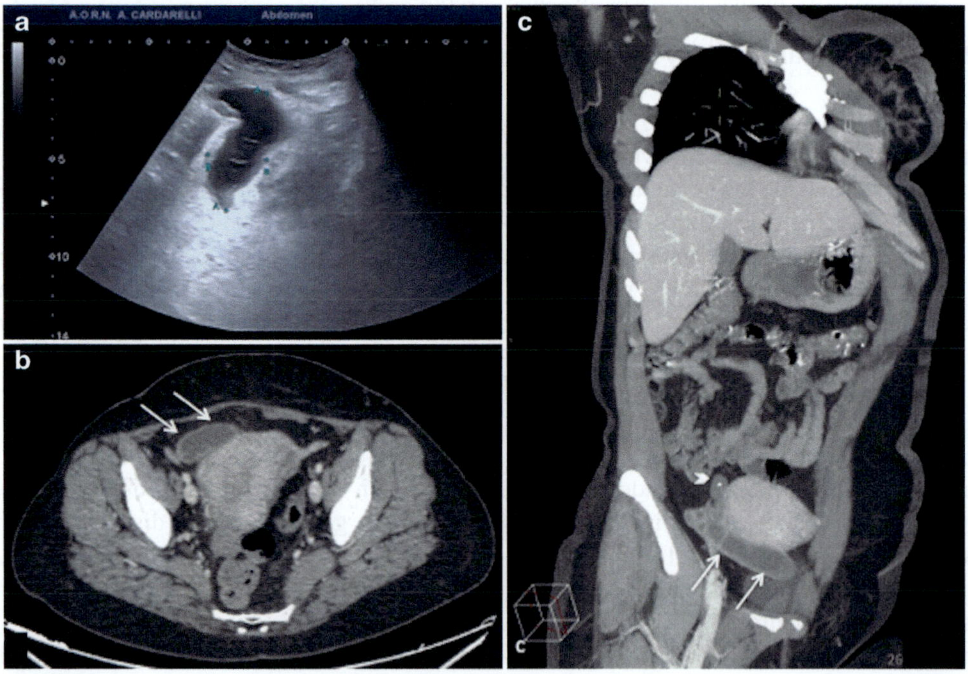

Fig. 1.28 Transabdominal sonography of the right adnexa (**a**) shows an anechoic oblong structure (**a**, calliper). Contrast-enhanced axial CT image (**b**) and maximum intensity projection (MIP) coronal-oblique reconstruction show tortuous and tubular fluid-filled structure seen in the right adnexa (**b, c** arrows). The right ovary cannot be seen separately from the structure (**c**, arrowhead). The typical convoluted shape size and site of the lesion is suggestive of dilated fluid-filled fallopian tube or hydrosalpinx

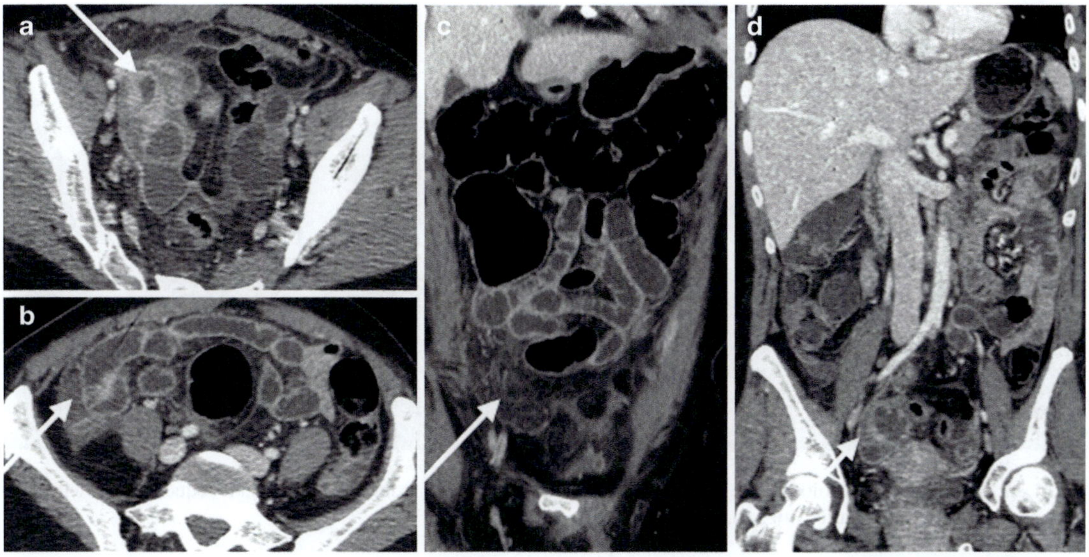

Fig. 1.29 Forty-nine-year old patient complaining of abdominal pain, mainly focused on the right iliac fossa, associated with fever and peritonism. There is a right ruptured tubo-ovarian abscess (**a**, straight arrow) with free peritoneal fluid (**b**, straight arrow) and fat stranding (**c**, straight arrow). (**d**) Coronal view of the ovarian abscess (straight arrow) [16]

valves within the ovarian veins, resulting in backflow to the pelvic veins. This causes the pelvic veins to swell and become tortuous, forming pelvic varicosities.

US findings include multiple enlarged (larger than 5 mm) veins adjacent to the ovary and uterus and enlarged (larger than 5 mm) arcuate veins that may cross the myometrium and connect to varicosities. An enlarged ovarian vein, greater than 6 mm in diameter, with retrograde flow, is a finding specific to PCS (Fig. 1.30) [1, 76].

Second-level investigations like CT and MRI play a role in excluding other causes of chronic pelvic pain, in diagnosing PCS, and in the planning of the treatment strategy (Fig. 1.31) [77].

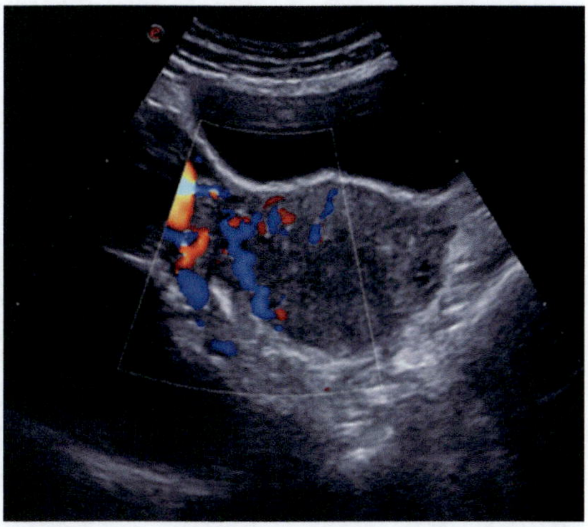

Fig. 1.30 Transabdominal sonography with colour-Doppler mode shows dilated veins in the right adnexa with reversed venous flow after Valsalva manoeuvre [16]

1.6.3 Thrombosis of the Gonadal Veins

Patients with gonadal vein thrombosis generally present with acute pelvic pain but additionally may present with a fever and leukocytosis. Septic thrombophlebitis may be present, but this is more common in postpartum patients, patients with PI, or patients undergoing pelvic surgery [78].

Thrombosis of the ovarian vein appears at US as a tubular or serpentine avascular structure, often devoid of echo or hypoechoic areas. It is commonly seen in the region of the right adnexa and iliopsoas muscle, corresponding to the vein subject to thrombosis (Fig. 1.32) [1, 78]. Extension into the inferior vena cava may occur.

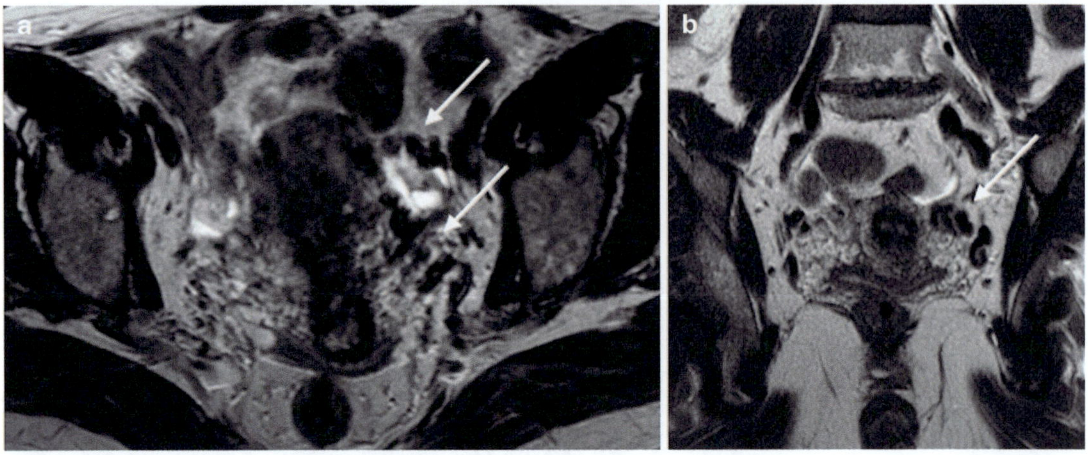

Fig. 1.31 Forty-three-year-old patient with pelvic pain. (**a**) MRI T2-W axial and (**b**) coronal sequences showing left varicocele with multiple varicosities (**a, b** arrows)

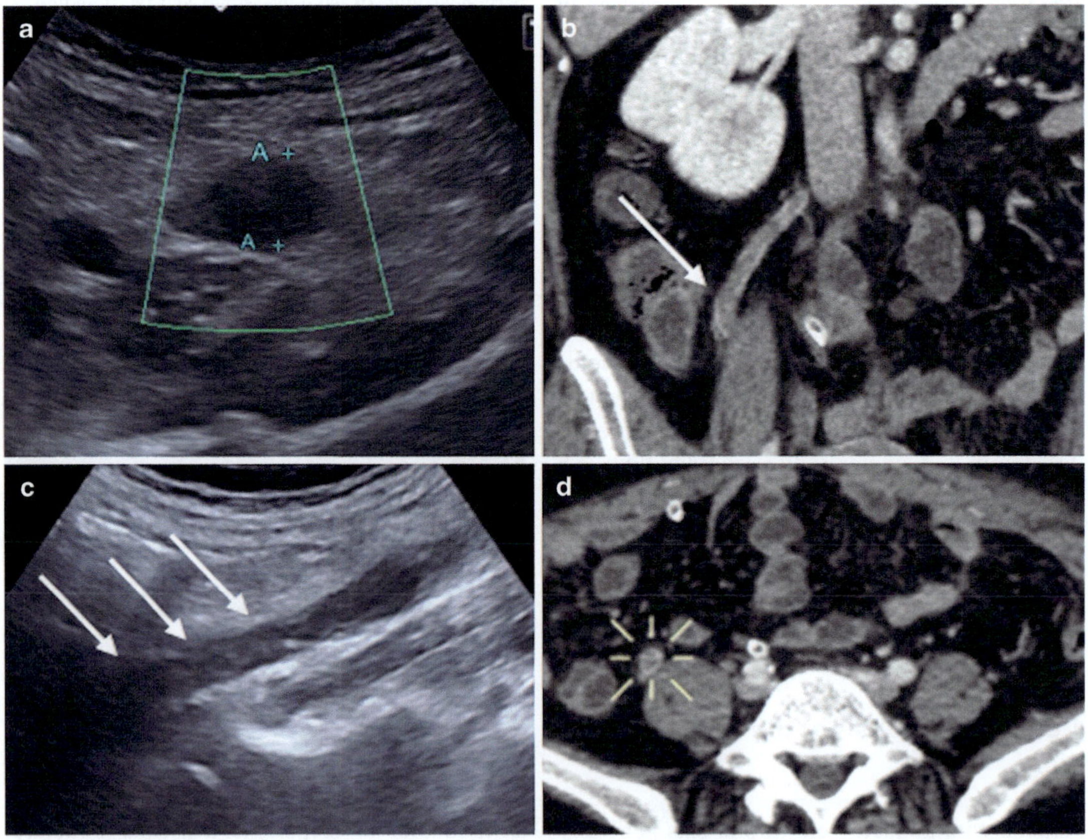

Fig. 1.32 Twenty-nine-year-old patient with post-partum right iliac fossa pain (**a, b**, US) and 34-year-old patient with right iliac fossa pain after ovarian cyst removal (**c, d** enhanced CT). At US there is distended lumen of the right ovarian vein (**a**, axial view) with hypoechoic content and lack of flow at Doppler evaluation, (**b**) longitudinal view of the ovarian vein thrombosis. CT is preferable in postoperative patient (**c, d**) offering a panoramic evaluation particularly useful for differential diagnostic purpose (**c**, coronal view of right ovarian vein thrombosis -arrow-; **d**, axial view) at [16]

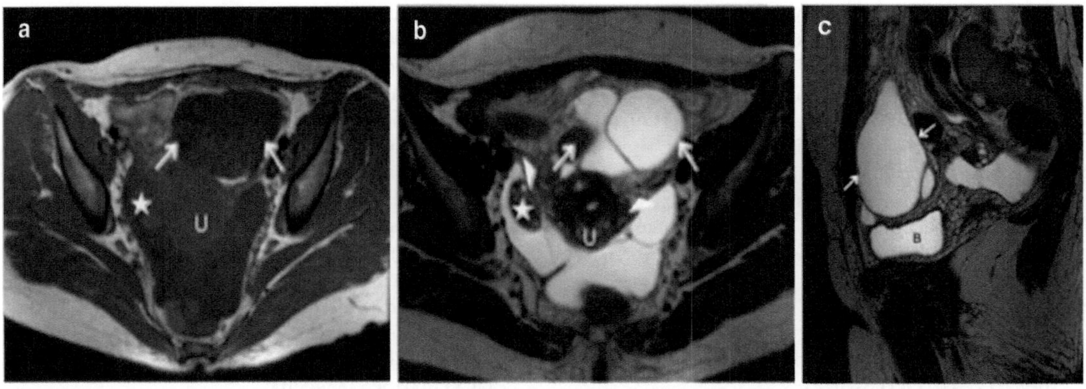

Fig. 1.33 Forty-eight-year-old woman with left-sided pelvic pain. Axial T1-W (**a**), T2-W (**b**), and sagittal T2-W (**c**) MRI show a large, well-defined multilocular cystic pelvic mass (arrows). Note several thin internal septa, radiating from the ovary, representing pelvic adhesions. The septa radiate from the ovary (star; **a, b**) with a classic 'spider in web' appearance (arrowheads; **b**). B, bladder; U, uterus. From: Di Serafino M, Pezzullo F, Iacobellis F, Angelini V, Barbuto L, Romano L Multilocular peritoneal inclusion cyst: a diagnostic challenge. EURORAD Case available at: https://www.eurorad.org/case/16913; doi: 110.35100/eurorad/case.16913

CT or MRI, both with contrast, must be performed to establish the diagnosis, assess the extent of thrombosis, and plan the treatment (Fig. 1.32).

1.6.4 Peritoneal Inclusion Cysts

Peritoneal inclusion cysts are benign lesions containing fluid that are located on the mesothelium of the abdominal area and pelvis. Although the pathogenesis is the subject of debate, with both hyperplastic and neoplastic origins, it is thought to develop from intra-abdominal inflammation with reactive mesothelial proliferation and impaired absorption of peritoneal fluid [73, 79, 80]. The imaging features of peritoneal inclusion cysts reflect their pathogenesis, and recognition of these features enables differentiation from an ovarian cystic mass (Fig. 1.33).

References

1. Norton ME, Scoutt LM, Feldstein VA. Callen—Ecografia in ostetricia e ginecologia (Italian Edition). 6th ed. Milano: Edra; 2018.
2. Mayer C, Deedwania P. Hysterosalpingogram. In: StatPearls [Internet]. Treasure Island, FL: StatPearls Publishing; 2021
3. Potter AW, Chandrasekhar CA. US and CT evaluation of acute pelvic pain of gynecologic origin in nonpregnant premenopausal patients. Radiographics. 2008;28(6):1645–59. https://doi.org/10.1148/rg.286085504.
4. Bennett GL, Slywotzky CM, Giovanniello G. Gynecologic causes of acute pelvic pain: spectrum of CT findings. Radiographics. 2002;22(4):785–801. https://doi.org/10.1148/radiographics.22.4.g02jl18785.
5. Cano Alonso R, Borruel Nacenta S, Díez Martínez P, María NI, Ibáñez Sanz L, Zabía GE. Role of multidetector CT in the management of acute female pelvic disease. Emerg Radiol. 2009;16(6):453–72. https://doi.org/10.1007/s10140-009-0808-8.
6. Swart JE, Fishman EK. Gynecologic pathology on multidetector CT: a pictorial review. Emerg Radiol. 2008;15(6):383–9. https://doi.org/10.1007/s10140-008-0732-3.
7. Boscak AR, Shanmuganathan K, Mirvis SE, Fleiter TR, Miller LA, Sliker CW, Steenburg SD, Alexander M. Optimizing trauma multidetector CT protocol for blunt splenic injury: need for arterial and portal venous phase scans. Radiology. 2013;268(1):79–88. https://doi.org/10.1148/radiol.13121370.
8. Takeda A, Koike W, Imoto S, Nakamura H. Three-dimensional computerized tomographic angiography for diagnosis and management of intractable post-partum hemorrhage. Eur J Obstet Gynecol Reprod Biol. 2014;176:104–11. https://doi.org/10.1016/j.ejogrb.2014.02.026.
9. Iraha Y, Okada M, Iraha R, Azama K, Yamashiro T, Tsubakimoto M, Aoki Y, Murayama S. CT and MR Imaging of gynecologic emergencies. Radiographics. 2017;37(5):1569–86. https://doi.org/10.1148/rg.2017160170.
10. Borders RJ, Breiman RS, Yeh BM, Qayyum A, Coakley FV. Computed tomography of corpus luteal

cysts. J Comput Assist Tomogr. 2004;28(3):340–2. https://doi.org/10.1097/00004728-200405000-00006.
11. Lucey BC, Varghese JC, Anderson SW, Soto JA. Spontaneous hemoperitoneum: a bloody mess. Emerg Radiol. 2007;14(2):65–75. https://doi.org/10.1007/s10140-007-0594-0.
12. Bazot M, Daraï E. Diagnosis of deep endometriosis: clinical examination, ultrasonography, magnetic resonance imaging, and other techniques. Fertil Steril. 2017;108(6):886–94. https://doi.org/10.1016/j.fertnstert.2017.10.026.
13. Smorgick N, Maymon R. Assessment of adnexal masses using ultrasound: a practical review. Int J Women's Health. 2014;6:857–63. https://doi.org/10.2147/IJWH.S47075.
14. Bonde AA, Korngold EK, Foster BR, Fung AW, Sohaey R, Pettersson DR, Guimaraes AR, Coakley FV. Radiological appearances of corpus luteum cysts and their imaging mimics. Abdom Radiol (NY). 2016;41(11):2270–82. https://doi.org/10.1007/s00261-016-0780-1.
15. Levine D, Brown DL, Andreotti RF, Benacerraf B, Benson CB, et al. Society of Radiologists in Ultrasound. Management of asymptomatic ovarian and other adnexal cysts imaged at US Society of Radiologists in Ultrasound consensus conference statement. Ultrasound Q. 2010;26(3):121–31. https://doi.org/10.1097/RUQ.0b013e3181f09099.
16. Di Serafino M, Iacobellis F, Schillirò ML, Verde F, Grimaldi D, Dell'Aversano Orabona G, Caruso M, Sabatino V, Rinaldo C, Cantisani V, Vallone G, Romano L. Pelvic Pain in Reproductive Age: US Findings. Diagnostics (Basel). 2022;12(4):939. https://doi.org/10.3390/diagnostics12040939. PMID: 35453987; PMCID: PMC9026765.
17. Tonolini M, Foti PV, Costanzo V, Mammino L, Palmucci S, Cianci A, Ettorre GC, Basile A. Cross-sectional imaging of acute gynaecologic disorders: CT and MRI findings with differential diagnosis-part I: corpus luteum and haemorrhagic ovarian cysts, genital causes of haemoperitoneum and adnexal torsion. Insights Imaging. 2019;10(1):119. https://doi.org/10.1186/s13244-019-0808-5.
18. Buy JN, Ghossain M, Gynecological imaging. In: Complications of adnexal masses. Springer-Verlag Berlin 2013, pp. 723-756 doi: https://doi.org/10.1007/978-3-642-31012-6.
19. Siegelman ES, Oliver ER. MR imaging of endometriosis: ten imaging pearls. Radiographics. 2012;32(6):1675–91. https://doi.org/10.1148/rg.326125518.
20. Foti PV, Farina R, Palmucci S, et al. Endometriosis: clinical features, MR imaging findings and pathologic correlation. Insights Imaging. 2018;9(2):149–72. https://doi.org/10.1007/s13244-017-0591-0.
21. Levine D. Ectopic pregnancy. Radiology. 2007;245(2):385–97. https://doi.org/10.1148/radiol.2452061031.
22. Kao LY, Scheinfeld MH, Chernyak V, Rozenblit AM, Oh S, Dym RJ. Beyond ultrasound: CT and MRI of ectopic pregnancy. AJR Am J Roentgenol. 2014;202(4):904–11. https://doi.org/10.2214/AJR.13.10644.
23. Lin EP, Bhatt S, Dogra VS. Diagnostic clues to ectopic pregnancy. Radiographics. 2008;28(6):1661–71. https://doi.org/10.1148/rg.286085506.
24. Parker RA 3rd, Yano M, Tai AW, Friedman M, Narra VR, Menias CO. MR imaging findings of ectopic pregnancy: a pictorial review. Radiographics. 2012;32(5):1445–60; ; discussion 1460–2. https://doi.org/10.1148/rg.325115153.
25. Litwicka K, Greco E. Caesarean scar pregnancy: a review of management options. Curr Opin Obstet Gynecol. 2011;23(6):415–21. https://doi.org/10.1097/GCO.0b013e32834cef0c.
26. Kirk E, Bourne T. Ectopic pregnancy. Obstet Gynaecol Reprod Med. 2011;21(7):207–11.
27. Wu R, Klein MA, Mahboob S, Gupta M, Katz DS. Magnetic resonance imaging as an adjunct to ultrasound in evaluating cesarean scar ectopic pregnancy. J Clin Imaging Sci. 2013;3:16. https://doi.org/10.4103/2156-7514.109758.
28. Lowe LH, Marchant TC, Rivard DC, Scherbel AJ. Vascular malformations: classification and terminology the radiologist needs to know. Semin Roentgenol. 2012;47(2):106–17. https://doi.org/10.1053/j.ro.2011.11.002.
29. Gloviczki P, Duncan A, Kalra M, Oderich G, Ricotta J, Bower T, McKusick M, Bjarnason H, Driscoll D. Vascular malformations: an update. Perspect Vasc Surg Endovasc Ther. 2009;21(2):133–48. https://doi.org/10.1177/1531003509343019.
30. Dahlgren LS, Effer SB, McGillivray BC, Pugash DJ. Pregnancy with uterine vascular malformations associated with hemorrhagic hereditary telangiectasia: a case report. J Obstet Gynaecol Can. 2006;28(8):720–3.
31. Grivell RM, Reid KM, Mellor A. Uterine arteriovenous malformations: a review of the current literature. Obstet Gynecol Surv. 2005;60(11):761–7. https://doi.org/10.1097/01.ogx.0000183684.67656.ba.
32. Rebarber A, Fox NS, Eckstein DA, Lookstein RA, Saltzman DH. Successful bilateral uterine artery embolization during an ongoing pregnancy. Obstet Gynecol. 2009;113(2 Pt 2):554–6. https://doi.org/10.1097/AOG.0b013e318193bfdf.
33. Thabet A, Kalva SP, Liu B, Mueller PR, Lee SI. Interventional radiology in pregnancy complications: indications, technique, and methods for minimizing radiation exposure. Radiographics. 2012;32(1):255–74.
34. Aziz N, Lenzi TA, Jeffrey RB, et al. Postpartum uterine arteriovenous fistula. Obstet Gynecol. 2004;103:1076–8.
35. Department of Reproductive Health and Research, World Health Organization. Maternal mortality in 2000: estimates developed by WHO, UNICEF, and UNFPA. Geneva: WHO; 2004.
36. Goldstein RB, Bree RL, Benson CB, Benacerraf BR, Bloss JD, Carlos R, Fleischer AC, Goldstein

SR, Hunt RB, Kurman RJ, Kurtz AB, Laing FC, Parsons AK, Smith-Bindman R, Walker J. Evaluation of the woman with postmenopausal bleeding: Society of Radiologists in Ultrasound-Sponsored Consensus Conference statement. J Ultrasound Med. 2001;20(10):1025–36. https://doi.org/10.7863/jum.2001.20.10.1025.
37. Vijayakumar A, Srinivas A, Chandrashekar BM, Vijayakumar A. Uterine vascular lesions. Rev Obstet Gynecol. 2013;6(2):69–79.
38. Gonsalves M, Belli A. The role of interventional radiology in obstetric hemorrhage. Cardiovasc Intervent Radiol. 2010;33(5):887–95. https://doi.org/10.1007/s00270-010-9864-4.
39. Ganguli S, Stecker MS, Pyne D, Baum RA, Fan CM. Uterine artery embolization in the treatment of postpartum uterine hemorrhage. J Vasc Interv Radiol. 2011;22(02):169–76.
40. Sellmyer MA, Desser TS, Maturen KE, Jeffrey RB Jr, Kamaya A. Physiologic, histologic, and imaging features of retained products of conception. Radiographics. 2013;33(3):781–96. https://doi.org/10.1148/rg.333125177.
41. Rath WH. Postpartum hemorrhage--update on problems of definitions and diagnosis. Acta Obstet Gynecol Scand. 2011;90(5):421–8. https://doi.org/10.1111/j.1600-0412.2011.01107.x.
42. Panelli DM, Phillips CH, Brady PC. Incidence, diagnosis and management of tubal and nontubal ectopic pregnancies: a review. Fertil Res Pract. 2015;1:15. https://doi.org/10.1186/s40738-015-0008-z.
43. Chetty M, Elson J. Treating non-tubal ectopic pregnancy. Best Pract Res Clin Obstet Gynaecol. 2009;23(4):529–38. https://doi.org/10.1016/j.bpobgyn.2008.12.011.
44. Vela G, Tulandi T. Cervical pregnancy: the importance of early diagnosis and treatment. J Minim Invasive Gynecol. 2007;14(4):481–4. https://doi.org/10.1016/j.jmig.2006.11.012.
45. Yu B, Douglas NC, Guarnaccia MM, et al. Uterine artery embolization as an adjunctive measure to decrease blood loss prior to evacuating a cervical pregnancy. Arch Gynecol Obstet. 2009;279:721–72.
46. Andreotti RF, Fleischer AC. The sonographic diagnosis of adenomyosis. Ultrasound Q. 2005;21(3):167–70. https://doi.org/10.1097/01.ruq.0000174751.34633.9a.
47. Chopra S, Lev-Toaff AS, Ors F, Bergin D. Adenomyosis: common and uncommon manifestations on sonography and magnetic resonance imaging. J Ultrasound Med. 2006;25(5):617–27; ; quiz 629. https://doi.org/10.7863/jum.2006.25.5.617.
48. Savelli L. Ultrasound evaluation of the female internal genitalia—EFSUMB course book. London: EFSUMB; 2012.
49. Cunningham RK, Horrow MM, Smith RJ, Springer J. Adenomyosis: a sonographic diagnosis. Radiographics. 2018;38(5):1576–89. https://doi.org/10.1148/rg.2018180080.
50. Leyendecker G, Bilgicyildirim A, Inacker M, et al. Adenomyosis and endometriosis. Re-visiting their association and further insights into the mechanisms of auto-traumatisation. An MRI study. Arch Gynecol Obstet. 2015;291(4):917–32. https://doi.org/10.1007/s00404-014-3437-8.
51. Buy JN, Ghossain M, Benign and malignant mesechymal tumors of the uterus, In: Gynecological imaging; Springer-Verlag Berlin; 597-638 2013.
52. Woźniak A, Woźniak S. Ultrasonography of uterine leiomyomas. Prz Menopauzalny. 2017;16(4):113–7. https://doi.org/10.5114/pm.2017.72754.
53. Wilde S, Scott-Barrett S. Radiological appearances of uterine fibroids. Indian J Radiol Imaging. 2009;19(3):222–31. https://doi.org/10.4103/0971-3026.54887.
54. Deshmukh SP, Gonsalves CF, Guglielmo FF, Mitchell DG. Role of MR imaging of uterine leiomyomas before and after embolization. Radiographics. 2012;32(6):E251–81. https://doi.org/10.1148/rg.326125517.
55. Maciel C, Tang YZ, Sahdev A, Madureira AM, Vilares MP. Preprocedural MRI and MRA in planning fibroid embolization. Diagn Interv Radiol. 2017;23(2):163–71. https://doi.org/10.5152/dir.2016.16623.
56. Khan AT, Shehmar M, Gupta JK. Uterine fibroids: current perspectives. Int J Women's Health. 2014;6:95–114. https://doi.org/10.2147/IJWH.S51083.
57. Salim S, Won H, Nesbitt-Hawes E, Campbell N, Abbott J. Diagnosis and management of endometrial polyps: a critical review of the literature. J Minim Invasive Gynecol. 2011;18(5):569–81. https://doi.org/10.1016/j.jmig.2011.05.018.
58. Buy JN, Ghossain M. Benign and malignant endometrium, In: Gynecological imaging; Springer-Verlag Berlin; 549-588 2013
59. Balcacer P, Cooper KA, Huber S, Spektor M, Pahade JK, Israel GM. Magnetic resonance imaging features of endometrial polyps: frequency of occurrence and interobserver reliability. J Comput Assist Tomogr. 2018;42(5):721–6. https://doi.org/10.1097/RCT.0000000000000765.
60. Buy JN, Ghossain M. Benign diseases of the cervix. In: Gynecological imaging; Springer-Verlag Berlin; 653-661 2013.
61. Barwick TD, Rockall AG, Barton DP, Sohaib SA. Imaging of endometrial adenocarcinoma. Clin Radiol. 2006;61(7):545–55. https://doi.org/10.1016/j.crad.2006.03.011.
62. Stamatellos I, Stamatopoulos P, Bontis J. The role of hysteroscopy in the current management of the cervical polyps. Arch Gynecol Obstet. 2007;276(4):299–303. https://doi.org/10.1007/s00404-007-0417-2.
63. Bhatla N, Berek JS, Cuello Fredes M, Denny LA, Grenman S, Karunaratne K, Kehoe ST, Konishi I, Olawaiye AB, Prat J, Sankaranarayanan R, Brierley J, Mutch D, Querleu D, Cibula D, Quinn M, Botha H, Sigurd L, Rice L, Ryu HS, Ngan H, Mäenpää J, Andrijono A, Purwoto G, Maheshwari A, Bafna UD, Plante M, Natarajan J. Revised FIGO staging for carcinoma of the cervix uteri. Int J Gynaecol Obstet. 2019;145(1):129–35. https://doi.org/10.1002/

ijgo.12749. Erratum in: Int J Gynaecol Obstet. 2019;147(2):279–280.
64. Merz J, Bossart M, Bamberg F, Eisenblaetter M. Revised FIGO staging for cervical cancer—a new role for MRI. Rofo. 2020;192(10):937–44. https://doi.org/10.1055/a-1198-5729. English, German.
65. Manganaro L, Lakhman Y, Bharwani N, Gui B, Gigli S, Vinci V, Rizzo S, Kido A, Cunha TM, Sala E, Rockall A, Forstner R, Nougaret S. Staging, recurrence and follow-up of uterine cervical cancer using MRI: updated guidelines of the European Society of Urogenital Radiology after revised FIGO staging 2018. Eur Radiol. 2021;31(10):7802–16. https://doi.org/10.1007/s00330-020-07632-9. Erratum in: Eur Radiol. 2021; Carcinoma and other tumors of the cervix, gynecological imaging, chapter 28, Springer.
66. Iacobellis F, Perillo A, Iadevito I, Tanga M, Romano L, Grassi R, Nicola R, Scaglione M. Imaging of oncologic emergencies. Semin Ultrasound CT MR. 2018;39(2):151–66. https://doi.org/10.1053/j.sult.2017.12.001.
67. Andreotti RF, Timmerman D, Strachowski LM, Froyman W, Benacerraf BR, Bennett GL, Bourne T, Brown DL, Coleman BG, Frates MC, Goldstein SR, Hamper UM, Horrow MM, Hernanz-Schulman M, Reinhold C, Rose SL, Whitcomb BP, Wolfman WL, Glanc P. O-RADS US risk stratification and management system: a consensus guideline from the ACR ovarian-adnexal reporting and data system committee. Radiology. 2020;294(1):168–85. https://doi.org/10.1148/radiol.2019191150.
68. Bhosale PR, Javitt MC, Atri M, Harris RD, Kang SK, Meyer BJ, Pandharipande PV, Reinhold C, Salazar GM, Shipp TD, Simpson L, Sussman BL, Uyeda J, Wall DJ, Zelop CM, Glanc P. ACR appropriateness criteria® acute pelvic pain in the reproductive age group. Ultrasound Q. 2016;32(2):108–15. https://doi.org/10.1097/RUQ.0000000000000200.
69. Sasaki KJ, Miller CE. Adnexal torsion: review of the literature. J Minim Invasive Gynecol. 2014;21(2):196–202. https://doi.org/10.1016/j.jmig.2013.09.010.
70. Moro F, Bolomini G, Sibal M, Vijayaraghavan SB, Venkatesh P, Nardelli F, Pasciuto T, Mascilini F, Pozzati F, Leone FPG, Josefsson H, Epstein E, Guerriero S, Scambia G, Valentin L, Testa AC. Imaging in gynecological disease (20): clinical and ultrasound characteristics of adnexal torsion. Ultrasound Obstet Gynecol. 2020;56(6):934–43. https://doi.org/10.1002/uog.21981.
71. Caprio MG, Di Serafino M, De Feo A, Guerriero E, et al. Ultrasonographic and multimodal imaging of pediatric genital female diseases. J Ultrasound. 2019;22(3):273–89. https://doi.org/10.1007/s40477-019-00358-5.
72. Lourenco AP, Swenson D, Tubbs RJ, Lazarus E. Ovarian and tubal torsion: imaging findings on US, CT, and MRI. Emerg Radiol. 2014;21(2):179–87. https://doi.org/10.1007/s10140-013-1163-3.
73. Sayasneh A, Ekechi C, Ferrara L, Kaijser J, Stalder C, Sur S, Timmerman D, Bourne T. The characteristic ultrasound features of specific types of ovarian pathology (review). Int J Oncol. 2015;46(2):445–58. https://doi.org/10.3892/ijo.2014.2764.
74. Curry A, Williams T, Penny ML. Pelvic inflammatory disease: diagnosis, management, and prevention. Am Fam Physician. 2019;100(6):357–64.
75. Kitaya K, Takeuchi T, Mizuta S, Matsubayashi H, Ishikawa T. Endometritis: new time, new concepts. Fertil Steril. 2018;110(3):344–50. https://doi.org/10.1016/j.fertnstert.2018.04.012.
76. Ney B, Diserens C, Vial Y, Mazzolai L. Syndrome de congestion pelvienne: une cause fréquente de douleur chronique [Pelvic congestion syndrome]. Rev Med Suisse. 2020;16(712):2042–5.
77. Osman AM, Mordi A, Khattab R. Female pelvic congestion syndrome: how can CT and MRI help in the management decision? Br J Radiol. 2021;94(1118):20200881. https://doi.org/10.1259/bjr.20200881.
78. Labropoulos N, Malgor RD, Comito M, Gasparis AP, Pappas PJ, Tassiopoulos AK. The natural history and treatment outcomes of symptomatic ovarian vein thrombosis. J Vasc Surg Venous Lymphat Disord. 2015;3(1):42–7. https://doi.org/10.1016/j.jvsv.2014.07.008.
79. Ho-Fung V, Jaimes CE, Pollock AN. Peritoneal inclusion cyst. Pediatr Emerg Care. 2011;27(5):430–1. https://doi.org/10.1097/PEC.0b013e3182184967.
80. Di Serafino M, Pezzullo F, Iacobellis F. et al. Multilocular peritoneal inclusion cyst: a diagnostic challenge. https://doi.org/10.35100/eurorad/case.16913

2 Imaging in Obstetrics

Valerio Di Paola, Francesco Lauriero, Federica Perillo, Luca Russo, Benedetta Gui, and Riccardo Manfredi

2.1 Introduction

Familiarity with the abnormal imaging features of obstetric pathology will potentially decrease fetal and maternal morbidity and mortality.

A first imaging approach is represented by abdominal or transvaginal ultrasound, thanks to its large availability. Magnetic resonance (MR) imaging is reserved for equivocal cases or when additional information is needed, especially in the first trimester. Computed tomography (CT) has a limited role in the evaluation of placental abnormalities because of ionizing radiation exposure and the relatively limited assessment of the fetus and fetal adnexa. However, CT can provide important information in specific circumstances, particularly on the evaluation of trauma and staging of malignant gestational trophoblastic disease.

An important aspect to consider is that the administration of iodinated or gadolinium contrast media should be avoided whenever a viable pregnancy is likely to be present.

2.2 Placental Pathology

Placenta is a maternal-fetal organ responsible for nutritive, respiratory, and excretory functions of the fetus during pregnancy. It is composed of maternal tissue (decidua), deriving from the endometrium, and fetal tissue (chorion), deriving from the trophoblast.

V. Di Paola (✉) · L. Russo · B. Gui
Dipartimento di Diagnostica per Immagini, Radioterapia Oncologica ed Ematologia, Policlinico Universitario Agostino Gemelli—IRCSS, Rome, Italy
e-mail: valerio.dipaola@policlinicogemelli.it; luca.russo@guest.policlinicogemelli.it; benedetta.gui@policlinicogemelli.it

F. Lauriero · F. Perillo
Istituto di Radiologia, Università Cattolica del Sacro Cuore, Rome, Italy
e-mail: francesco.lauriero@guest.policlinicogemelli.it

R. Manfredi
Dipartimento di Diagnostica per Immagini, Radioterapia Oncologica ed Ematologia, Policlinico Universitario Agostino Gemelli—IRCSS, Rome, Italy

Istituto di Radiologia, Università Cattolica del Sacro Cuore, Rome, Italy
e-mail: riccardo.manfredi@policlinicogemelli.it

R. Niola et al. (eds.), *Diagnostic and Interventional Radiology in Gynecological and Obstetric Diseases*, https://doi.org/10.1007/978-3-031-11910-1_2

The formation of the placenta takes place 7–8 days after fertilization, and by week 12 of gestation, the placenta is usually formed. At approximately day 7 after fertilization, the blastocyst attaches to the endometrial epithelium at the embryonic pole, and the outer trophectoderm layer (trophoblast) differentiates into syncytiotrophoblasts and cytotrophoblasts. Syncytiotrophoblast cells start to penetrate and invade the endometrial connective tissue. After the blastocyst implants in the endometrium, the syncytiotrophoblast cells erode into the endometrial glands and the blood vessels, establishing lacunar networks, which are the primordia of the intervillous spaces of the placenta. Cytotrophoblasts form a stem cell column for villous development and differentiate along a villous and an extra-villous pathway. Villous cytotrophoblastic cells remain attached to the villous basement membrane, whereas extravillous cytotrophoblastic cells, also referred to as intermediate trophoblast, break through the syncytium at selected sites and infiltrate the decidua, the myometrium, and the arteries of the implantation site and establish the maternal/fetal circulation [1].

Ultrasound (US) is the first line of imaging for placental assessment. The placenta is visible by 10 weeks gestation appearing as a thickened echogenic rim of tissue surrounding the gestational sac. Intervillous flow can be detected with color-Doppler by 12–14 weeks gestation. By 15 weeks gestation, the retroplacental clear space can be detected as a 1–2 cm thick hypoechoic area behind the placenta, composed of decidua, myometrium, and uterine vessels [2]. The normal US appearance of the placenta is a disc-shaped structure with uniform echogenicity and rounded edges, usually located along the anterior or posterior uterine walls. The midportion of the placenta typically measures between 2 and 4 cm in thickness. Sometimes focal hypoechoic areas with a slow flow can be detected corresponding to venous lakes. When the placenta shows an increased echogenicity, placental hemorrhage or hypoxia should be suspected, whereas reduced echogenicity and a jelly-like appearance of the placenta can be associated with pre-eclampsia. Placental calcification may be due to vascular insufficiency which increases the risk of adverse outcome.

MR imaging is indicated in the diagnostic workup when the ultrasound evaluation is equivocal or if additional information is required, thanks to the advantage of high soft-tissue contrast resolution and a large field of view. It is important to request that the patient not void for at least 1 h before the examination, to achieve the moderate bladder distension needed for evaluating the vesical-uterine interface. This is crucial, especially for cases of suspected *placenta accreta spectrum* (PAS).

The accuracy of the interpretation of PAS depends on the placental evolution throughout pregnancy. Before the 23rd week of gestation, as the placenta may not be mature, an MRI to evaluate abnormal placentation would not produce satisfactory results. However, between the 24th and 30th weeks of gestation, the optimal time to perform an MRI examination to assess PAS, the normal placenta shows a homogeneous intermediate signal intensity and is usually clearly differentiated from the myometrium, which is more hyperintense and heterogeneous [2]. After the 30th week of gestation, the placenta has a more heterogeneous signal intensity on the T2-weighted image. This is because the placenta has matured and the uterine wall has thinned, which diminishes the specificity of many of the documented MRI findings of PAS. Therefore, the optimal window for performing MRI in this clinical setting is between 24th and 30th weeks of gestation. It should be noted that performing MRI later than 30th weeks is not contraindicated because we still can rely on the integration of MRI signs or its correlation with US findings.

Dedicated imaging of the placenta should be divided into two parts: (1) maternal multiplanar imaging based on maternal anatomy and (2) placental multiplanar/multi-sequence imaging obtained orthogonal to the placental location, regardless of the maternal axis. Initially, images orthogonal to the maternal pelvis are helpful to evaluate the relationship of the placenta and uterus with the rest of the maternal anatomy.

MRI protocol should include multiplanar T2-weighted (both HASTE/SSFSE and FISP/FIESTA/balanced-FFE sequences) on the pelvis in the sagittal, coronal, and axial planes. Those sequences should be obtained also in the axial oblique plane perpendicularly to the placenta-myometrium interface with a recommended slice thickness ≤4 mm. T1-weighted TSE sequence with fat suppression, in the axial or sagittal plane, is recommended for detection of any intra- or retroplacental hemorrhage/abruption. Sagittal T1-weighted images without fat saturation over the bladder-lower uterine segment interface are highly recommended to evaluate for a normal line of bright fat between the bladder dome and the lower uterine segment. In the setting of other abnormal signs of the placenta accreta spectrum, the absence of bright T1 fat in this area can imply an extension of the placenta beyond the borders of the uterine wall (placenta percreta) [3].

Optional sequences are multiplanar steady-state free precession (SSFP) sequences for the distinction of vascularity and placental margins and diffusion-weighted imaging (DWI), with lower b values ranging from 0 or 50 s/mm^2 and upper b values ranging from 600 to 1000 s/mm^2, for the delineation of the placental boundaries in patients with severely engorged myometrium [4].

In the first trimester and up to approximately 24 weeks of gestational age, the placenta is immature and relatively thin (2–2.5 cm), showing a homogeneous high T2 signal intensity and relatively low T1 signal intensity. Between 24 and 31 weeks gestation, the placenta becomes slightly lobulated and develops internal signal heterogeneity. Multiple thin, hypointense lines crossing the perpendicular axis of the placenta progressively appear, representing the interlobular septa, that are better distinguished on SSFSE than SSFP sequences. Beyond 30 weeks of gestation, the placenta is thicker (3–4 cm) and its heterogeneity is easily identified, perhaps because of the clear visualization of the interlobular septae and expected senescence. Even in normal third-trimester pregnancies, it is not unusual to see more prominent regions of mild T2 hyperintensity near the basal membrane, which likely represents changes of the normal aging of the placenta and should not be confused with placental hydrops.

The interface between the maternal side of the placenta and the uterine wall should be evaluated on T2 SSFSE sequences because the inner myometrial line is typically hypointense and can be a useful imaging landmark. The contrast between the mildly hyperintense placental signal, the hypointense inner myometrium, and the hyperintense serosal and peri-uterine vessels gives a trilaminar "bright-dark-bright" appearance and enables optimal visualization of the placental–uterine interface. The peri-uterine vessels are also quite valuable as a secondary means to evaluate the uterine wall (particularly in suspected placentation anomalies). These commonly enlarged and tortuous vessels collected just external to the myometrium have been described as a "worm sign" because they look like serpiginous tangled areas of hyperintensity (on SSFP sequence) with mixed flow void artifact (on SSFSE sequence). Myometrial contractions are commonly imaged incidentally, visible as rounded or lentiform regions of transient myometrial thickening, demonstrating the low signal intensity typical of smooth muscle on T2-weighted images [5].

CT may be used in selected circumstances, particularly in trauma or, less frequently, in the evaluation of known or suspected metastatic disease. Because of CT low tissue contrast resolution normal placenta is not clearly distinguishable from the myometrium.

2.2.1 Placental Morphology

A variation in placental morphology may be the presence of an accessory small lobe as in the *succenturiate* placenta (Fig. 2.1). When the accessory lobe is equal in size to the main lobe, a bilobed placenta can be detected. The succenturiate placenta is associated with an increased risk of vasa previa, rupture of the

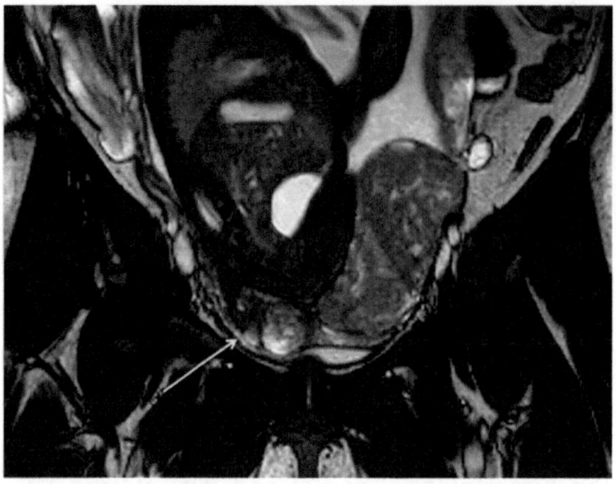

Fig. 2.1 Succenturiate placenta in a 35-year-old woman at 30° weeks of gestation with placenta percreta. T2-weighted coronal MRI image shows an accessory placental lobe with similar signal intensity of the main body of the placenta (*yellow* arrow)

vessels connecting lobes, and retained placenta, which can result in postpartum hemorrhage. Additionally, there can be abnormalities in the relationship between the placenta and chorioamniotic membranes, leading to higher rates of complications. These include the circumvallate placenta that occurs when the fetal chorionic plate of the placenta is too small and the chorionic membranes do not insert at the edge of the placenta but at some distance inward from the margins, giving an appearance of a ring of doubled membranes and fibrin surrounding the perimeter of the placenta. This variant may be complete if it included the entire placental circumference, or partial. It is associated with an increased risk of chronic placental abruption, preterm delivery, and small for gestational age status. At US a linear band or shelf-like structure isoechoic to the placental tissue, corresponding to the raised edge of the placenta, can be detected.

2.2.2 Placental Thickness and Location

The placental thickness should be measured in the midportion of the placenta. The average thickness of a normal placenta ranges from 2 to 4 cm, and the anterior placentas are approximately 7 mm thinner than posterior or fundal placentas so that an anterior placenta greater than 3.3 cm and a posterior placenta of greater than 4 cm should be considered thickened. A thickened placenta has been described in association with TORCH infections, gestational diabetes, and fetal hydrops. If cysts are present in the thickened placenta, molar pregnancy or triploidy should be suspected. A thin placenta can be related to pre-eclampsia and intrauterine growth restriction (IUGR).

Placental location may be anterior or posterior, fundal, left or right. Early in gestation, the placenta starts low in the uterus and as the pregnancy progresses, it moves up ("migrates") and away from the internal cervical os, in relation to the increase in the uterine volume. By about 30 weeks (early third trimester), the placenta reaches its final location. Initial interpretation for each case requires identification of the cervix and endocervical canal, which appears as a well-defined central hyperintense line of mucosa (this includes the mucosa and the mucus secreted by the endocervical glandular epithelium), surrounded by hypointense bands of cervical stroma (smooth muscle and fibroelastic tissue). The relationship of the internal cervical os and the placental margin should be evaluated, and any degree of *placenta previa* identified. Low-lying placenta occurs when the placental edge is located in the lower uterine segment within 2 cm or less of the internal cervical os, while placenta previa occurs when the placental edge covers partially (*partial placenta previa*) or completely (*complete or central placenta previa*) the internal cervical os. If placental tissue reaches the margin of the internal cervical os but does not cover it, placenta previa is called *marginal* (Fig. 2.2). Cesarean delivery is indicated when the distance of the placental edge from the internal cervical os is lower than 10 mm. Transvaginal US is superior to transabdominal US for the detection of the low-lying placenta. When placenta previa is detected early in pregnancy, follow-up US in the third trimester is recommended to reassess the position of the placenta.

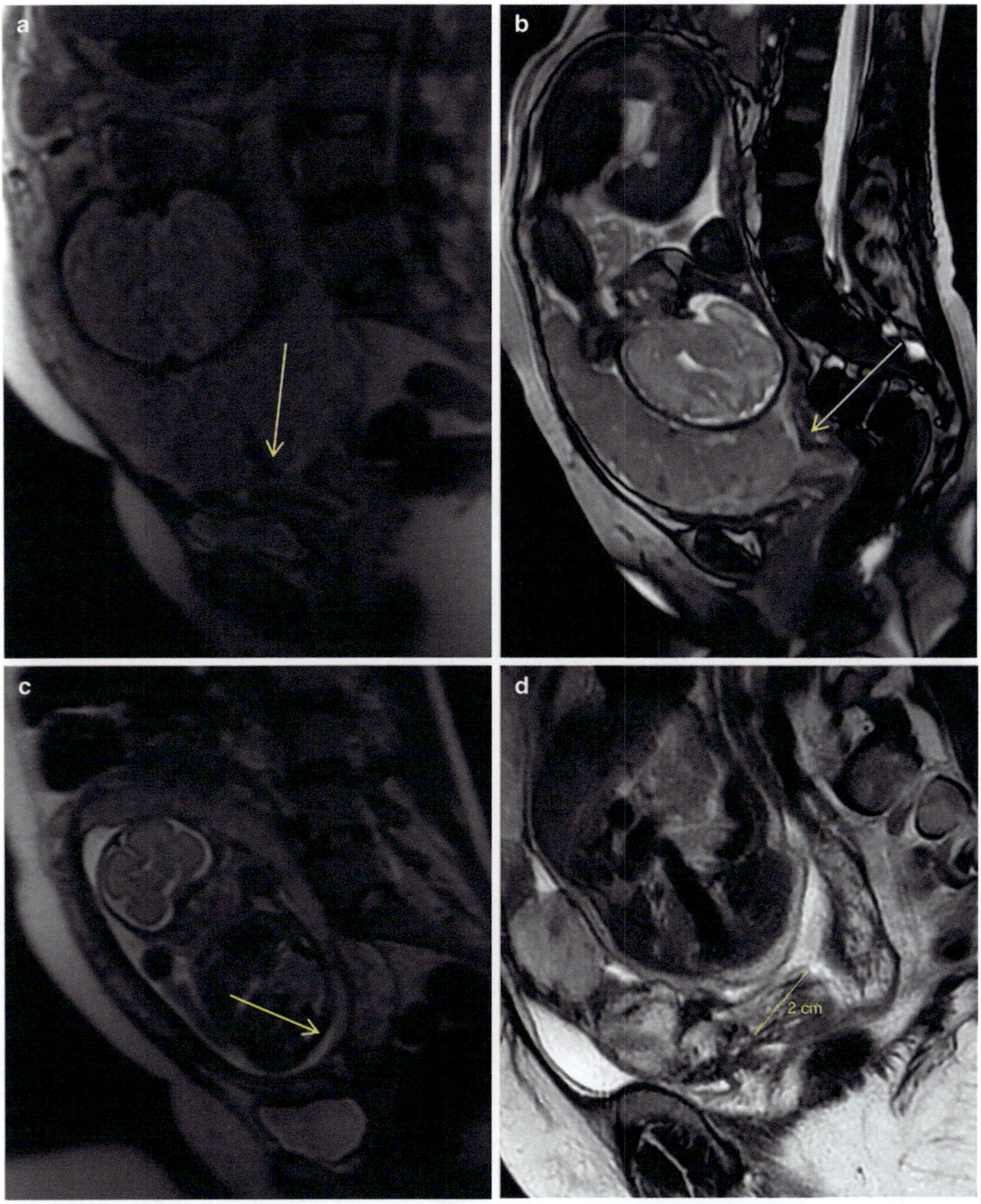

Fig. 2.2 T2-weighted sagittal MRI images show different patterns of placenta previa according to its relationship with inner cervical os: in *complete or central placenta previa*, placenta totally covers inner cervical os (**a**); in *partial placenta previa*, placenta partially covers the inner cervical os (**b**); in *marginal placenta previa*, placental tissue reaches the margin of the internal cervical os but does not cover it (**c**); in *low-lying placenta*, the placental edge is located in the lower uterine segment within 2 cm or less of the internal cervical os (**d**)

2.2.3 Cord Insertion Abnormalities

The umbilical cord is visualized at US by 42 days of gestation and is well established by 8–9 weeks of gestation. At US, the umbilical cord appears as a twisted, ropelike, echogenic structure that connects the fetus at its umbilicus to or near the center of the placenta. Abnormal cord insertion is associated with IUGR, fetal heart rate abnormalities, placental abruption, preterm labor, low Apgar scores, and neonatal demise. The umbilical cord insertion site should be routinely evaluated at all obstetric US examinations. Marginal cord insertion occurs when the umbilical cord inserts within 2 cm of the placental edge and is best diagnosed using Doppler US. This condition is not associated with an increased risk of growth impairment or preterm delivery, though marginal cord insertion less than 0.5 cm from the placental edge may progress to velamentous cord insertion later in pregnancy. In velamentous insertion, the umbilical vessels diverge from each other, and run between the chorion and the amnion, inserting into these membranes but not reaching the placenta. Therefore, the umbilical vessels are not supported by the placenta or by Wharton jelly. Diagnosis of velamentous cord insertion is made at Doppler US by findings of splayed umbilical vessels at the periphery of the placenta and an absence of central cord insertion.

Velamentous cord insertion is associated with cord compression and a higher risk of IUGR, congenital anomalies, preterm labor, placental abruption, vasa previa, low Apgar scores, and abnormal intrapartum fetal heart rate patterns [6]. When velamentous cord insertion is detected at routine obstetric US examination, patients should be evaluated with serial US examinations to monitor for complications. The prevalence of marginal cord insertion is 7–9% in singleton pregnancies and 24–33% in twins, while the prevalence of velamentous cord insertion is 1% in singleton pregnancies and about 15% in monochorionic twin gestations.

2.2.4 Vasa Previa

Vasa previa refers to umbilical vessels, unsupported by Wharton jelly or placental tissues, that cross or run in the proximity (<2 cm) of the internal cervical os. Its prevalence is low, approximately 0.04%, but it carries a significant risk of fetal death when the membranes break with 60% of mortality if it is misdiagnosed before the delivery. Correct diagnosis of vasa previa before rupture of the membranes increases fetal survival from a rate of 44% to 97%. The key to preventing an adverse fetal outcome is to perform a cesarean delivery before rupture of the fetal membranes occurs. Color Doppler US is the imaging modality of choice and shows hypoechoic tubular structures overlying the internal cervical os with a fixed position during maternal repositioning. Power-Doppler US shows fetal-type flow, with a fetal heart rate, within these vessels. Differential diagnosis includes funic presentation, defined as one or several loops of the umbilical cord located above the cervix and between the fetal presenting parts and the fetal membranes that overlie the cervix. Repositioning the mother during the US examination or serial scans may help differentiate these entities. The umbilical cord segment with funic presentation will move, whereas in the case of vasa previa the location of the cord segment will not change. Another potential US mimic is marginal sinus previa, prominent maternal vessels at the edge of the placenta.

2.2.5 Placental Cyst

True cysts, also called chorionic plate cysts, are anechoic thin-walled structures with an estimated prevalence of 2–7%. They are usually benign and small and frequently go unnoticed; very rarely, if larger than 4.5 cm, they have been reported to be associated with IUGR. Placental lakes or intervillous spaces are usually hypoechoic with swirling echoes and demonstrate low-velocity laminar flow at B-mode or Doppler imaging. They are usually seen in the late second trimester or third trimester. They are not associated with uteroplacental complications or adverse pregnancy outcomes.

2.2.6 Placental Abruption

Placental abruption occurs when there is a partial or complete detachment of the placenta from the underlying myometrium before the expected delivery time. Placental abruption complicates approximately 1% of pregnancies and most frequently occurs between 24 and 26 weeks of gestation. Risk factors for abruption include chronic hypertension, trauma, and advanced maternal age.

Imaging appearance of placental abruption can be classified based on the location of the hematoma as retroplacental, marginal subchorionic, preplacental, and intraplacental [7]. Retroplacental hematoma is located behind the basal plate and usually results from disruption of small arterioles. Marginal subchorionic hematomas are the most common type and are usually due to rupture of the uteroplacental veins. They are located near the placental margin, with an extension between the chorio-amniotic membranes and the placenta proper. Preplacental hematoma is less common and located behind the amnion above the chorionic plate, while intraplacental hematoma is a bleeding in the intervillous space of the placenta.

US remains the initial modality of choice for placental assessment despite its low sensitivity in the detection of placental abruption, with reported sensitivity as low as 25%, as acute and subacute hematomas are frequently isoechoic to placental tissue. Despite low sensitivity (as low as 24%), imaging findings when present are highly specific for abruption (92–96%). Ultrasound has a high positive predictive value (88–100%) and a low negative predictive value (14–53%) [8]. Acute or subacute hematomas usually have a subtle appearance since they may have echogenicity similar to or slightly higher than the adjacent placenta, while chronic hematomas usually are hypoechoic. Hematomas tend to be isoechoic acutely, have mixed echogenicity subacutely, then are hypo- to anechoic when chronic, appearing similar to amniotic fluid. Retroplacental hematoma should be suspected at US if the retroplacental hypoechoic zone is thickened to more than 2 cm. An ultrasound maneuver has been described to identify acute and sub-acute preplacental hematomas. Gently pushing the transducer on the hematoma shows some mobility or softness in the hematoma, which is not present in the normal adjacent placental tissue. This phenomenon has been termed the "jello effect" of hematoma. Preplacental hematoma may be associated with mass effect on the placental cord insertion and consequently result in ischemia and abnormal umbilical cord Doppler signal with increased risk of fetal demise. Additionally, a thickened placenta with rounded bulging and heterogeneous echotexture with loss of the placental-myometrial interface can also be present. A positive finding of a hematoma at US is associated with worse neonatal outcome since visualization of a blood clot likely indicates a large-volume hemorrhage that would be more likely to manifest signs and symptoms.

Differential diagnosis on MRI includes uterine contractions, which are usually transient, and uterine fibroids, which demonstrate internal vascularity at color-Doppler imaging.

Placental assessment with CT is usually performed in the setting of trauma, when CT is performed for assessment of maternal injuries. The reported sensitivity in the detection of placental abruption after trauma is as high as 100% and specificity ranges from 79.5% to 82%. At CT, the placenta appears homogeneous in the first and early second trimesters, becoming increasingly heterogeneous in the second and third trimesters. Placental cotyledons begin to form in the second trimester and can be seen as foci of rounded low attenuation surrounded by enhancing placenta. After a trauma, on contrast-enhanced CT, placental abruption may present as a partial or full-thickness area of low attenuation, which usually forms acute angles with the myometrium. Myometrial contractions can appear as low-attenuation areas and resemble infarction; however, myometrial contractions have obtuse angles with the adjacent myometrium. Detection of the placental hematoma is challenging on non-contrast CT, because hematoma may have the same attenuation as the pla-

Table 2.1 Traumatic abruption placenta scale (TAPS): CT-based placental enhancement grading system

Grade	Placental enhancement (%)	Imaging findings
0	100	Homogeneous high attenuation
1	>50	Heterogeneous placenta with low-attenuation geographic areas due to normal variants
2a	>50	Full thickness areas of low attenuation with acute angles with myometrium
2b	25–50	Contiguous or full thickness areas of low attenuation with acute angles with myometrium
3	<25	Large perfusion defects with <25% overall residual placental enhancement

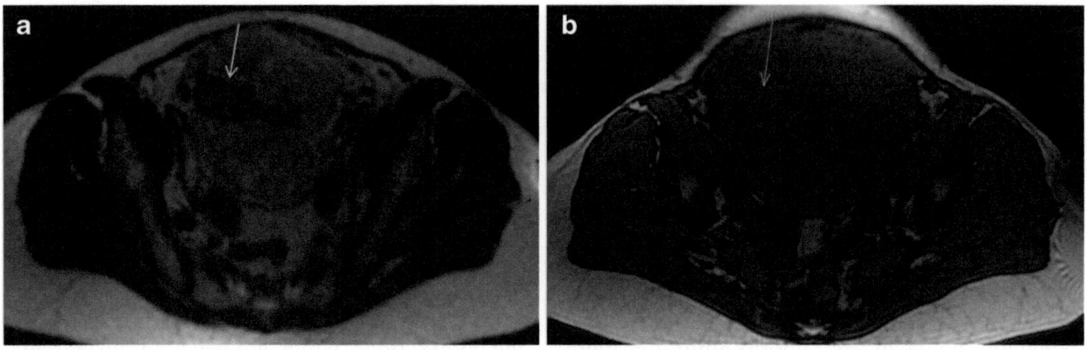

Fig. 2.3 Placenta increta in a 36-year-old woman at 33° weeks of gestation, with history of previous cesarian section. T2-weighted axial image shows a hyperintense area delined by a hypointense rim on the anterior right side of the placenta (*green* arrow in **a**), which corresponds to the hyperintense area on the T1-weighted axial image (*green* arrow in **b**), representing an intraplacental hematoma in a subacute phase

centa. Hyperattenuating amniotic fluid from placental bleeding into the amniotic cavity may occasionally be seen. An abnormal elevation of the placental edge should raise a concern about the presence of undermining hematoma. As placental heterogeneity increases with gestational age, detection of placental injury becomes more challenging. For this reason, a standardized CT grading system has been proposed for the evaluation of the placenta in the setting of trauma, called the Traumatic Abruption Placental Scale (TAPS), which has five grades (Table 2.1) [9]. When a grade 2a or higher is estimated, extended clinical observation is necessary and cesarean section is mandatory if clinical symptoms and signs of abruption occur.

MR imaging is superior to US in the evaluation of placenta hemorrhage, likely owing to the improved soft tissue contrast and a wider field of view. MR imaging can accurately depict placental abruption, with an excellent interobserver agreement and with a reported high sensitivity of 95–100% and high specificity of 100%. However, since management of abruption is based on clinical findings, not on imaging findings, MR imaging is not routinely performed and can be considered after negative US results if the diagnosis of abruption would potentially change management.

At MR imaging, hematomas are diagnosed on the basis of the identification of a well-marginated intrauterine blood collection, the signal intensity of which varies according to onset. T1- and T2-weighted sequences are complementary, and both are required for complete tissue characterization. By considering the signal intensity changes on T1- and T2-weighted imaging with special reference to the paramagnetic effects of methemoglobin, it is possible to estimate the age of the bleeding and intrauterine hematomas can be accurately classified into hyperacute, acute, early subacute, late subacute, and chronic hematomas (Fig. 2.3). Diffusion-weighted imaging

(DWI) is an excellent sequence for detecting intrauterine hemorrhagic lesions. Blood breakdown products cause susceptibility effects and can be accurately demonstrated with the diffusion-weighted sequence [10]. Therefore, T2-weighted half-Fourier RARE and true FISP are useful sequences, which are highly sensitive in detecting acute ischemia and can easily identify hematomas.

2.2.7 Placenta Accreta Spectrum Disorders

Placenta accreta spectrum (PAS) represents the abnormal invasion of the placental chorionic villi beyond the decidua basalis. PAS should be considered as a disease resulting from a combination of many factors such as a defective decidua, abnormal trophoblastic attachment, abnormal angiogenesis and vascular remodeling, and progressive uterine scar dehiscence. At the beginning of the twentieth century, the first studies on placenta accreta reported the estimated incidence to be 1 in 30,000 deliveries in the US. By contrast, recent publications from all over the world reported a notable increase in the prevalence of this condition, with an incidence of 1 in 533 births and even 1 in 321 births in populations with higher rates of cesarean section [11]. In the presence of placenta previa, the history of one cesarean section confers a risk of almost 24% for PAS disorders. This risk reaches up to 64% when there is a history of multiple (≥3) cesarean sections. Prior cesarean section, placenta previa, advanced maternal age, high gravidity and parity, multiple abortions with curettage, and anterior low location of the placenta have all been established as risk factors for placenta accrete [12]. PAS is classified according to the depth of placental invasion into the uterine wall (i.e., placenta accreta, increta, and percreta), with increasing degrees of invasion into and outside the uterine wall. In *placenta accreta*, the placenta is in direct contact with the myometrium, with partial or complete absence of the decidua basalis; in *placenta increta*, the placenta invades the myometrium but not the serosa; in *placenta percreta*, the placental invasion extends beyond the uterine serosa and into surrounding structures.

US remains the first line of imaging for the detection of PAS disorders. The transvaginal approach provides higher resolution and therefore enhances visualization. First and most importantly, it confirms the presence of placenta previa when suspected on a transabdominal ultrasound examination. Second, the transvaginal approach allows to evaluate the eventual placental invasion of the cervix, the posterior bladder wall, and internal aspects of the bladder. Tertiary centers are also using MRI for preoperative diagnosis and surgical planning. MR imaging is a complementary imaging examination when US findings are equivocal, or the placenta is located on the posterior wall of the uterus. Overall sensitivity and specificity of MR imaging for this condition are 75–100% and 65–100%, respectively. Uniform US and MRI lexicon has been proposed.

US features of PAS may be present as early as the first trimester. The three main markers include a gestational sac (GS) implanted in the lower uterine segment, a GS that is embedded in a cesarean section scar, and the presence of multiple vascular spaces (lacunae) within the placental bed. If the pregnancy continues, the lacunae become more prominent and are well-recognized markers for PAS in the second and third trimesters of pregnancy. In the second and third trimesters, multiple ultrasound findings have been associated with PAS such as multiple vascular lacunae, loss of the normal hypoechoic retroplacental zone, abnormality of the uterine serosa-bladder interface, thinning of the retroplacental myometrium, bulging of the lower uterine segment, and increased placental vascularity on color-Doppler.

Multiple vascular lacunae within the placenta, or a "Swiss-cheese" appearance is one of the most important sonographic findings of PAS in the second and third trimester. Lacunae are typically located deep within the placenta, have an irregular border, and a turbulent flow with high velocity and low impendence on color-Doppler. Multiple vascular lacunae within the placenta are correlated with high sensitivity and low false-positive rate for PAS; their positive predictive value varies by study and ranges from 73% to 100% and their negative predictive value is between 88% and 100%. However, it is important to remember that lacunae may be present in normal placentas. Moreover, PAS has been reported in the absence of multiple vascular lacunae.

Multiple vascular lacunae are defined on MR imaging as dilated tortuous signal void (>6 mm) or clump of intraplacental vessels on T2 SSFSE sequences within the placental parenchyma, which becomes high signal intensity on SSFP sequence, consistent with abnormal vascularity (Fig. 2.4). These disorganized vessels are frequently located near the areas of dark intraplacental banding on T2-weighted images, and they may occasionally extend beyond the placenta to the underlying myometrium. The resulting subplacental vascularity can cross the uterine serosa and may be associated with extensive neovascularity around the uterus, cervix, vagina, and bladder. This has led to the recent proposal of a sign termed the "stripped fetal vessel sign," defined as a large caliber intraplacental vessel that extends between the maternal and fetal placental surface without a change in vessel caliber.

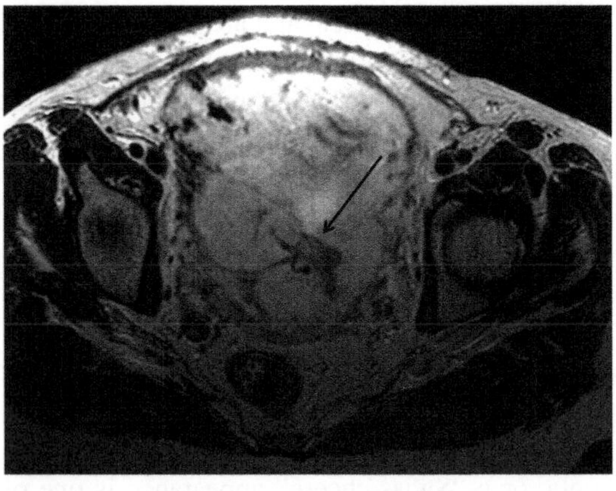

Fig. 2.4 Placenta percreta in a 37-year-old woman at 27° weeks of gestation. T2-weighted axial image shows dilated intraplacental tortuous signal void (*black* arrow), consistent with multiple vascular lacunae suggesting abnormal placental vascularity. In the same patient, dark intraplacental bands with irregular margins can be seen, representing areas of fibrin deposition due to repetitive intraplacental hemorrhage or infarcts. The patient underwent significant intraoperative bleeding during the cesarian section and consequent hysterectomy

Dark intraplacental bands on T2-weighted MR imaging is the most sensitive MRI feature for the diagnosis of PAS. They are characterized by irregular margins and a maximum diameter ranging from 6 to 20 mm or more. They are thought to represent areas of fibrin deposition due to repetitive intraplacental hemorrhage or infarcts. The sensitivity values of this sign for the diagnosis of placenta accreta, increta, and percreta are 89.7%, 89.7%, and 82.6%, respectively; specificity, however, is only moderate with corresponding values of 49.5%, 63.4%, and 58.5%. Furthermore, intraplacental dark bands have been shown to be a significant predictor of a poor maternal outcome as they were associated with increased intraoperative blood loss and hysterectomy.

Loss of the normal retroplacental zone between the placenta and the uterus is another second- and third-trimester marker for PAS. At US, loss of the normal hypoechoic (clear) retroplacental zone has a reported detection rate of 93%, a sensitivity of 52%, and a specificity of 57%. Furthermore, the loss of the clear space between the placenta and uterus is angle-dependent and can be seen in normal anterior placentas. Thus, this marker should not be used alone, but rather in combination with other markers. On MRI focal defects and myometrial thinning in the uteroplacental interface and disruption of the inner layer of the uteroplacental interface on T2-weighted images can be predictive of PAS with high sensitivity (97.4%) but, like at US imaging, with poor specificity (36.4%).

On US, the normal serosal-bladder interface is an echogenic smooth line without irregularities of vascular signals. If interruption of the serosal line, thickening of the line, or increased vascularity on color-Doppler are detected, PAS should be suspected. This marker is helpful particularly in cases of placenta percreta but less diagnostic when there is no bladder invasion. However, the sensitivity ranges from 70% to 90% and the specificity is about 99%. The positive and negative predictive values are 96% and 92%, respectively. On MRI, invasion of the bladder may be suspected in case of interruption, irregularity, or "tenting" of the bladder wall (Fig. 2.5). Direct visualization of placental tissue in the bladder lumen on MRI is highly specific (100%) for bladder involvement. The "bladder vessel sign," defined as visualization of numerous tortuous signal voids traversing the space from the uterus to the bladder, seems to be another accurate predictor of bladder wall involvement (including bladder serosa) with high diagnostic values up to 96%.

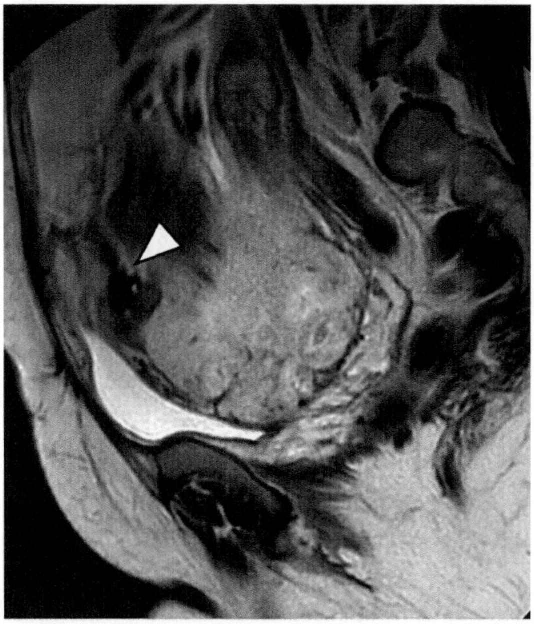

Fig. 2.5 Placenta percreta in a 35-year-old woman at 30° weeks of gestation. T2-weighted sagittal image shows tenting of the superior wall of the bladder, stretched and infiltrated by abnormal placental tissue. A flow void was also present in the adjacent placental tissue (arrowhead). The patient had acute vaginal bloody discharge at 35° weeks of gestation and underwent emergency cesarian section and successive subtotal hysterectomy

The presence of a *focal exophytic mass* is highly specific for PAS disorders and depicts placenta percreta and usually is located anteriorly toward the bladder or laterally toward the parametrium (Fig. 2.6).

Another marker for PAS is a retroplacental *myometrial thickness of <1 mm* (Fig. 2.7). Myometrial thinning has been described as an early sign suggesting placenta accreta. However, on US, determination of myometrial thickness in the lower uterine segment is difficult to assess and a cut-off for irregularity is controversial, since the lower uterine segment myometrium is thinner in patients with previous cesareans. One study reports a median lower uterine segment myometrial thickness of 2.4 mm in the third trimester. The sensitivity and specificity for this marker are very variable on US and range from 22% to 100% and 100% to 72%, respectively. On MRI, myometrial thinning can be present even in normal placentas, but it is highly unlikely to display total loss or disruption of the hypointense outer myometrial wall on T2-weighted images in the absence of PAS disorder. Thus, focal interruption of the myometrium is a moderately sensi-

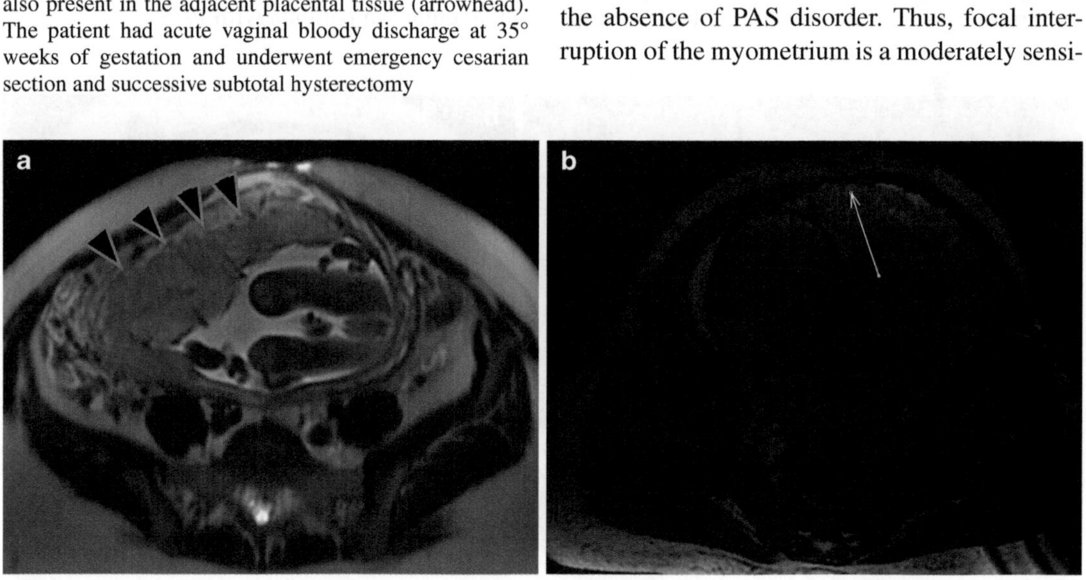

Fig. 2.6 Placenta percreta in a 24-year-old woman at 26° weeks of gestation with placenta percreta T2-weighted TSE axial image (**a**) shows the infiltration of the periuterine fat by placental tissue on the right antero-lateral uterine wall (arrowheads), with irregular interface. T2-weighted FIESTA axial image (**b**) better depicts the infiltration of the rectus abdominis muscles (arrow), which appear pinched by placental tissue. The patient underwent hysterectomy after the cesarian section

tive (63.6%) and specific (72.2%) sign for the detection of PAS disorders. Because extreme thinning can occur in late gestation, this sign should not be used as an independent sign but used in conjunction with other signs of PAS disorder.

Another proposed sign of PAS is *bulging of the lower uterine segment* (Fig. 2.7). Deviation of the uterine serosa can cause the placenta to bulge and impinge the bladder. On MRI, this finding can be best delineated on coronal and/or sagittal images. This bulging of the uterine contour has been suggested as a useful sign in the assessment of myometrial invasion with a sensitivity and specificity for the diagnosis of placenta increta and percreta of 76.7% and 62.5%, respectively. Where a bulge in the uterine contour is accompanied by focal disruption of the myometrium, the specificity of the sign increases.

Lumpy contour and rounded edge can be identified in PAS, resulting from placental tethering. Conversely, the normal placenta has a smooth contour and tapering, angled edges. These findings are frequently observed with a placental bulge (Fig. 2.7).

In case of abnormal placentation, the vascular architecture at the placental bed exhibits major alterations, with the vessels becoming nonuniformly distributed and very heterogeneous in size. On color-Doppler, the normal sub-placental venous complex should appear non-pulsatile with low-velocity venous blood flow waveforms. Identification of the *abnormal vascular architecture* on MRI exhibited the greatest accuracy for the diagnosis of PAS with sensitivity, specificity, PPV, and NPV equal to 81.6%, 100.0%, 100.0%, and 61.1%, respectively. The presence of uterine serosal hypervascularity on prenatal MRI (Fig. 2.8) is associated with increased intraoperative blood loss as well as with other complications during delivery, including hysterectomy or the need for bladder repair. In addition, the presence of bridging vessels linking the placenta and bladder with high diastolic arterial blood flow also suggests PAS. The sensitivity of color-Doppler for the diagnosis of invasive placenta ranges from 86% to 100% and the specificity is between 92% and 94%. On MRI, an extensive flow-void network extending from the uterine serosa to the bladder-uterine space ("bladder vessel" sign) or within the parametrial adipose tissue ("parametrial vessel" sign) is a highly accurate feature for the diagnosis of bladder and parametrial involvement in patients with PAS.

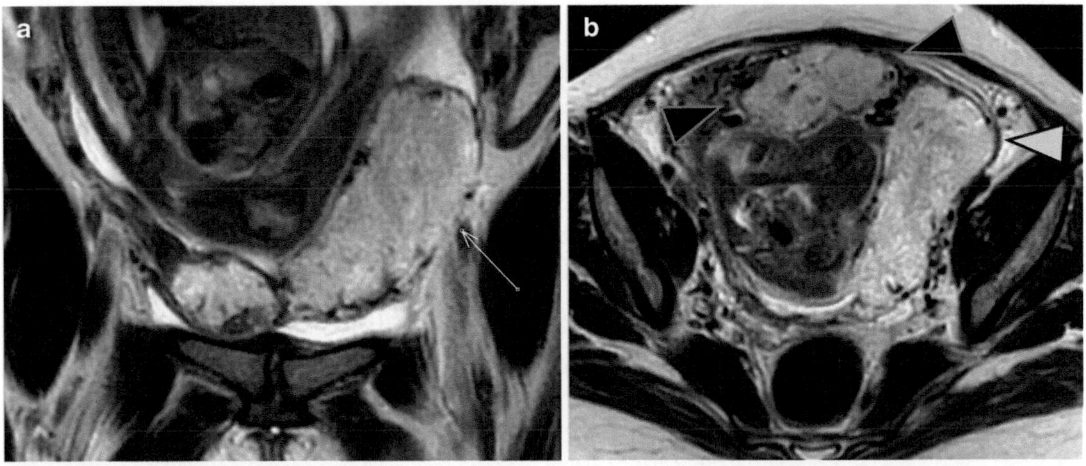

Fig. 2.7 Placenta percreta in a 35-year-old woman at 30° weeks of gestation. T2-weighted coronal image (**a**) shows myometrial thinning, which appears focally disrupted (*yellow* arrow in **a**). T2-weighted axial image (**b**) demonstrates bulging of the lower uterine segment (*yellow* arrowhead in **b**) and lumpy contour and rounded edge of placenta (*black* arrowheads in **b**)

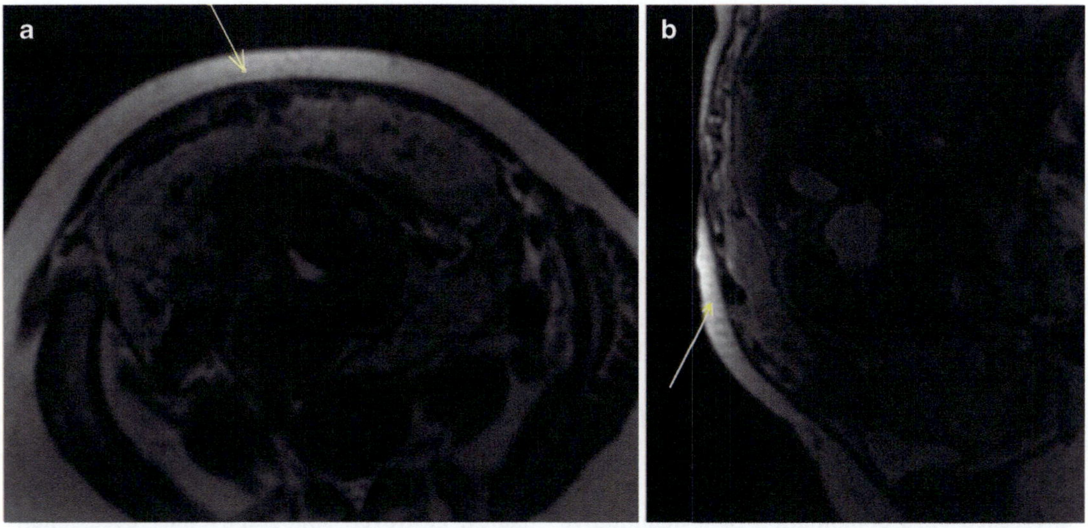

Fig. 2.8 Placenta increta in a 39-year-old woman at 30° weeks of gestation. T2 axial (**a**) and sagittal (**b**) images show an extensive flow-void network extending from the uterine serosa to the muscular abdominal wall, representing abnormal vascular architecture (yellow arrows)

Table 2.2 Main MRI signs of placenta accreta spectrum (PAS)

Spectral MRI findings of PAS	
Placenta accreta/increta	Placenta percreta
Dark intraplacental band	Myometrial thinning
Heterogeneous placenta	Focal disruption of myometrium
Placental bulge	Bladder or adjacent structural invasion
Lumpy contour and rounded edge	Focal exophytic mass sign
Abnormal/disorganized placental vascularity	
Thinning or loss of retroplacental T2 dark zone	

In conclusion, the MRI signs mentioned above are more specific than others. Placental heterogeneity, asymmetric thickening of the placenta, placental ischemic infarction, and abnormal intraplacental vascularity are reported as non-specific findings. Furthermore, the presence of only one specific MRI sign cannot be sufficient to diagnose PAS disorders, while the presence of at least two specific signs sensibly improves MRI accuracy [13]. A schematic summary of the main MRI signs of PAS is reported in Table 2.2.

2.3 Ectopic Pregnancy

Ectopic pregnancy refers to the abnormal implantation of blastocyst outside the endometrium of the uterine cavity [14, 15]. Ectopic pregnancy has an incidence of 1–2% in the general population, and of 2–5% among patients who have utilized assisted reproductive technology [16, 17], with a 9–14% mortality rate, representing the most common cause of pregnancy-related mortality in the first trimester [18, 19]. Major risk factors for ectopic pregnancy include a history of ectopic pregnancy, pelvic inflammatory disease, and gynecologic surgery. Other risk factors include a history of infertility, placenta previa, use of an intrauterine device, congenital uterine anomalies, endometriosis, history of smoking, exposure to diethylstilbestrol, and pregnancy conceived by assisted reproduction.

Patients with ectopic pregnancy present non-specific symptoms, such as crampy abdominal or pelvic pain, which can be unilateral or diffuse and range from mild to debilitating. However, up to 50% of patients do not report symptoms. Typical signs include first-trimester vaginal bleeding, which is typically intermittent, light, and either bright or dark red and rarely exceeds the normal menstrual flow. Sometimes a tender adnexal mass may be present. As an ectopic pregnancy enlarges, the risk for rupture increases and it should be suspected in patients with signs of shock, sometimes associated to shoulder pain due to the diaphragm irritation. Hemorrhage from ectopic pregnancy is the leading cause of pregnancy-related maternal death in the first trimester so that it should be treated on an emergency basis. The intensity of pelvic pain does not always correspond with the size of an ectopic pregnancy, and sometimes pain can even decrease after tubal rupture.

The diagnosis of ectopic pregnancy is typically based on a combination of a quantitative serum human chorionic gonadotropin (β-hCG) test and findings on transvaginal ultrasound (TVUS).

Usually, normal intrauterine pregnancies are associated with an early increase in β-hCG levels with a curvilinear trend. The rate of increase is at least 53% in 2 days, until β-hCG values reach a plateau at 9–11 weeks of gestational age and begin to decrease at approximately 20 weeks. In ectopic pregnancies, serum β-hCG values increase at a much slower rate, although up to 21% of cases present a doubling time not significantly different from that of viable intrauterine pregnancies. However, if β-hCG levels rise less than 50% during a 48-h period, a non-viable pregnancy (intra- or extra-uterine) must be suspected, and an associated early β-hCG plateau is highly suggestive of an ectopic pregnancy.

As TVUS is able to detect a gestational sac when β-hCG levels are higher than 2000 mIU/mL, it is preferred to transabdominal ultrasound, which can demonstrate intrauterine pregnancy when β-hCG levels exceed 6500 mIU/mL.

TVUS is highly accurate in the diagnosis of normal intrauterine pregnancy and ectopic pregnancy, with a sensitivity for the diagnosis of ectopic pregnancy that ranges from 73% to 93% and is dependent on the gestational age and the expertise of the ultrasonographer. In normal intrauterine pregnancies, approximately 4.5 weeks after the last menstrual period, TVUS shows the *intradecidual sign*, a small fluid collection (0.2–0.5 cm in diameter) located within the endometrium, surrounded by a hyperechoic ring. After a few days, the *double decidual sac* is identifiable, with two concentric hyperechoic rings that surround the anechoic gestational sac. At about 5.5 weeks of gestational age, *the secondary yolk sac* can be detected into the gestational sac and intrauterine pregnancy can be confirmed. Embryonic cardiac activity should be demonstrated at 5–6 weeks, when the gestational sac measures more than 18 mm.

In patients suspected to have an ectopic pregnancy, because of subthreshold β-hCG levels, the lack of an intrauterine gestational sac must lead to a detailed search for an ectopic pregnancy. However, sonography may occasionally fail to delineate even a more advanced ectopic pregnancy because of its inherent limited resolution and field of view, particularly in patients with severe pain or with non-ideal body habitus. In other cases, TVUS may reveal an adnexal mass which may be not typical for ectopic pregnancy.

MR imaging may be helpful in these situations by providing a larger field of view and an opportunity for additional anatomic localization in difficult cases, as it can provide images with high soft-tissue contrast in any plane and a more specific characterization of tissues and fluids. Fat-suppression techniques can also increase the conspicuity of inflammatory lesions. In addition, ascites and complex fluid can be easily identified on T2-weighted images. T2*-weighted images are useful for the identification of hemorrhage and air bubbles. Furthermore, contrast-enhanced imaging is useful in the evaluation of lesion vascularity and location in relation to pelvic vessels, as well as for the presence and site of active bleeding [20]. However, if an intrauterine gestation is a diagnostic possibility, gadolinium-based contrast agents should be avoided, since gadolinium crosses the placenta and appears in the fetal bladder shortly after maternal intravenous administration, and the long-term effects on the fetus are unknown [21]. Hence, MRI should be reserved for situations in which patients are hemodynamically and clinically stable and for whom additional information is necessary to guide patient care decisions and cannot be obtained using US.

CT is not the imaging modality of choice for the diagnosis of ectopic pregnancy, but it is occasionally performed in the evaluation of abdominal or pelvic pain of unknown cause or in a trauma setting. CT is certainly not an appropriate modality to be used for the purpose of the diagnosis of ectopic pregnancy. Strict urine or serum β-HCG screening before imaging is mandatory to avoid such an unexpected CT diagnosis.

Tubal pregnancy is the most frequent ectopic pregnancy (95% of cases), predominantly in the ampullary region (70%) and less commonly in the isthmus (12%) or fimbria (11.1%). The most common ultrasonographic sign of a tubal pregnancy detected in up to 89–100% of patients is the presence of an *adnexal mass* separated from the ovary (Fig. 2.9). This sign is more specific when the mass contains a yolk sac or when it moves independently from the ovary. The second typical sign of tubal pregnancies is the *tubal ring sign*, a hyperechoic ring surrounding an extrauterine gestational sac. The hypervascularity of the hyperechoic ring, detected at color-Doppler US, is defined "ring of fire" *sign*. However, the latter sign is not specific for ectopic pregnancy, because it can be documented surrounding a normal maturing follicle or a corpus luteal cyst, and so it is important to determine if this type of flow is within the ovary or outside it.

On MR imaging the most specific finding of ectopic pregnancy is the identification of the extrauterine gestational sac, a sac-like cystic

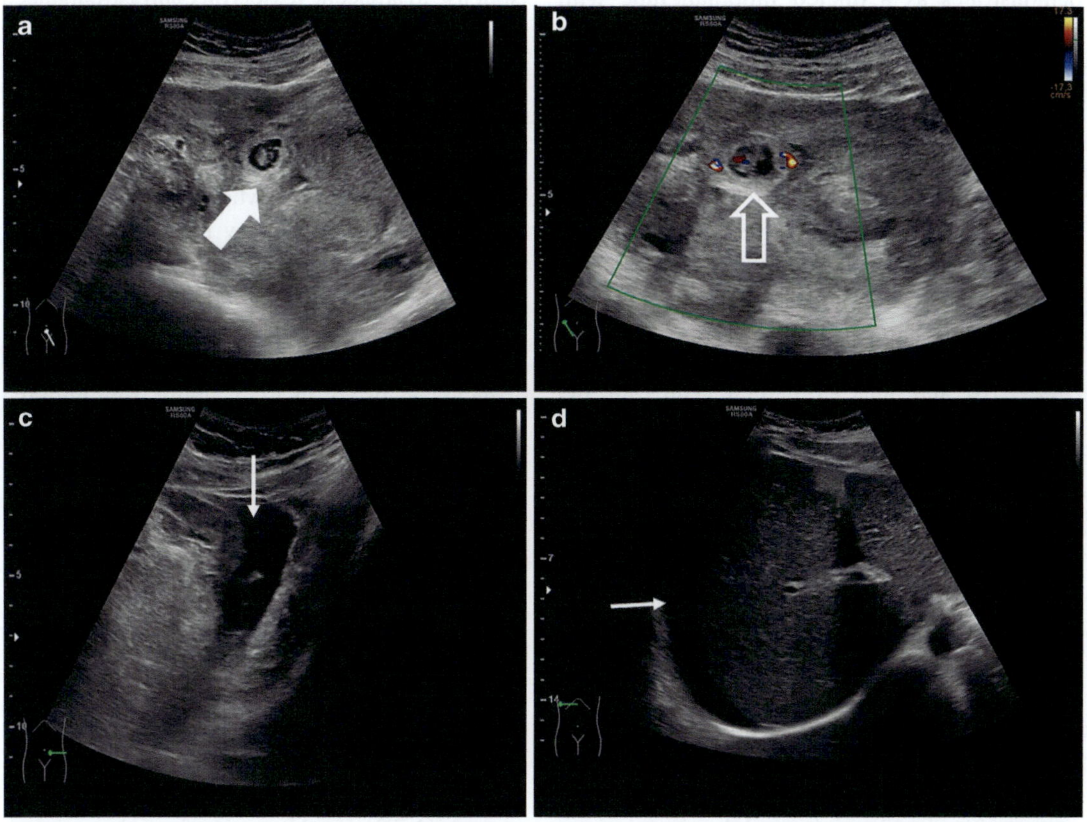

Fig. 2.9 Tubal pregnancy in a 23-year-old woman. Transabdominal US axial images show an extrauterine gestational sac separated from the ovary on the right side of the uterus (thick arrow in **a**), surrounded by a peripheral hyperechoic rim with hypervascularity (ring of fire sign) at color-Doppler US images (empty arrow in **b**). A large volume of fluid is seen throughout the abdomen, especially in the pelvis and around the liver (thin arrows in **c** and **d**, respectively)

tubal structure surrounded by a thick wall, corresponding to the tubal ring sign seen on US. The wall typically demonstrates high signal intensity on T2-weighted MR images and frequently is associated with an adjacent area of hemorrhage showing distinct low T2-weighted signal intensity and intermediate or high signal intensity on T1-weighted images. The cystic gestational sac-like component has been reported to frequently contain foci of acute hemorrhage characterized as regions of intermediate or high signal intensity on T1-weighted MR images. If contrast medium is administrated, enhancing *treelike solid components* representing fetoplacental tissues within mass may also be seen [22]. Another MRI finding is the *hematosalpinx* with tubal dilatation after implantation of the embryo into the epithelium of the fallopian tube. It typically demonstrates as a dilated fallopian tube with high signal intensity fluid on T1-weighted images.

CT findings similarly include a *pelvic cystic mass* with or without *hemoperitoneum*. On CT or MRI, the cystic mass may show some degree of peripheral enhancement, corresponding to the classic sonographic "ring of fire" sign.

An intrauterine finding of ectopic pregnancy is the *pseudo-gestational sac*, a thick decidual reaction surrounding intrauterine fluid, that is centrally located within the endometrial canal (Fig. 2.10), and must be distinguished from the double decidual sac of a viable pregnancy, which is located eccentrically within the endometrial canal. Another intrauterine finding is the presence of *thin-walled decidual cysts*, located at the junction of the endometrium and myometrium.

Extrauterine findings of ectopic pregnancy include *pelvic free fluid*, not very specific, *hematosalpinx*, and *hemoperitoneum* that is a more specific finding, with an 86–93% positive predictive value when β-hCG levels are abnormal. The presence of echogenic fluid within the Morrison pouch could be a sign of ruptured ectopic pregnancy with significant intra-abdominal hemorrhage. On MRI, disruption of tubal wall enhancement may be seen in a ruptured tubal pregnancy, and the demonstration of acute or recent hematoma (showing distinct low signal intensity on T2-weighted sequences) outside the enhancing implantation site may suggest tubal rupture in symptomatic patients. MRI can also help in the detection of hemoperitoneum, which appears as a fluid characterized by high signal intensity on T1-weighted images with fat suppression, and by mixed signal intensity on T2-weighted images. On CT, the appearance of hemorrhage varies with its age and location. Acute hemorrhage has an attenuation of 30–45 HU on unenhanced images because of its high proteinaceous content. Clotted blood appears hyperdense (>60 HU) because the concentration of hemoglobin increases in the first few hours after hemorrhage. The *sentinel clot sign* refers to the finding of a hyperdense clot near the site of bleeding. Active hemorrhage can be detected as high-attenuation foci nearly isodense to adjacent vessels on contrast-enhanced CT (Fig. 2.11).

Interstitial pregnancy is uncommon (2–4% of cases) and is based on the presence of trophoblastic tissue in the intra-myometrial segment of the fallopian tube. Its rate increases after in vitro fertilization or in patients who undergo salpingectomy. Interstitial pregnancy may be recognized later than the other ectopic pregnancies (even in the 16th week) because of the greater distensibility of this segment of the fallopian tube, and can lead to uterine rupture and life-threatening hemorrhage because of its high supply from both the ovarian and uterine vessels. The most specific US finding is the *interstitial line sign*, an echogenic line that extends into the upper region of the uterine horn and borders the margin of the intramural gestational sac. Another finding is the eccentric location of the gestational sac surrounded by a thin layer of the myometrium. These findings can be wrongly detected in some cases such as in uterine distortion due to the presence of leiomyomas. The diagnosis may be confirmed on MRI by the presence of an uninterrupted junctional zone separating the gestational sac, with heterogeneous high T2-signal intensity, from the endometrium. MRI may also be helpful in differentiating an interstitial from a normal intrauterine pregnancy in an anomalous uterus, such as a bicornuate uterus.

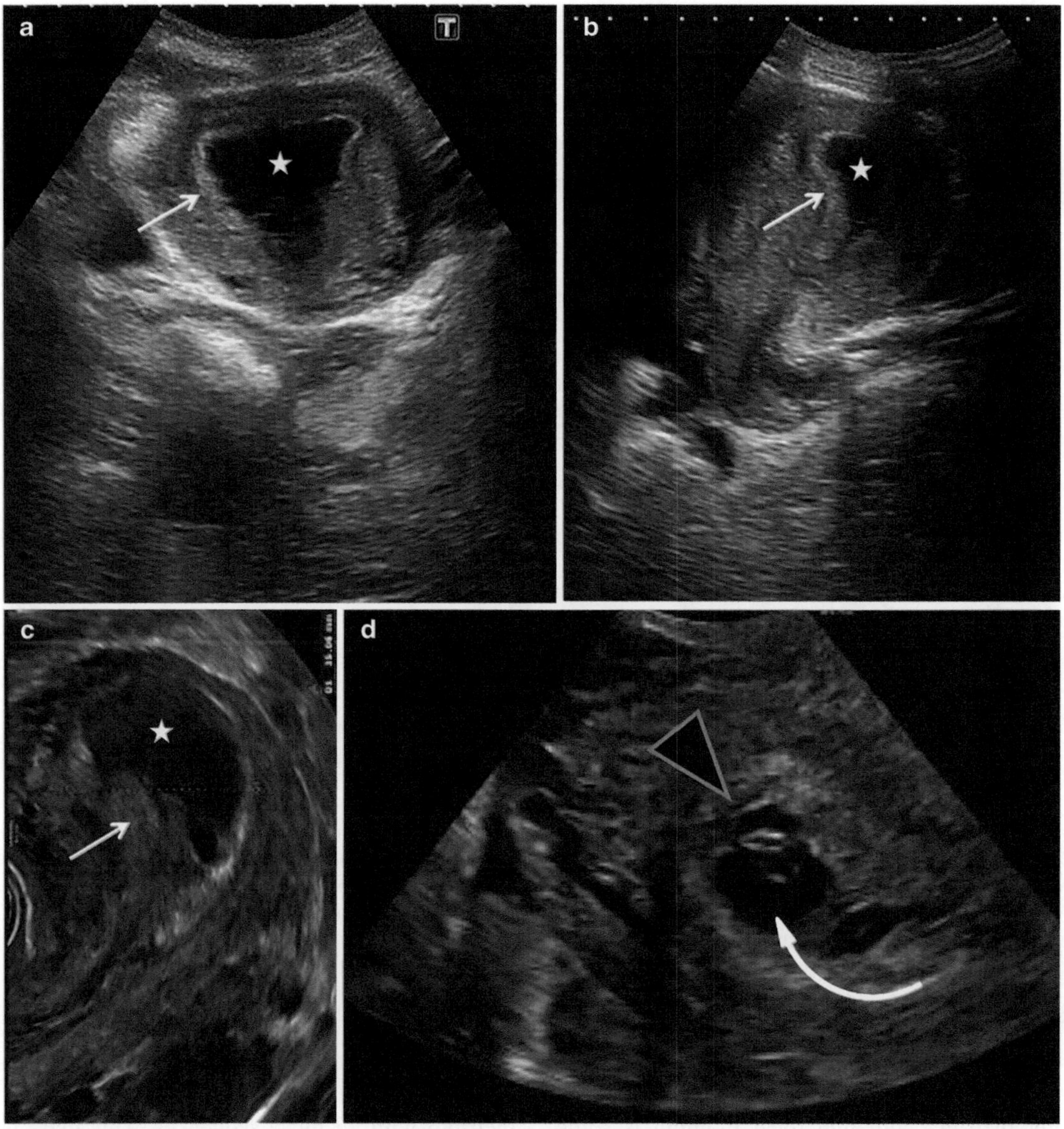

Fig. 2.10 Tubal pregnancy in a 41-year-old woman who underwent FIVET 1 month before; β-HCG levels 5,600 mU/mL. Axial (**a**) and sagittal transabdominal ultrasound images show a thick decidual reaction (arrows in **a** and **b**) surrounding intrauterine fluid (asterisks in **a** and **b**), which is centrally located within the endometrial canal and not eccentrically such as in a viable pregnancy and without embryo (pseudogestational sac sign). Sagittal transvaginal (**c**) ultrasound image better depicts the decidual reaction (arrow) and the pseudogestational sac (asterisk). Axial transvaginal (**d**) ultrasound image shows an adnexal mass with a hyperechoic ring (arrowhead) surrounding the extrauterine gestational sac with a yolk sac (curved arrow) inside it

On CT, a rounded ring-enhancing mass can be seen abutting the uterine fundus in the cornual region. The myometrium may sometimes be seen to partially surround the gestational sac.

Interstitial pregnancy must be distinguished from the *angular pregnancy*, which refers to the implantation in one of the lateral angles of the uterus, medially to the uterine-tubal junction and the round ligament of the uterus, and sometimes can be carried to term. At MR imaging, angular pregnancies appear as gestational sacs implanted in the lateral angle of the uterus and can be con-

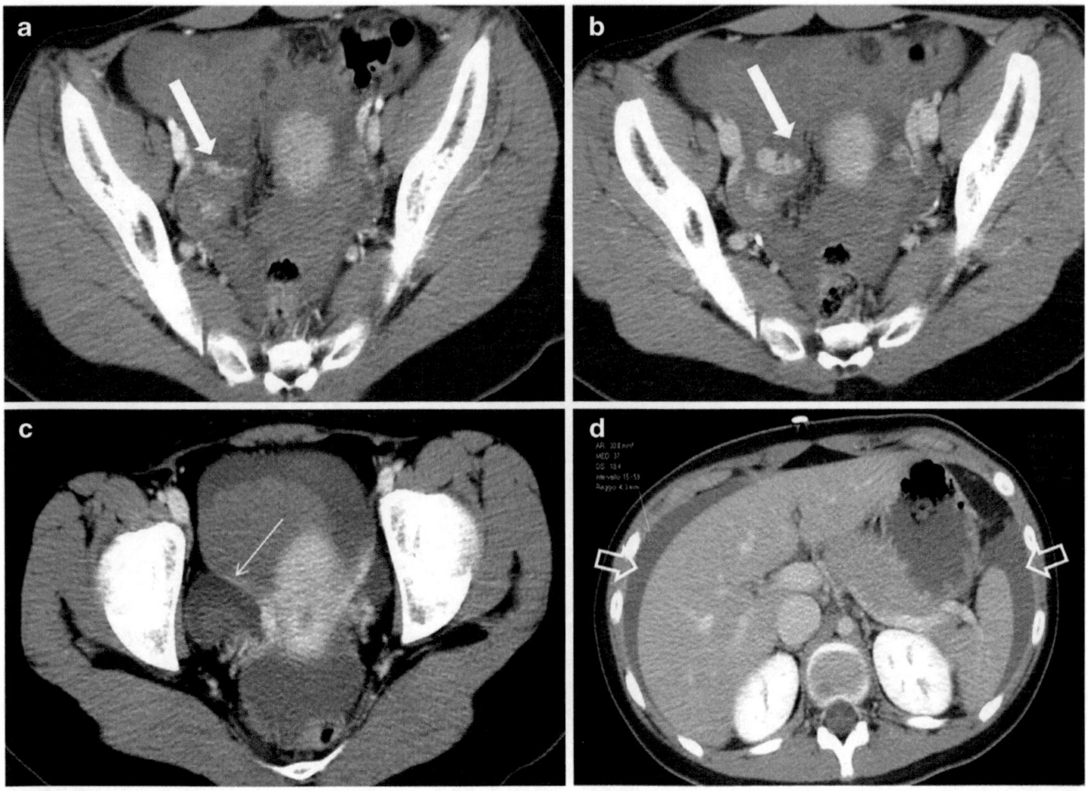

Fig. 2.11 Hemoperitoneum in a 14-year-old woman with tubal pregnancy (β-HCG levels: 13,082 mU/mL). The axial CT images in the arterial (**a**) and venous (**b**) phase depict an active bleeding on the anterior side of the hypervascular adnexal mass (thick arrows); these findings are consistent with ruptured left tubal pregnancy. The axial late phase (**c**) better shows the peripheral enhancement of the adnexal mass (thin arrow). Venous phase CT image of the upper abdomen (**d**) shows also a large volume of high-density fluid throughout the abdomen, suggesting the presence of hemoperitoneum (empty arrow in **d**). The patient underwent right salpingectomy and drainage of 3000 cc of hemoperitoneum

fused with normal pregnancies. These gestational sacs will be completely surrounded by uterine myometrium, although focal thinning is sometimes seen. High signal intensity in the uterine wall itself can represent intramural hemorrhage. It is also important to look for placental invasion of the myometrium because placenta accreta is frequently seen in these patients.

Cornual pregnancy occurs when the blastocyst abnormally implants in a horn of an anomalous uterus (i.e., unicornuate, bicornuate, didelphys, or septate uteri). As in the interstitial pregnancy, in cornual pregnancy the gestational sac is in an eccentric position surrounded by a thin layer of the myometrium (<5 mm). At MR imaging, a cornual ectopic pregnancy will appear as a gestational sac surrounded by a wall that should match the signal intensity of normal myometrium with all pulse sequences. This mass is located along the lateral margin of the dominant horn. The contralateral dominant, or non-rudimentary, horn will be laterally displaced and has been described as a "banana-shaped uterus" [23].

Ovarian pregnancy refers to the retention of a fertilized ovum within the ovary. It is uncommon, accounting for 3% of all ectopic pregnancies, and a risk factor for ovarian pregnancies is the use of intrauterine devices. US diagnosis of an ovarian ectopic pregnancy may be difficult to distinguish from ovarian germ cell tumors or other ovarian pathology. A suggestive US finding is the pres-

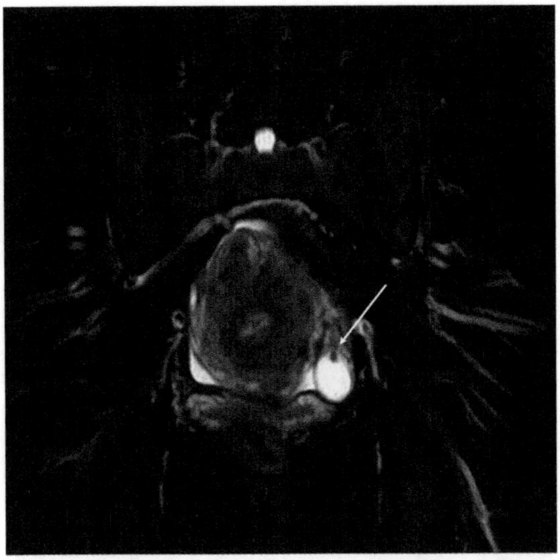

Fig. 2.12 Ovarian pregnancy in a 38-year-old woman. Coronal T2-weighted image with fat suppression shows a fluid hyperintense mass in the left ovary, representing a gestational sac-like structure with an empty uterine cavity. A small fetal pole on the upper side of the sac is also seen (arrow)

ence of a gestational sac with a wide hyperechoic outer ring within the ovary. An MRI finding is a gestational sac-like structure on or within the ovary that may contain fetal components or acute hemorrhage, with distinct low signal intensity on T2-weighted image (Fig. 2.12). On CT, a heterogeneous mass arising from the ovary can similarly be seen.

Cervical pregnancy is rare (less than 1%) and refers to the abnormal implantation of the embryo in the endocervical canal. Risk factors are a history of dilatation and curettage and in vitro fertilization. The *hourglass* or *barrel shape* of the uterus due to the distention of the cervix by the fetus is typical and the presence of cardiac activity below the internal uterine orifice is suggestive of cervical pregnancy. The *sliding sign* refers to the sliding of the gestational sac against the endocervical canal after pressure is applied to the cervix using a transducer probe and indicates an occurring miscarriage allowing to exclude cervical pregnancy [24]. As on US, MRI findings include a normal *endometrial stripe*, a *gestational sac* occupying the cervix, and the *hourglass-shaped uterus* with an *enlarged cervical canal*. A suggestive MRI finding may be the presence of a *lobulated mass*, with heterogeneous mixed signal intensity and a complete or partial dark rim on T2-weighted images can be observed. Early detection and treatment of cervical pregnancy with Methotrexate may prevent the need for hysterectomy.

Scar pregnancy is also called cesarean section scar ectopic pregnancy (CSEP). It has been estimated to occur in 0.15% of pregnant women with prior cesarean deliveries. Probably a tract connecting the endometrial cavity and myometrium facilitates the implantation of the blastocyst so that the gestational sac can successively be visualized in the anterior wall of the inferior aspect of the uterus, surrounded by myometrium and fibrous tissue. MRI is able to demonstrate gestational sac localization and its relationship with adjacent organs, and it can assess eventual myometrial invasion and bladder involvement (Fig. 2.13). A key MRI finding is the *absence* or *thinning of myometrium* between the bladder wall and the gestational sac on T2-weighted imaging. The most important complication in CSEP is uterine rupture, usually secondary to the thinning of the anterior myometrium due to the compression by the gestational sac. Although successful births have been described with expectant management, many recommend interruption of the pregnancy when the diagnosis is certain because of the significant risk of an emergency hysterectomy.

Intra-abdominal pregnancy is very rare (1.4%) and is usually seen in patients who have utilized assisted reproductive technology (ART). It is defined as implantation within the intraperitoneal cavity excluding tubal, ovarian, and intraligamentous locations. MRI and CT can be helpful in confirming the diagnosis, determining anatomic relationships and potential vascular connections, and assessing placental adherence (Fig. 2.14). Findings of abdominal ectopic pregnancy at MR imaging include the presence of a gestational sac outside the reproductive tract, with or without signs of hemorrhage. The lack of myometrium surrounding the sac can be an important finding. Enhancement of the peritoneum around the sac-like structure may also be

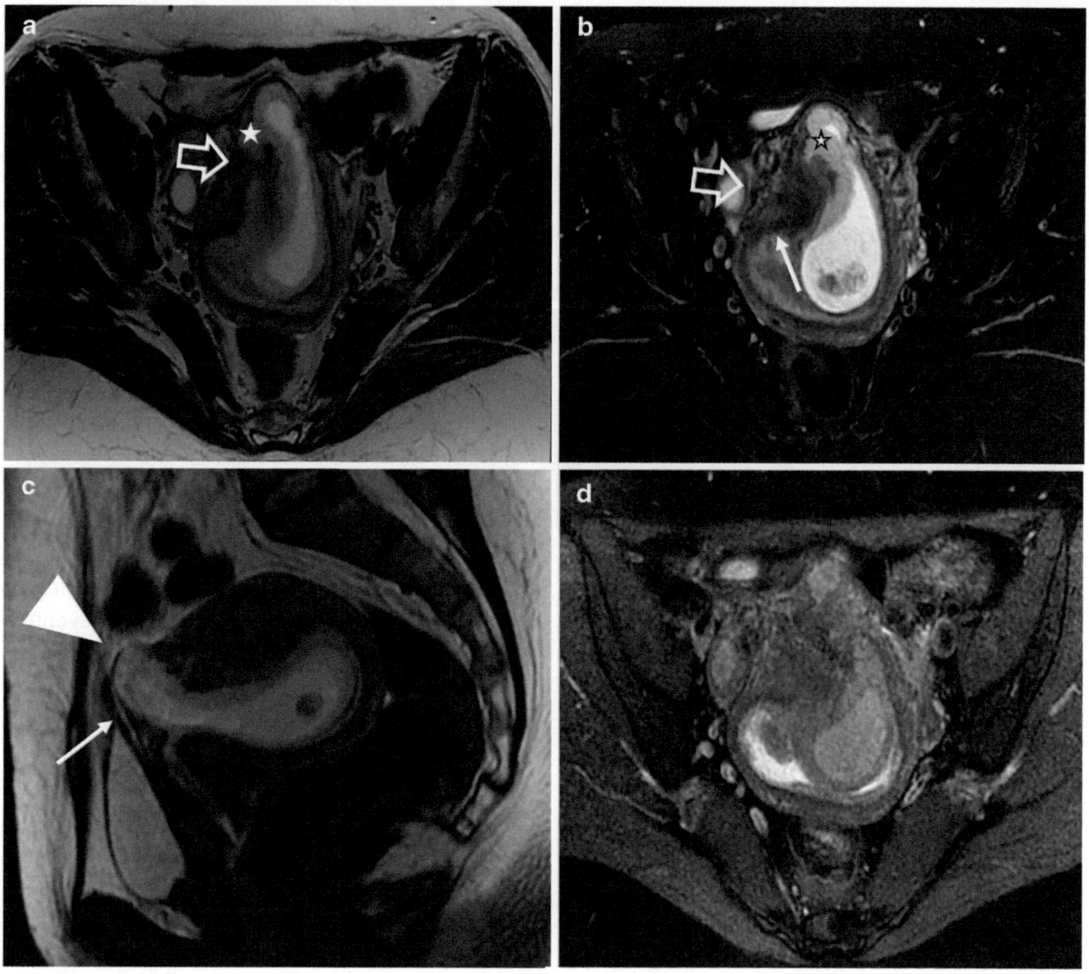

Fig. 2.13 Scar pregnancy in a 35-year-old woman. Axial T2-weighted image (**a**), even with fat suppression (**b**), shows the implantation of gestational sac with a well-formed fetus within it (thin arrows in **b**) on the anterior wall of the lower uterine segment, in the region of the scar of the previous cesarean section (empty arrows in **a** and **b**), where placental tissue is seen (asterisks in **a** and **b**). The sagittal T2-weighted image (**c**) shows better as the gestational sac bulges throughout the cesarean scar, where the myometrium is very thin or focally absent, and the bulging gestation sac appears to be covered only by thin hypointense serosa (arrowhead in **c**). However, the urinary bladder wall appears to be preserved, with a separating hyperintense fat plane (thin arrow in **c**). The axial T1-weighted image with fat suppression (**d**) shows the hyperintensity of the content of the endometrial cavity, suggestive of recent bleeding

seen in abdominal pregnancies. Important considerations at imaging include the identification of sites of placental implantation, because this information has deep implications for treatment planning. On CT an *intra-abdominal extrauterine gestational sac-like structure* with an *enhancing rim* can be seen. However, CT generally provides a less detailed placental evaluation. Because of the elevated risk of hemorrhage, maternal mortality associated with intra-abdominal pregnancy is higher than 20%.

Heterotopic pregnancy refers to the coexistence of an intrauterine and extrauterine pregnancy and has been reported in 1–3% of patients who have utilized ART, so it should be considered in these patients with pelvic pain. If a patient undergoes a spontaneous or elective abortion of intrauterine pregnancy but continues to experi-

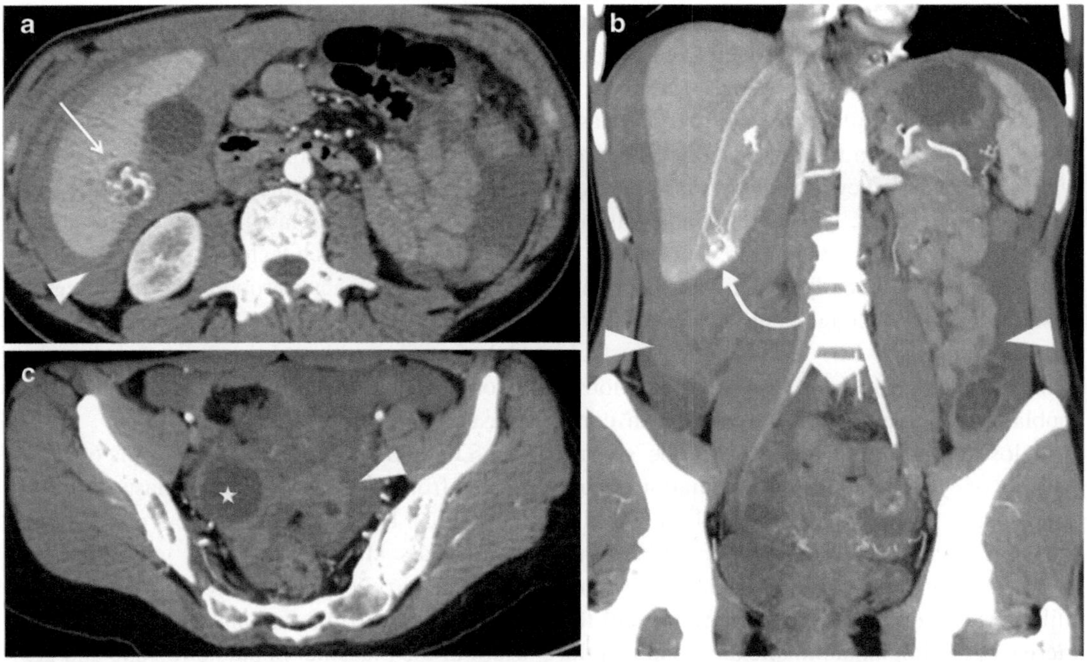

Fig. 2.14 Liver pregnancy in a 25-year-old woman, presenting with abdominal pain and acute anemia. (**a**) Axial CT image in the arterial phase shows a hypervascular round lesion (arrow) on the posterior surface of the segment VI, with large and tortuous vessels with a pseudo-decidual pattern. Hemoperitoneum is also present, especially in the perihepatic space (arrowhead). Maximum Intensity Projection (MIP) reconstruction on the coronal plane (**b**) better shows the aberrant feeding vessels to the hypervascular lesion, with activation of abnormal shunts with right hepatic veins (curved arrow) and a large amount of hemoperitoneum in the abdominal and pelvic cavity (arrowheads). Axial CT image (**c**) in the arterial phase shows a corpus luteum (asterisk) in the right ovary, with hemoperitoneum in the pelvic cavity (arrowhead)

ence persistent pelvic pain with abnormal β-hCG levels, heterotopic pregnancy should be suspected. MRI is the imaging tool used to detect both intrauterine and extrauterine pregnancy in cases with high clinical suspicion for this condition. Findings on MRI include *heterogeneous mass-like extrauterine gestational sac* and *intrauterine embryo* with or without hematosalpinx and hemoperitoneum.

2.4 Gestational Trophoblastic Disease

Gestational trophoblastic disease (GTD) encompasses a range of pregnancy-related disorders, consisting of *premalignant disorders*, such as *complete* and *partial hydatidiform mole* (CHM and PHM), and of *malignant disorders*, such as *invasive mole* (IM), *choriocarcinoma* (CC), *placental-site trophoblastic tumor* (PSTT), and *epithelioid trophoblastic tumor* (ETT). The malignant gestational tumors are also known as *gestational trophoblastic neoplasia* (GTN) and can metastasize or lead to death if untreated [25, 26].

According to American Cancers Society's most recent estimates, GTD occurs in about 1 out of every 1000 pregnancies in the United States. Most of these are molar pregnancies. Choriocarcinoma occurs in about 2 to 7 pregnancies out of every 100,000 pregnancies in the United States, with a higher incidence among African American women. Overall, GTD is more common in Asia and Africa. The prevalence rates of both hydatidiform mole and choriocarcinoma have declined over the past 30 years in all groups, possibly related to improved economies and diet as well as a decline in the total birth rates.

GTD take their origin from the trophoblastic epithelium of the placenta, derived from the outermost layer of the blastocyst that originates in early embryonic differentiation. Trophoblasts can be classified into three distinct populations: cytotrophoblasts, syncytiotrophoblasts, and intermediate trophoblasts. The cytotrophoblasts are the germinative cells situated on the surface of the chorionic villi. In early gestation, cytotrophoblasts differentiate along a villous and an extravillous pathway. On the villous surface, cytotrophoblasts differentiate into syncytiotrophoblasts, a polynucleated structure with complete loss of proliferative activity. The second pathway of cytotrophoblast differentiation occurs in the placental bed where the embryo invades into the endometrium. The cytotrophoblasts differentiate into intermediate trophoblasts that infiltrate the decidua, the myometrium, and the arteries of the implantation site and establish the maternal/fetal circulation [1]. Hydatidiform moles and choriocarcinoma take origin from cytotrophoblasts and syncytiotrophoblasts, while PSTTs and ETTS arise from intermediate trophoblasts.

CHM is characterized by diffuse hydropic swelling and trophoblastic hyperplasia and in most of the cases (about 90%) arises when an anuclear ovum is fertilized by a haploid sperm, which then undergoes duplication resulting in a 46XX androgenetic karyotype. About 10% of complete moles result from fertilization of an empty ovum by two sperm, resulting in a 46XY or 46XX karyotype.

PHM presents two populations of chorionic villi, one with normal morphology and the other with scattered hydropic villi and focal trophoblastic hyperplasia and is almost always triploid, arising from fertilization of a haploid ovum (23X) by two sperm or by one sperm that reduplicates itself, which results in a zygote with a total of 69 chromosomes (69XXX, 69XXY, 69XYY). Sometimes partial hydatidiform moles can be tetraploid.

IM or CC can occur after CHM in 15–20% of cases and after PHM in less than 5% of cases. In particular, IM is the most common of the two types of GTN that follows almost always CHM and usually has a diploid karyotype of paternal origin. CC can arise after any type of pregnancy, in particular after hydatidiform mole in about 50% of cases, and less commonly after a normal pregnancy or an abortion. It is a malignant β-hCG-producing epithelial tumor with central necrosis, cytotrophoblast-like cells with a characteristic biphasic architecture and multinucleate, pleomorphic syncytiotrophoblast-like regions. Intra-placental choriocarcinoma can metastasize to distant sizes and rarely can neonatal choriocarcinoma occur resulting from the metastatic spread from choriocarcinoma.

PSTT and ETT are the rarest forms of tumor, arising from intermediate trophoblasts, with similar clinical behavior. Both tumors may manifest many years after a non-molar gestation. They present microscopically as trophoblastic infiltration confined to the endometrium and myometrium of the placental implantation site and grow more slowly, metastasize later, more commonly involve lymph nodes, and produce less β-hCG than do choriocarcinomas.

2.4.1 Complete and Partial Hidatiform Mole

Early diagnosis of CHM is made with the combination of serial β-hCG levels measurements and transvaginal ultrasonography (TVUS) often in asymptomatic patients. However, common presenting symptoms include vaginal bleeding, enlarged uterus, and hyperemesis. Rarely, only in untreated patients complications can occur, such as anemia, preeclampsia, hyperthyroidism, and respiratory distress. Diagnosis of PHM is more challenging before uterine evacuation, so that it is usually made with histologic analysis. Vaginal bleeding is the most common presenting symptom of PHM, and usually occurs later than those with CHM. Another difference between the two types of hydatidiform mole is the β-hCG level that is markedly elevated in CHM (>100,000 mIU/mL), while less than 10% of patients with PHM present such high β-hCG values.

A typical TVUS finding in CHM is the *snowstorm sign*, which is the presence of a heterogeneous echogenic mass within several hypoechoic foci in a large-for-date uterus, with the absence of fetus. Another finding is the so-called *bunch of grapes sign* due to hydropic chorionic villi that appears as multiple small anechoic cystic spaces from 1 to 30 mm, that often are associated with irregular fluid collection in the uterine mass. The cysts in molar pregnancy are caused by hydropic swollen villi and do not show blood flow on color-Doppler images. In the second trimester the cystic spaces become larger and grow in number. In about 20% of patients, an extrauterine TVUS finding is detectable: It consists of the presence of *theca lutein cysts*, which appears as multiple large functional cysts in both ovaries secondary to the ovarian stimulation by the elevated β-hCG values. In PHM there are multiple TVUS findings such as an empty gestational sac or containing amorphous hyperechoic fetal parts, ovoid gestational sac, fetal anomalies, oligohydramnios, and enlarged placenta with internal cystic change determining a typical Swiss cheese pattern.

The performance of US in detecting all types of hydatidiform moles is poor, with a sensitivity and specificity respectively of 44% and 74% and positive predictive value and negative predictive value respectively of 88% and 23%. Furthermore, detection rates improved significantly beyond 14 weeks of gestation, compared to when the scan was carried out in the first trimester [27].

US performance in detecting CHM (58–95%) is better compared to PHM (17–29%). False negatives are common, therefore the correlation with β-hCG levels is helpful as they are markedly elevated in molar pregnancies compared to anembryonic gestation or miscarriage in which there are normal or decreasing β-hCG values. Because of the low performance of US in diagnosing molar pregnancies, it is necessary that all products of conceptions from nonviable pregnancies undergo histologic analysis as well as obtain β-hCG-levels 3–4 weeks after the evacuation.

CT is generally used to stage a suspected malignancy and evaluate for metastatic disease in GTN. Moles appear as a hypodense intrauterine mass relative to the enhancing myometrium, with thin intralesional enhancing septa. Ovaries are enlarged and show the typical "spoke-wheel" pattern due to the presence of multiple fluid cysts, separated by thin septa.

MR imaging is used when sonography is not clear enough because of non-ideal body habitus or the presence of multiple leiomyomas. In CHM and PHM little or no abnormalities may be present in the first trimester, although sometimes a heterogenous mass that distends the uterine cavity may be detected, with high intensity in T2-weighted images and low intensity T1-weighted images relative to the adjacent myometrium. Successively, multiple small cysts may appear within the mass and T2-weighted images show a thin rim of hypointense myometrium surrounding the mass (Fig. 2.15). Areas of high-intensity signal on T1-weighted images, suggesting hemorrhage, may be present within the mass. Multiple dilated vessels due to tumor neovascularity can be also seen within the ovaries and myometrium. After administration of gadolinium contrast medium moles typically demonstrate enhancing heterogeneous tissue containing multiple small cystic spaces.

In about 1.5/1,000,000 deliveries, molar pregnancies may occur as ectopic molar pregnancies [28] or, more rarely, as twin pregnancy with a CHM and a coexisting normal fetus. The latter condition is equally rare and often (40% of cases) results in live births. It should be suspected when is present a normal alive fetus together with an abnormal cystic placenta. A typical US finding is the *twin peak sign*, due to the presence of a triangular echogenic chorionic tissue that separates the normal twin gestational sac from that of molar pregnancy.

Twin pregnancy with a CHM should be differentiated from PHM and placental mesenchymal dysplasia (PMD), as also in these conditions a cystic placenta is present. In PHM, the presence of cystic placenta is associated with an anomalous or dead fetus. In PMD the cystic spaces within the enlarged placenta correspond to dilated vessels, which result in increased vascularity at color-Doppler US, described as the *stained-glass sign* [29]. Furthermore, PMD occurs in a singleton pregnancy and the placenta is located in the gestational sac compared to a twin pregnancy

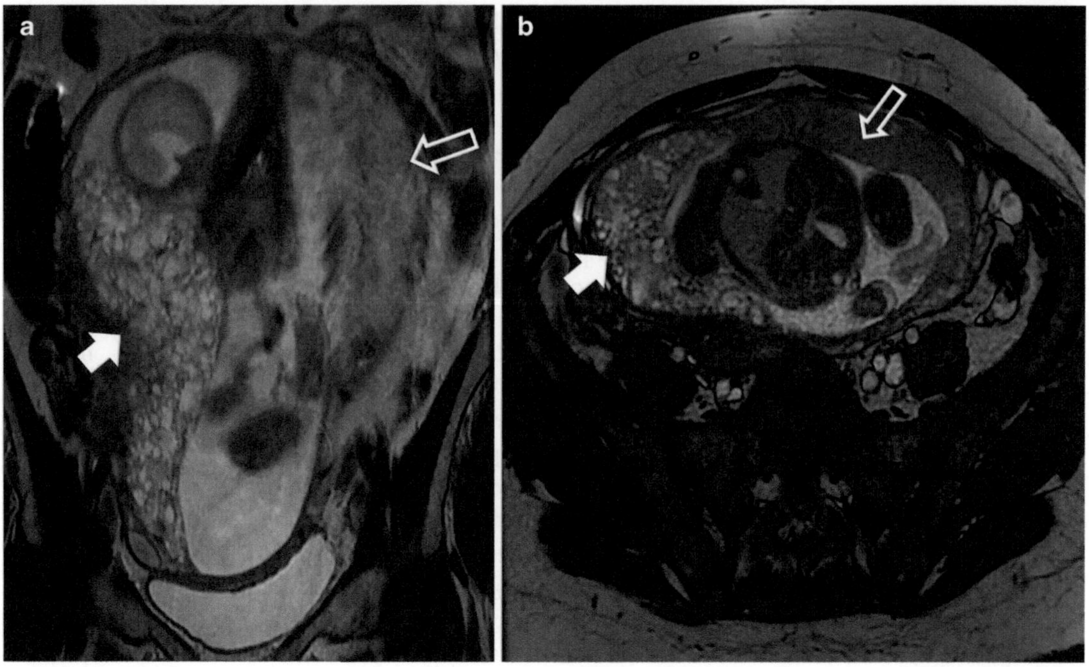

Fig. 2.15 Complete hydatidiform mole in a 51-year-old woman at 22° weeks of gestation with twin pregnancy obtained after heterologous ICSI and regular development of only one of the two fetuses; β-HCG levels (511,118 mU/mL). Coronal T2-weighted TSE image (**a**) and axial FIESTA image (**b**) show a heterogeneous mass with well-defined cystic spaces on the right side of the uterus (thick arrow in **a** and **b**), which is in contact with the normal placenta located on the left side (empty arrow in **a** and **b**). The normal fetus (arrowhead in **a** and **b**) is also seen

with a CHM and a coexisting normal fetus in which the cystic placenta is located in a gestational sac different from that containing the fetus.

Ectopic molar pregnancies may occur in the fallopian tubes, in the cervix, and ovaries. There are no clinical differences from ectopic non-molar pregnancies, although ectopic molar pregnancy tends more to present with hemoperitoneum, due to the higher tendency to rupture. US findings include an empty uterus and a complex adnexal mass with or without a live embryo.

2.4.2 Gestational Trophoblastic Neoplasia

Gestational trophoblastic neoplasia (GTN) follows hydatidiform mole (60%), previous spontaneous abortion/abortion (30%), and normal pregnancy or ectopic gestation (10%). Post-molar GTN must be suspected in asymptomatic patients with β-hCG levels that fail to normalize after molar pregnancy. According to International Federation of Gynecology and Obstetrics (FIGO), the agreed criteria to diagnose GTN include: (1) four or more plateaued β-hCG concentrations over 3 weeks (days 1, 7, 14, and 21); (2) increase of β-hCG concentrations for three or more consecutive measurements for at least 2 weeks (days 1, 7, and 14); (3) a histologic diagnosis of choriocarcinoma; and (4) elevated β-hCG concentrations for 6 months or longer [30].

Both patients with molar or non-molar GTN should present abnormal uterine bleeding months to years after evacuation or delivery. β-hCG levels are usually elevated in choriocarcinoma and only modestly elevated in PSTT and ETT. If possible, persistently elevated β-hCG values should be supported by histologic or radiologic evidence; in particular, TVUS is mandatory to exclude a new pregnancy, measure uterine volume, and assess for the spread of disease within the pelvis. At grey-scale US, the endometrial mass has not a specific appearance, as it may be hyperechoic or hypoechoic and homogeneous or heterogeneous, showing small cystic spaces which represent hemorrhage, necrosis, or vascular spaces. Color-Doppler US is also not specific, as GTN may present minimal or high vascularity. However, trophoblastic vessels show a high-velocity and low-resistance waveform, and resistive index (RI) and uterine artery pulsatility index (PI) could help in the evaluation of GTN, showing lower RIs in invasive moles (0.28) and choriocarcinoma (0.25) compared to CHM (0.55) and PHM (0.56). Low PI levels are indicative of increased uterine blood flow and arteriovenous shunting.

ETT is sometimes described as a well-circumscribed mass with sharp borders and peripheral hypoechoic halo at grey-scale US with peripheral increased vascularity at color-Doppler US, although this pattern is not typical of all cases of ETT, and these lesions may present decreased vascularity.

At CT primary tumor appears as a focal low-attenuation mass within an enlarged uterus (Fig. 2.16), although CT is usually used only for evaluation and staging of metastatic disease.

MR imaging findings are not specific for the differentiation between the various types of GTN. Usually, MRI shows an ill-defined mass within the myometrium that displaces the junctional line, characterized by isointensity on T1-weighted images and hyperintensity on

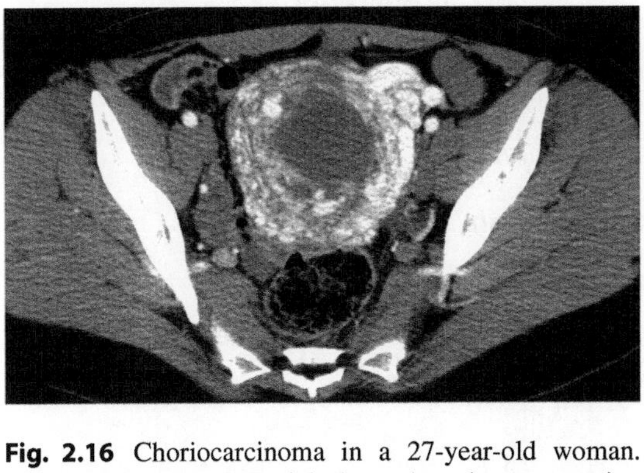

Fig. 2.16 Choriocarcinoma in a 27-year-old woman. Axial CT image on arterial phase show low-attenuation mass within an enlarged uterus surrounded by enlarged and tortuous vessels reproducing decidual reaction and chorioinic villi

T2-weighted images, compared to the adjacent myometrium, with marked enhancement after intravenous administration of gadolinium contrast medium. The lesion may show hemorrhagic areas, with increased intensity on T1-weighted images, and numerous vessels can be seen within the myometrium because of the increased vascularity. Obviously, MRI is preferred to TVUS in the evaluation of pelvic tumor extension and pelvic lymph nodes.

On MR imaging, PSTT has been described with a hypervascular pattern, that is similar to that of other types of GTN, and with a hypovascular pattern that occurs when the mass is poor of vessels and is characterized by isointensity to adjacent myometrium on T1-weighted images and isointensity to slight hyperintensity on T2-weighted images. After intravenous administration of gadolinium contrast medium, a central non-enhanced area, due to necrosis and colliquation, can be detected. In most cases, ETT appears as a well-circumscribed mass with high signal intensity on T2-weighted images, low signal intensity on T1-weighted images compared to normal myometrium, and heterogeneous enhancement after intravenous administration of gadolinium enhancement medium.

Approximately 30% of patients with GTN have metastasis at the time of diagnosis, most commonly to the lungs (80%), so that when the diagnosis of GTN is made, lung CT is strictly recommended. If lung metastases are detected, the risk of brain or abdominal solid organ metastasis is markedly increased. Brain metastases usually occur in patients with a previous diagnosis of lung metastasis with a prevalence that ranges from 3.4% to 8.8%. In women with non-molar choriocarcinoma, the risk to develop brain metastasis is approximately 20%, so in this group it is important to perform brain imaging. Liver metastases are rare, with a prevalence that ranges from 1.8% to 3.4%, and more frequently occur in patients with non-molar GTN (75% of cases).

Thus, in absence of lung metastasis, brain MRI or abdominal CT are not required, unless choriocarcinoma or suspected GTN after non-molar pregnancy is histologically diagnosed.

The most frequent pattern of pulmonary metastatic disease is that of multiple well-defined and rounded nodules, although some patients may present with a single nodule. Metastasis with surrounding ground-glass opacities (the "halo" sign) are commonly seen on thin-section CT images and reflect alveolar hemorrhage surrounding these highly vascular lesions [31]. Less frequent is the pattern characterized by cavitated and bulla-forming lung metastasis or the endobronchial tumor diffusion that results in obstructive atelectasis and may manifest as an intrabronchial mass at CT.

Brain metastasis from GTN may be single or multiple and appear as hyperdense lesions at non-enhanced CT and with a variable signal intensity at MR imaging, due to the presence of intralesional hemorrhage, as these lesions tend to spontaneously hemorrhage.

Liver metastases are typically multiple and rounded and may be heterogeneous because of the possibility of intralesional hemorrhage. They are hypervascular lesions characterized by marked enhancement during the arterial phase that should be part of the screening protocol in these patients. Other sites of GTN metastasis reported are the spleen, kidneys, ovaries, gastrointestinal tract, spine, and skin. Lymphatic spread (to pelvic lymph node) is usually seen with PSTTs.

Management of GTN depends on the FIGO staging and classification (Table 2.3) and on FIGO/WHO scoring system based on prognostic factors (Table 2.4), according to which a score of 6 or below is considered low-risk, while a score above 6 is considered high-risk. Patients with low-risk GTN and with no metastasis (Stage I) should be treated with a single chemotherapeutic agent, having cure rates approximatively of 100%. A score of 7 or greater is high-risk disease that requires combination chemotherapy with or without radiation therapy or surgery; the cure rate ranges from 80% to 90%. In patients with PSTT or ETT, simple hysterectomy is the most appropriate treatment, since both tumors are less chemo-sensitive than other types of GTN.

Table 2.3 FIGO staging and classification for GTN

FIGO stage	Description
I	Gestational trophoblastic tumors strictly confined to the uterine corpus
II	Gestational trophoblastic tumors extending to the ovaries or to the vagina, but limited to the genital structures
III	Gestational trophoblastic tumors extending to the lungs, with or without genital tract involvement
IV	All other metastatic sites

Table 2.4 FIGO/WHO scoring system for GTN based on prognostic factors

FIGO/WHO risk factor scoring with FIGO staging	0	1	2	3
Age	<40	>40	–	–
Antecedent pregnancy	Mole	Abortion	Term	–
Interval from index pregnancy (months)	<4	4–6	7–12	>12
Pretreatment hCG mIU/mL	$<10^3$	$>10^3$, $<10^4$	$>10^4$, $<10^5$	$>10^5$
Largest tumor size including uterus (cm)	–	3–4	≥5	–
Site of metastasis including uterus	Lung	Spleen, kidney	Gastrointestinal tract	Brain, liver
Number of metastasis identified	–	1–4	5–8	>8
Previous failed chemotherapy	–	–	Single drug	Two or more drugs

2.4.3 Placental Nontrophoblastic Tumors

Chorioangioma is the most common nontrophoblastic placental tumor and is identified in 1% of placentas at histopathologic analysis. Chorioangioma is a benign vascular tumor supplied by fetal circulation. Most chorioangiomas are small, while large chorioangiomas greater than 4 cm are uncommon with a variable prevalence of 1 in 9000 to 1 in 16,000. At gray-scale US, chorioangioma is seen as a well-circumscribed tumor with mixed echogenicity different from the adjacent placental tissue. Chorioangioma commonly arises from the fetal surface of the placenta near the cord insertion. Tiny calcifications may be seen at US and suggest a favorable prognosis. Color-Doppler US and spectral Doppler waveforms can help differentiate chorioangioma from other placental masses or processes, including placental hemorrhage, hematoma, teratoma, and infarction. Chorioangioma has abundant internal vascularity with a low-resistance arterial flow and in some cases may show turbulent venous flow or a single feeding vessel. Large chorioangiomas are associated with high fetal morbidity and mortality of up to 30–40%. Fetal complications include polyhydramnios, fetal anemia, and fetal hydrops.

Placental teratoma is a rare tumor composed of all three germ cell layers. It has been described as benign and is essentially never associated with congenital abnormalities in the fetus. The US features of this tumor include a placental soft-tissue mass of varied echogenicity due to calcifications, fat, and fluid.

Maternal melanoma has been reported as the most common tumor to metastasize to the placenta.

References

1. Altieri A, Franceschi S, Ferlay J, Smith J, La Vecchia C. Epidemiology and aetiology of gestational trophoblastic diseases. Lancet Oncol. 2003;4(11):670–8.
2. Fadl S, Moshiri M, Fligner CL, Katz DS, Dighe M. Placental imaging: normal appearance with review of pathologic findings. Radiographics. 2017;37(3):979–98.
3. Meyers ML, Brown BP. Placental magnetic resonance imaging part I: the normal placenta. Pediatr Radiol. 2020;50(2):264–74.
4. Jha P, Pōder L, Bourgioti C, Bharwani N, Lewis S, Kamath A, et al. Society of Abdominal Radiology (SAR) and European Society of Urogenital Radiology (ESUR) joint consensus statement for MR imaging of placenta accreta spectrum disorders. Eur Radiol. 2020;30(5):2604–15.
5. Allen BC, Leyendecker JR. Placental evaluation with magnetic resonance. Radiol Clin N Am. 2013;51(6):955–66.
6. Moshiri M, Zaidi SF, Robinson TJ, Bhargava P, Siebert JR, Dubinsky TJ, et al. Comprehensive imaging review of abnormalities of the umbilical cord. Radiographics. 2014;34(1):179–96.
7. Trop I, Levine D. Hemorrhage during pregnancy: sonography and MR imaging. AJR Am J Roentgenol. 2001;176(3):607–15.
8. Fadl SA, Linnau KF, Dighe MK. Placental abruption and hemorrhage-review of imaging appearance. Emerg Radiol. 2019;26(1):87–97.
9. Saphier NB, Kopelman TR. Traumatic abruptio placenta scale (TAPS): a proposed grading system of computed tomography evaluation of placental abruption in the trauma patient. Emerg Radiol. 2014;21(1):17–22.
10. Masselli G, Brunelli R, Di Tola M, Anceschi M, Gualdi G. MR imaging in the evaluation of placental abruption: correlation with sonographic findings. Radiology. 2011;259(1):222–30.
11. Morlando M, Collins S. Placenta accreta spectrum disorders: challenges, risks, and management strategies. Int J Women's Health. 2020;12:1033–45.
12. Berkley EM, Abuhamad A. Imaging of placenta accreta spectrum. Clin Obstet Gynecol. 2018;61(4):755–65.
13. Valentini AL, Gui B, Ninivaggi V, Miccò M, Giuliani M, Russo L, et al. The morbidly adherent placenta: when and what association of signs can improve MRI diagnosis? Our experience. Diagn Interv Radiol. 2017;23(3):180–6.
14. Panelli DM, Phillips CH, Brady PC. Incidence, diagnosis and management of tubal and nontubal ectopic pregnancies: a review. Fertil Res Pract. 2015;1:15.
15. Rana P, Kazmi I, Singh R, Afzal M, Al-Abbasi FA, Aseeri A, et al. Ectopic pregnancy: a review. Arch Gynecol Obstet. 2013;288(4):747–57.
16. Barnhart KT. Clinical practice. Ectopic pregnancy. N Engl J Med. 2009;361(4):379–87.
17. Practice Committee of the American Society for Reproductive Medicine. Medical treatment of ectopic pregnancy: a committee opinion. Fertil Steril. 2013;100(3):638–44.
18. Lin EP, Bhatt S, Dogra VS. Diagnostic clues to ectopic pregnancy. Radiographics. 2008;28(6):1661–71.
19. Centers for Disease Control and Prevention. Ectopic pregnancy: United States, 1990–1992. MMWR Morb Mortal Wkly Rep. 1995;44(3):46–8.
20. Kao LY, Scheinfeld MH, Chernyak V, Rozenblit AM, Oh S, Dym RJ. Beyond ultrasound: CT and

MRI of ectopic pregnancy. AJR Am J Roentgenol. 2014;202(4):904–11.
21. Parker RA, Yano M, Tai AW, Friedman M, Narra VR, Menias CO. MR imaging findings of ectopic pregnancy: a pictorial review. Radiographics. 2012;32(5):1445–60.
22. Srisajjakul S, Prapaisilp P, Bangchokdee S. Magnetic resonance imaging in tubal and nontubal ectopic pregnancy. Eur J Radiol. 2017;93:76–89.
23. Ozeren S, Caliskan E, Corakci A, Ozkan S, Demirci A. Magnetic resonance imaging and angiography for the prerupture diagnosis of rudimentary uterine horn pregnancy. Acta Radiol. 2004;45(8):878–81.
24. Winder S, Reid S, Condous G. Ultrasound diagnosis of ectopic pregnancy. Australas J Ultrasound Med. 2011;14(2):29–33.
25. Seckl MJ, Sebire NJ, Berkowitz RS. Gestational trophoblastic disease. Lancet. 2010;376(9742):717–29.
26. Shaaban AM, Rezvani M, Haroun RR, Kennedy AM, Elsayes KM, Olpin JD, et al. Gestational trophoblastic disease: clinical and imaging features. Radiographics. 2017;37(2):681–700.
27. Fowler DJ, Lindsay I, Seckl MJ, Sebire NJ. Histomorphometric features of hydatidiform moles in early pregnancy: relationship to detectability by ultrasound examination. Ultrasound Obstet Gynecol. 2007;29(1):76–80.
28. Gillespie AM, Lidbury EA, Tidy JA, Hancock BW. The clinical presentation, treatment, and outcome of patients diagnosed with possible ectopic molar gestation. Int J Gynecol Cancer. 2004;14(2):366–9.
29. Kuwata T, Takahashi H, Matsubara S. "Stained-glass" sign for placental mesenchymal dysplasia. Ultrasound Obstet Gynecol. 2014;43(3):355.
30. FIGO Oncology Committee. FIGO staging for gestational trophoblastic neoplasia 2000. Int J Gynaecol Obstet. 2002;77(3):285–7.
31. Martínez-Jiménez S, Rosado-de-Christenson ML, Walker CM, Kunin JR, Betancourt SL, Shoup BL, et al. Imaging features of thoracic metastases from gynecologic neoplasms. Radiographics. 2014;34(6):1742–54.

Part II

Interventional Radiology in Woman

3 Embolic Agents in Interventional Radiology in Gynecological and Obstetric Diseases

Pierleone Lucatelli, Leonardo Teodoli, and Mario Bezzi

3.1 Embolic Materials

Recently, the number of embolic agents has increased significantly; however, it must be kept in mind that a combined approach using multiple agents is often most useful. To choose the embolic agent needed, the anticipated end result of the embolization procedure must be understood. For instance, embolization for bleeding from a post-traumatic pseudoaneurysm has a different goal from embolization of a tumor mass. Similarly, embolization for bleeding from a neoplastic mass has a purpose different from that of preoperative embolization of the same pathology. Large embolic agents such as coils and Gelfoam pledgets may be used for embolization of large vessels; proximal vessels can be occluded safely without risk of tissue infarction due to the extensive collateral network. Large agents may be also used in tissues with an end-organ vascular supply in which the entire blood supply to the area of interest is to be occluded; however, large agents should not be used in vessels in which future embolization or transcatheter therapy is anticipated.

By occlusion of the only vascular supply to a region, future selective catheterization will be precluded by occluding the sole vascular access to the pathology. In contrast to large agents, liquid agents such as alcohol or glue will embolize to the most distal vascular supply and cause infarction by occluding the smallest arterioles supplying a lesion. Because collateral supply occurs at a site proximal to the embolization, liquid embolization is effective in destroying tissue even when there is significant parasitization or collaterization of blood supply from an adjacent source; however, it should not be used unless cell death and necrosis are the desired end results.

A second characteristic that must be considered when choosing an embolic agent is the desired degree of permanence of the occlusion. In particular, some materials are biodegradable, and recanalization of the embolized vessel should be anticipated.

Embolic materials are categorized into two general classes, according to whether they provide permanent or temporary occlusion. Permanent occlusion is generally required for progressive disease (i.e., tumors), whereas a temporary embolic agent is appropriate for self-limited processes that may heal with time (i.e., traumatic lesions).

Most vessels embolized with Gelfoam pledgets and powder will recanalize within 2 to 3 weeks. Absorbable gelatin sponge is not radiopaque but is injected as a mixture with iodinated contrast material. Starch microspheres represent another biodegradable agent with an in vivo half-life of 20–30 min. Autologous blood clots,

P. Lucatelli (✉) · L. Teodoli · M. Bezzi
Policlinico Umberto I, Department of Radiological, Oncological and Pathological Sciences, Sapienza University of Rome, Rome, Italy

R. Niola et al. (eds.), *Diagnostic and Interventional Radiology in Gynecological and Obstetric Diseases*, https://doi.org/10.1007/978-3-031-11910-1_3

another biodegradable agent, are currently used infrequently because of the ready availability of other agents.

Polyvinyl alcohol (PVA) particles are a commonly used permanent agent, with sizes ranging from approximately 50 to 2800 lm. Embolization with PVA particles usually causes a permanent occlusion of vessels that corresponds to the size of the particles used. Other materials that have been used experimentally or in clinical trials include polylactic acid microspheres, ethylene vinylacetate copolymer particles dissolved in PVA, and human dura mater.

Embolization with particulate agents is considered complete when slowing of flow, not complete statis, is visualized. Because all arteries will tend to "back thrombose" to the previous bifurcation point when a distal occlusion is encountered, excessive embolization will decrease outflow enough that the entire feeding artery may thrombose. Fluoroscopically noted reflux is another indicator that the embolization procedure should be stopped [1–6].

3.1.1 Temporary Embolic Agents

Temporary embolic agent is an absorbable gelatin sponge (Gelfoam; Upjohn, Kalamazoo, Mich), a water-insoluble gelatin that allows vessel recanalization within several weeks after placement.

3.1.1.1 Absorbable Gelatin Sponge (Gelfoam)

Gelfoam is a medical device intended for application to bleeding surfaces as a hemostatic. It is a water-insoluble, off-white, nonelastic, porous, and pliable product prepared from purified porcine skin. It may be cut without fraying and is able to absorb and hold within its interstices, many times its weight of blood and other fluids. Gelfoam is absorbed completely, with little tissue reaction. This absorption is dependent on several factors, including the amount used, the degree of saturation with blood or other fluids, and the site of use. It is usually absorbed completely within 4 to 6 weeks.

Gelfoam Sterile Compressed Sponge is a water-insoluble, hemostatic device prepared from purified porcine skin gelatin, and capable of absorbing up to 45 times its weight of whole blood. The absorptive capacity of Gelfoam is a function of its physical size, increasing as the size of the gelatin sponge increases. The mechanism of action of hemostatic devices is supportive and mechanical, arresting bleeding by the formation of an artificial clot and by producing a mechanical matrix that facilitates clotting (Fig. 3.1).

It was the first embolic particle used in humans. Gelfoam induces hemostasis by accelerating development and providing structural support to the thrombus. The use of Gelfoam is primarily related to its temporary effect; it is primarily used to stop bleeding or to devascularize a lesion before surgical deletion. Gelfoam is usually completely reabsorbed (depending on the amount used, the degree of saturation with blood, and the site where it is used), with little tissue reaction. When used as an embolic material, the vessel recanalizes within a few weeks.

Gelfoam can be administered in numerous ways, depending on the indication for embolization. "Torpedoes" can be created by tightly rolling up small strips of Gelfoam and injecting them through a catheter placed at or slightly proximal to the intended level of embolization. Gelfoam torpedoes are also useful for the embolization of needle or catheter tracts. Alternatively, less selective embolization can be performed with Gelfoam

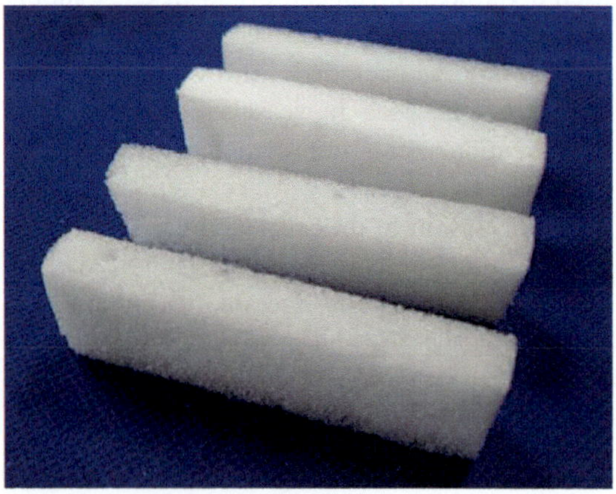

Fig. 3.1 Absorbable gelatin sponge

suspension. The slurry can be created by cutting strips and loading them into a syringe connected via a three-way tap to another syringe filled with contrast. The materials are pumped back and forth between the syringes to create a suspension of smaller Gelfoam particles. Gelfoam powder is no longer commercially available.

Jenkins et al. have theorized that the clotting effect of Gelfoam may be due to the release of thromboplastin from platelets, occurring when platelets entering the sponge become damaged by contact with the walls of its myriad of interstices. Thromboplastin interacts with prothrombin and calcium to produce thrombin, and this sequence of events initiates the clotting reaction. The authors suggest that the physiologic formation of thrombin in the sponge is sufficient to produce the formation of a clot, by its action on the fibrinogen in the blood.

In the meaning of adverse effects, there have been reports of fever associated with the use of Gelfoam, without demonstrable infection. Gelfoam may form a nidus of infection and abscess formation and has been reported to potentiate bacterial growth.

Gelfoam is not radiopaque and is typically mixed with iodinated contrast material before injection.

There have been few reports on the use of gelatin sponge as an embolic agent for uterine artery embolization (UAE). Most of the studies regarding UAE are for symptomatic fibroids. A recent study reports experience in 60 patients using gelatin sponge particles to treat symptomatic fibroids and shows a high clinical success rate of 98.0% (49 of 50 patients) with improvement in menorrhagia, 95.7% (45 of 47 patients) with improvement in bulk-related symptoms, 98.2% with increased satisfaction (54 of 55 patients), and 47.8% (95% CI: 39.2–55.8) with good fibroid volume reduction 12 months after the procedure. These symptom-related improvement rates were correlated with the volume reduction of the dominant fibroid.

In these reports, the menorrhagia symptoms improved in 89.5% (95% CI: 76.1–100%) of the patients, and the dominant fibroid volume was reduced by 65.1% (95% CI: 57.7–72.5%) 12 months after the procedure. Gelatin sponge, a water-insoluble, hemostatic material prepared from purified gelatin (a nonantigenic protein), has been used for embolization for over 30 years as a bio-degradable, intravascular embolic agent in interventional radiology with specific use as a temporary embolic agent in hemorrhage.

The absorbable feature of the gelatin sponge reveals that arteries that were previously sealed with a gelatin sponge could be recanalized within several weeks. However, recanalization has been shown to cause no disadvantage for embolized fibroids, as follow-up enhanced MRI showed that most fibroids were infarcted and reduced in volume without any regrowth, while the blood flow of the intact uterine myometrium was conserved.

Furthermore, gelatin sponge is much cheaper and more cost-effective than other embolic agents, which might reduce the cost of UAE procedures. In contrast, the drawbacks of gelatin sponge include its tedious preparation and the variable fragment sizes achieved. Gelatin sponge particles are often hand-prepared and cut from sheets of gelatin sponge to make a slurry.

In their report, gelatin sponge particles were not shown to be inferior to nPVA particles in terms of improvement of mean hemorrhage score and rate of volume reduction of the dominant fibroid (60.2 ± 18.1%) at the 3-month follow-up after UAE, while only 33.4% of the size decrease in the dominant fibroid was seen.

Further examinations should be needed to standardize reporting of technical and clinical outcomes to guide practice. Regarding adverse events, no angiography-related complications occurred, and postprocedural complications including fibroid rupture, infection, permanent amenorrhea, and deep venous thrombosis were observed in 11 (18.3%) of 60 patients, four of whom had multiple complications. Three of five fibroid ruptures occurred 1–2 months after UAE, which was consistent with a previous report describing the greatest frequency of fibroid ruptures within 3 months. The remaining two occurred after 6 and 7 months, respectively, which suggests that fibroid ruptures can occur at any time after UAE and patients should be advised of this late complication.

Of the five infective complications, three (60%) exhibited fibroid rupture suggesting that fibroid rupture is a component of a spectrum of infections in UAE.

Two patients with a history of previous surgery experienced a tubo-ovarian abscess. UAE probably causes ischemia of the fallopian tubes that rise the tendency of germs to soar the tract easily and trigger endothelial damage, leading to a tubo-ovarian abscess.

The incidence of infectious complications was 8.3%, which was a little higher compared to the comprehensive review report (1–3%).

Since the use of gelatin sponge agents has been reported to be associated with infectious complications, this high incidence might not be an insignificant disadvantage to use gelatin sponge particles in the clinical setting.

Since this potential risk, early articles proposed using as little Gelfoam as possible, avoiding prolonged exposure of Gelfoam to contaminated air, and thoroughly compressing the Gelfoam so that large air bubbles are removed and not introduced into a patient. These recommendations remain important when using Gelfoam as an embolic agent.

The incidence of permanent amenorrhea after UAE is highly age-dependent, and the reported amount of permanent amenorrhea in women whose age is >45 years is 20–40%, while at <45 years of age, the occurrence is 0–3%.

When patients of motherhood age think about undergoing UAE, the question of fertility preservation is often at the forefront of the decision-making process. Some guidance may be obtained by reviewing the results of pelvic embolization procedures performed for different indications and by determining if embolization affects the ability of patients to maintain an intrauterine gestation to full term. Stancato-Pasik et al. reported 12 patients who underwent UAE with Gelfoam because of obstetric hemorrhage and found that 11 of 12 patients returned normal menses and all patients wanting a subsequent pregnancy (3/12) delivered healthy neonates. McIvor and Cameron studied three successful pregnancies in seven patients who underwent UAE to control hemorrhage caused by gestational trophoblastic tumors.

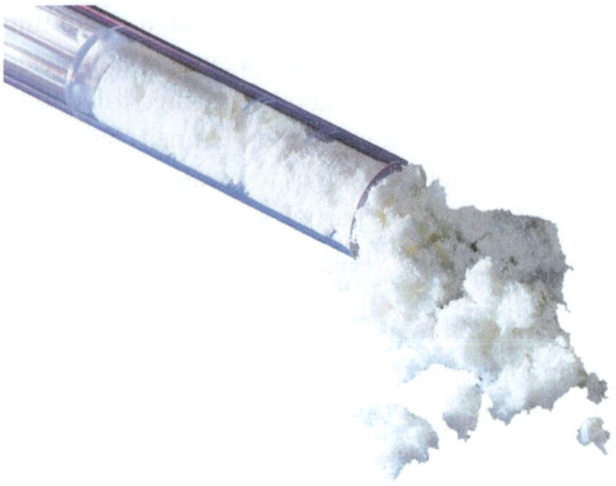

Fig. 3.2 Avitene

Dickey et al. explained six pregnancies in 18 patients who underwent UAE for control of postpartum bleeding. Several case reports have described successful pregnancies after Gelfoam embolization for post-operative hemorrhages, cervical ectopic pregnancy, and other indications. Given these findings, it does appear that UAE using Gelfoam is effective at controlling abnormal pelvic bleeding while maintaining a patient's ability to maintain a full-term intrauterine gestation [5–10].

3.1.1.2 Avitene

Avitene (Davol, Inc., Cranston, RI) is a microfibrillar collagen preparation supplied in the form of a powder. In arteries embolized with Avitene, moderate recanalization occurs within 2 weeks and total recanalization within 2 months. It is a useful agent for tumor necrosis and organ ablation (101), as it can be administered through a microcatheter (Fig. 3.2).

3.1.2 Permanent Embolic Agents

Particulate agents are manufactured in different sizes and establish mechanical occlusion also activating thrombin and promoting fibroblast growth. The level of vascular occlusion is controlled by the diameter of the particles selected, typically from 150 to 1200 μm. Five spherical particulate embolic agents are currently available: tris-acryl gelatin microspheres (Embosphere; BioSphere Medical, Rockland, Mass), PVA-based micro-spheres (Contour SE; Boston Scientific, Natick, Mass), PVA-based hydrogel microspheres (Bead Block; Biocompatibles, Farnham, England), super-absorbing polymer microspheres (Quadrasphere; BioSphere Medical), and hydrogel microspheres covered with a polymer coating (Embozene; Celo-Nova BioSciences, Newnan, Ga).

3.1.2.1 Polyvinyl Alcohol

Initially recognized for its use in domestic sponges and other household and industrial products, PVA is also a frequently used embolic agent (Fig. 3.3). Its biocompatibility has been established since its first medical application by Grindlay and Claggett, who used it as a sealing material after pneumonectomy. Then it has been applied in burn patients as a skin replacement, in patients with rectal prolapse, and for resolution of cardiac defects including tetralogy of Fallot. In this setting, PVA is readily incorporated into tissue by the ingrowth of granulation tissue.

The preparation of PVA for use as an embolic agent first involves its transformation into a foam that can absorb water and become instantly compressible. Once the compressed foam is dried, it preserves its compressed shape but when placed into solution, it returns to its original shape. Particles are prepared by rasping or blending a compressed block of PVA or punching out PVA plugs. The resulting shavings or particles are passed through filters with sequentially smaller holes to separate them into various sizes. One potential problem with this method is that the irregular shape of the PVA particles may permit large particles to pass through small holes depending on the orientation of a particular particle as it passes through the holes. This problem was responsible for the variability in size and shape that was seen in early particle preparations before changes were made in the industrial process to guarantee size uniformity. PVA, like Gelfoam, is not radiopaque and is typically mixed with iodinated contrast material before injection (Fig. 3.4).

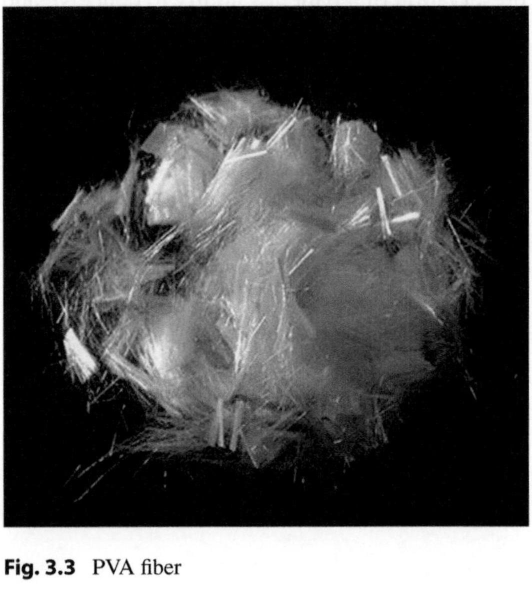

Fig. 3.3 PVA fiber

PVA has historically been used in cements, packaging materials, water-resistant adhesives, cosmetics, and household sponges. The original PVA embolic particles (Cook, Bloomington, IN; Boston Scientific, Natick, MA) are still in use. They are irregularly shaped chips from blocks or sheets and are available in sizes from 50 to 1200 m. PVA is also supplied in the form of microspheres (Contour SE, Boston Scientific, Natick, MA). PVA particles produce mechanical occlusion of the vessel in addition to thrombin activation and induction of internal fibroblast growth, leading to a relatively permanent occlusion. While the permanence of PVA as an embolic agent is well established, it is also clear that occlusion caused by PVA particles is not always permanent. Proposed mechanisms for recanalization include angioneogenesis and capillary regrowth caused by vascular proliferation within the organized thrombus and resorption of thrombus found between PVA clumps in the lumen of an embolized vessel after resolution of inflammation.

PVA particles are distributed either dry or in solution. They must be mixed in a contrast solution and saline to be used. PVA particles tend to clump together, leading to occlusion of vessels that are larger than the diameter of the individual particles. As a result, these particles can be used to occlude vessels ranging from arterioles to

Fig. 3.4 PVA mixed with contrast material

larger arteries. The level of occlusion can be controlled to some extent by the dilution of the particles used. Several maneuvers exist to minimize, or at least make more predictable, the tendency for agglomeration.

The first successful use of PVA as an embolic agent was reported by Tadavarthy et al. in two studies of patients with different pathologies such as cervical carcinoma, hemangiosarcoma of the liver, hemangioendothelioma of the neck and forehead, and an arteriovenous malformation of the spine. Since then, PVA has been successfully used to embolize vessels in patients with a variety of conditions such as gastrointestinal bleeding, hypervascular bone metastases, head and neck arteriovenous malformations and tumors, hepatic neoplasms, and hemoptysis caused by cystic fibrosis. Before its use in uterine fibroid embolization procedures, PVA was not routinely used during pelvic embolization.

In men, PVA has been successfully used in the treatment of both high-flow and low-flow priapism. In women, Pisco et al. reported the use of PVA in the treatment of bleeding caused by pelvic tumors; the researchers discovered that when compared with Gelfoam, PVA particles resulted in better control of hemorrhage and fewer relapses. Poppe et al. reported the effective use of PVA particles to control hemorrhage associated with a uterine arteriovenous malformation and preservation of a patient's ability to conceive and carry a pregnancy to term.

Depending on the disease course and the engaged organ, the required level of occlusion (i.e., proximal or distal) will determine the particle size selected for a given embolization procedure. Generally, the use of small particles will result in a more distal occlusion, boosting the risk for end-organ infarction. Nevertheless, the inclination of PVA particles to cluster together often makes the effective size of this agent larger than that of the individual particles, which may account for a proximal occlusion during embolization. Decreasing the tendency for particulate aggregation, with dilution and slow infusion, may lead to a more distal embolization. The optimum particle size for uterine fibroid embolization has not been recognized, but most centers are using particles measuring 350–500 μm or 500–710 μm in diameter. The histologic effects of PVA on embolized blood vessels have been exposed in several studies. Firstly, PVA particles adhere to the vessel wall, leading to slow flow in the vessel. Finally, this leads to thrombosis and inflammatory reactions, foreign body reactions, and focal angionecrosis of the vessel wall. Angionecrosis manages to be confined to where particles are in contact with the vessel wall and can theoretically lead to perivascular extravasation of PVA particles; however, this finding has not been constantly detected. The foreign body reaction induced by PVA has been described to endure as long as 28 months after embolization. PVA is considered by many to be a permanent embolic agent because it is not biodegradable. The long-term appearance of intravascular PVA particles was studied by Davidson and Terbrugge in a patient with a facial vascular malformation that was resected 8 years after embolization. In this patient, no evidence of particle fragmentation was found, and the only change in particle morphology was small calcification. Nevertheless, PVA particles are not regularly found in samples gained after embolization. Some reports have theorized that this may be caused by the distal migration of particles. Other researchers have said that conflicting findings may be caused by using H&E staining during the preparation of pathologic slides; PVA particles are best seen with the Verhoeff-van Gieson stain. The reported duration of vascular occlusion generated by PVA has been variable. Some investigators reported occlusions continuing for at least several months. A persistent occlusion will occur with the organization of thrombus, vanishing of inflammatory infiltrate, and growth of connective tissue into the particles, resulting in fibrosis. Luminal recanalization after embolization with PVA has been reported as well. Proposed mechanisms for recanalization have included angioneogenesis and capillary regrowth caused by vascular proliferation inside the organized thrombotic clot and resorption of the thrombus found between clumps of PVA in the lumen of an embolized vessel after the resolution of inflammation. Recanalization does seem to occur in the part of the vessel lumen previously containing thrombus and not in the portion containing PVA particles.

Complications relating to the use of PVA particles as an embolic agent have been described.

The presence of small particles in the first part of preparations of PVA enhanced the risk for inadvertent end-organ damage. Manufacturing techniques were modified to minimize the number of particles smaller than the sizes specified for a given preparation of PVA.

The use of PVA particles for UAE was first explained by Ravina et al. in 1995. In that report, 16 patients underwent UAE as a primary treatment for uterine fibroids. With a mean follow-up of 20 months, 14 of 16 patients described resolution or improvement of the presenting symptoms; two patients needed surgery because of continuing symptoms after embolization. Since 1997, published articles have validated the initial results of Ravina et al. The most common indication for uterine fibroid embolization is abnormal or heavy menstrual bleeding. Improvement of symptoms has been reported in 80–96% of patients undergoing UAE with PVA particles. This technique has also been related to uterine volume reductions of 40–48% and fibroid volume reductions of 46–78%. Recently, midterm results have shown the continued success of this procedure, with 81% of patients reporting improvement of their symptoms at a mean follow-up of 16 months after embolization. Complications resulting in significant patient morbidity or requiring additional therapeutic procedures are rare, with an expected rate of occurrence of less than 2%. Siskin et al., Aziz et al., and McLucas et al. specifically studied the histologic effects observed after UAE with PVA particles. Both Aziz et al. and McLucas et al. noted that the particles did not fill the entire lumen of the embolized vessel. A foreign body reaction introduces platelet aggregation and thrombus development in the intraluminal matrix of PVA particles. It is the thrombus formation that results in arterial occlusion and ultimately conducts to interstitial edema within the fibroid followed by ischemic necrosis and hyalinization. The myometrium tissue nearby to a fibroid embolized with PVA particles has been noted to be viable but edematous and chronically inflamed. Luminal recanalization may represent one of the possible causes of treatment failure after UAE according to the fact that the particles do not occupy the entire vessel lumen, partial recanalization of the thrombus is possible and has been reported. Aziz et al. also noted that after UAE particles can be found in the arteries of the parametrium and outer myometrium, which would likely permit continued endometrial function after the recanalization of larger vessels. However, inadvertent end-organ damage, in this case involving the uterus, can possibly result in uterine ischemia or endometrial infection, both of which may potentially need a hysterectomy for treatment. Particles may also be found in the mesovarium and mesosalpinx after UAE, which may cause possible ovarian or tubal dysfunction after UAE. Permanent amenorrhea is a rare event occurring in fewer than 2% of patients after UAE with PVA particles, and it has been attributed to reduced ovarian perfusion or infarction. Nevertheless, without a detailed change in follicle-stimulating hormone levels before and after UAE, the relationship between a PVA embolization and premature menopause remains unverified currently. Other rare complications of UAE with PVA particles include transcervical expulsion of an embolized fibroid, a small-bowel infection caused by necrosis of an adjacent pedunculated fibroid after embolization, and fatal pulmonary.

It is not yet clear whether fertility and the ability of the uterus to successfully maintain an intrauterine gestation are preserved when PVA is used for UAE.

UAE achieved with PVA does not definitively preclude future pregnancy. The problem with studying absolute numbers of pregnancies after uterine fibroid embolization is that the true number of patients wishing and actively attempting to become pregnant after this procedure is small compared with the number of patients undergoing this procedure.

Patients considering treatment for symptomatic uterine fibroids are often perimenopausal and do not wish for children. Because of this fact and the reluctance of many centers to perform this procedure on patients desiring future children, the pregnancy rate after uterine fibroid embolization with PVA is difficult to ascertain [6, 7, 11–17].

3.1.2.2 Microsphere

Compared with conventional PVA, the main advantages of spherical embolic agents are ease of injection and less catheter clogging, resulting in more predictable occlusion levels. Several spherical embolic agents have been developed.

The first to be used in patients, Embosphere microspheres (BioSphere Medical, Rockland, MA), are biocompatible, hydrophilic, nonabsorbable, and precisely calibrated trisacrylic gelatin particles. Embospheres have FDA approval for use in hypervascular tumors and uterine fibroid embolization (Fig. 3.5).

Currently, five spherical embolic agents are available including Embosphere, Contour SE PVA microsphere (Boston Scientific Corporation, Natick, MA); PVA Bead Block hydrogel microsphere (Terumo Interventional Systems, Tokyo, Japan); QuadraSphere, super absorbent polymer microspheres (BioSphere Medical); and Embozene, Polyzene-F coated hydrogel microspheres (CeloNova BioSciences, Inc., Newnan, GA). The microspheres are available in sizes

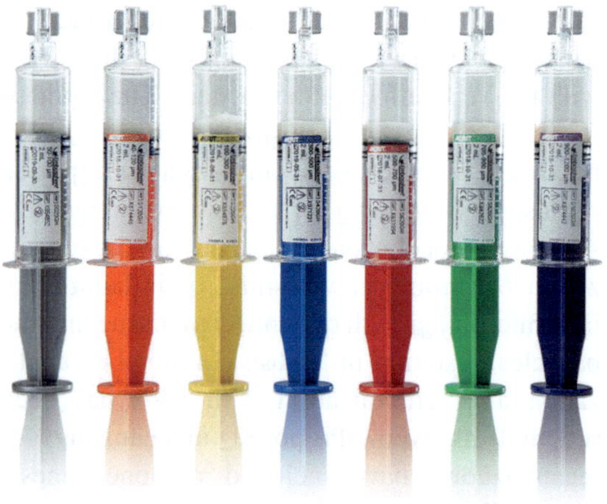

Fig. 3.5 Embosphere, different colors indicate different microsphere dimensions

from 40 to 1200 μm and are supplied in sterile apyrogenic sodium chloride solution. There are physical and mechanical differences between each of the spherical embolization agents that can significantly affect clinical outcomes. For any given embolization procedure, each type of microsphere differs in the particle size used and the angiographic end point. It is essential to know the specifics of each type of spherical embolic agent before use [15, 18].

3.1.2.3 Liquid Embolic Agents

Glue

Glue (cyanoacrylate) is a fast and efficient non-resorbable, non-radiopaque embolic material (Fig. 3.6).

Liquid monomeric cyanoacrylate is converted to a solid long-chain polymer immediately upon contact with anionic substances such as plasma, blood cells, endothelium, or saline. The reaction proceeds so rapidly that the glue will solidify in a catheter unless a substance is added to extend the polymerization time. The most commonly used agent is ethidized oil (Ethiodol, Lipiodol), typically in cyanoacrylate to oil ratios ranging from 1: 5 to 2: 5 depending on the time required until polymerization. Some operators also add powdered tantalum to increase radiopacity during injection, particularly for intracranial procedures. It is critical that this preparation takes place in an ion-free environment to prevent premature polymerization, preferably on a side table separate from that used for the rest of the angiographic procedure. The glue bolus is introduced into the catheter after it has been washed with D5W solution and is ejected from the catheter with another bolus of D5W. The catheter is typically changed after each injection. Histopathologic studies of the glue show that cyanoacrylate causes a more intense inflammatory reaction than that caused by PVA and involves the vessel wall and adjacent interstitial areas. This inflammatory reaction eventually leads to vessel necrosis, fibrous growth, and permanent occlusion. The most common applications of glue are the treatment of vascular malformations, particularly intracranial, although it has been applied throughout the body for virtually every embolic indication. Risks of using cyanoacrylates include rapid polymerization and reflux resulting in the catheter sticking in place or occlusion of the feeding vessel without nidal penetration. If the polymerization time is too long, cyanoacrylate can pass into the venous circulation, causing pulmonary emboli [19].

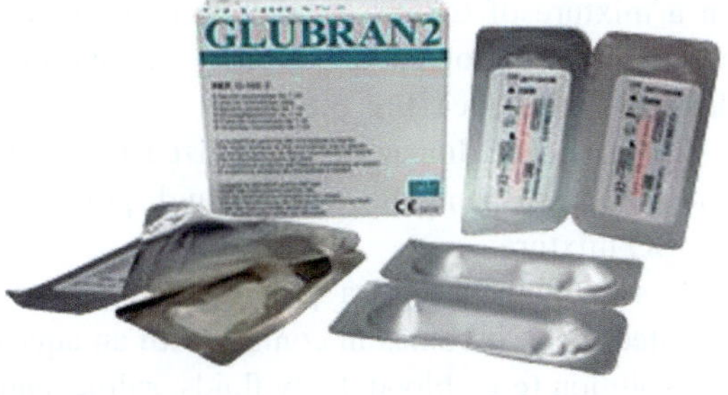

Fig. 3.6 Glue

Liquid Polymers

These agents have been used off label in the pelvic circulation, where they are particularly useful for treating AVMs or when a catheter cannot be passed to a sufficiently distal location for adequate embolization with another agent. Unlike particulate embolic agents, metallic devices and liquid embolic agents are radiopaque.

Several types of liquid embolic agents are available on the market. These embolic agents were designed for the treatment of vascular pathologies of the central nervous system and later have also been used for the treatment of pathologies of the extra-neurological territory.

Some liquid embolizing agents are composed of an embolizing material dissolved in a solvent that is typically dimethyl sulfoxide (DMSO). DMSO traces its roots to the nascent German chemical industry of the late nineteenth century. In the search for cheaper, more efficient methods to produce paper from wood pulp, a process was developed in which its by-products included a variety of sulfide-containing compounds. These malodorous sulfides were converted to less-noxious sulfoxides, including DMSO. This colorless liquid found immediate application as a polar, aprotic solvent miscible with water and able to dissolve an enormous catalog of polar and nonpolar small molecules. Since the 1860s, DMSO has been extensively studied in the chemical literature. DMSO was soon recognized to have the unique ability to "carry" small molecules through a variety of barriers. It was noted that DMSO spilled onto the hands would quickly cause a distinctive garlic taste on the tongue, which led to the systematic investigation of DMSO as a transport agent that could be used to deliver small molecules through skin and mucosa.

In the body, DMSO rapidly oxidizes to dimethyl sulfone (methlysulfonylmethane-MSM) and dimethyl sulfide. Both DMSO and MSM are soluble in both oil and water-based liquids. However, dimethyl sulfide is hydrophobic and tends to be insoluble in water and soluble in oil-based liquids. Clearance of DMSO and MSM is achieved by both excretion in the urine and feces and by elimination through the lungs and skin in the form of dimethyl sulfide.

The various devices on the market differ in the composition of the embolizing component, in the different concentrations, and in the different radiopaque component that makes the material visible during embolization procedures and during subsequent controls [19–26].

Phil

The Phil liquid embolic device (Precipitating Hydrophobic Injectable Liquid, MicroVention Terumo, Tustin, CA, USA) is composed of a non-adhesive copolymer (polylactideco-glycolide and polyhydroxyethylmethacrylate) dissolved in DMSO with an iodine component (triiodophenol) covalently bound to the copolymer, causing radiopacity. Phil is supplied in pre-filled 1 mL sterile syringes (Fig. 3.7).

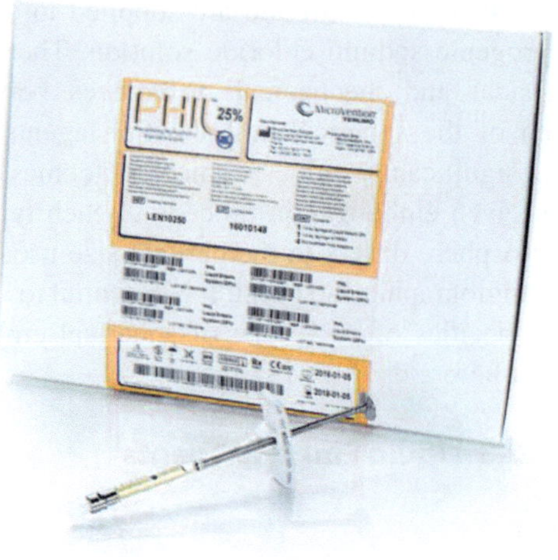

Fig. 3.7 Phil system

Phil solidifies through a process of precipitation initiated when it encounters an aqueous solution (e.g., blood, body fluids, normal saline, and water), and the solvent DMSO rapidly diffuses out of the polymer mass, causing in-situ precipitation of a soft radiopaque polymeric embolus. Complete precipitation occurs within 3 to 10 min. The microcatheter must be primed with the DMSO solvent to fill its dead space. Afterwards, Phil is first slowly injected to displace the DMSO, and then the injection is continued at a slow steady rate (recommended rate 0.16 mL/min). The iodine component allows visualization of Phil under fluoroscopy, with no risk of microcatheter blockage, at the same time minimizing artifacts at follow-up imaging studies and facilitating staged procedures or repeated treatments. It is compatible with surgical resection with no reported hazards related to sparking/combustion and no tattoo effect in the treatment of superficial malformation. Phil is available in a range of liquid viscosities (25%, 30%, and 35%): Lower viscosities, achieved by reducing the polymer/dimethyl sulfoxide ratio, are indicated for the embolization of arteriovenous malformations where depth penetration in small diameter vessels is required [27].

Onyx

Onyx liquid embolic device is a premixed radiopaque injectable embolic agent that is not a true glue and has no adhesive properties. It is based on a mixture of EVOH (ethylene vinyl alcohol copolymer) dissolved in DMSO (anhydrous dimethyl sulfoxide) (Fig. 3.8).

To provide radiopacity, micronized tantalum powder is suspended in the liquid polymer/DMSO mixture.

It solidifies through a precipitation process initiated when it comes in contact with an aqueous solution (e.g., blood, body fluids, saline, and water) and the DMSO solvent rapidly diffuses

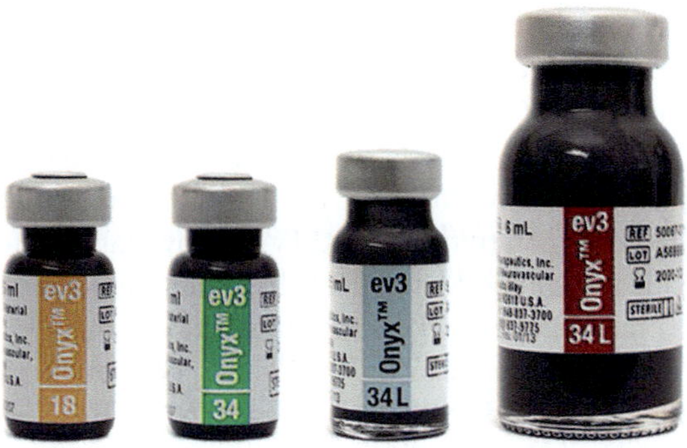

Fig. 3.8 Onyx

from the polymer mass causing in situ precipitation of a soft radiopaque polymer embolus. Complete precipitation occurs within minutes (range: 3–10 min).

When this mixture encounters aqueous media such as blood, the DMSO diffuses rapidly, resulting in in situ precipitation and solidification of the polymer. It forms a soft elastic embolus without adhesion to the vascular wall or catheter. The polymerization process is primarily influenced by the amount of ethylene vinyl acetate (EVOH) copolymer in the mixture.

Onyx is commercially available with different viscosities (18-20-34-500): Lower viscosities are indicated for more distal, low-flow areas, while higher viscosities are more useful for high-flow conditions. The lower the EVOH concentration, the less viscous the solution will be and the longer it will take to precipitate. Because the polymer will solidify upon contact with aqueous media, the release catheter must be pre-rinsed with DMSO.

A DMSO-compatible catheter is required. Onyx is non-adhesive, allowing easy removal of the release catheter and the polymer itself. Unfortunately, it is quite expensive. It is primarily used for intracranial aneurysms; however, in peripheral embolization Onyx has been used successfully to treat conditions such as endoleak and AVM [1, 3, 22, 28–31].

Alcohol

Absolute alcohol is a very effective embolizing agent although it must be used with great care. It can be injected intravascularly or by direct percutaneous puncture. In contact with the vessel wall, ethanol denudes the endothelium, which leads to thrombosis and eventual fibrosis. In addition, upon contact with the blood, ethanol induces further thrombosis. Both actions lead to complete and permanent vascular occlusion. This effective occlusion can be used to advantage for tumor or organ ablation, particularly renal embolization, and by very experienced practitioners for the treatment of vascular malformations. It is important to consider the risk of toxicity when using alcohol.

The main disadvantage of absolute ethanol is the risk of necrosis of nearby tissues (including nerves) or skin. Methods to reduce the risk of nontarget embolization include occlusion balloons used in some cases to control reflux.

The risk of systemic toxicity increases with doses greater than 1 mL/kg or if the total volume exceeds 60 mL. The patient should be monitored closely. Some practitioners advocate the use of pulmonary arterial pressure monitoring during procedures involving ethanol [32].

3.1.2.4 Metal Coils and Plugs

They can achieve permanent arterial occlusion; coils are made of stainless steel or platinum wire covered with thrombogenic fibers and are available in many sizes and shapes. Typically, these devices are used to occlude vessels larger than 2 mm in diameter, and they are most useful for the occlusion of focal arterial abnormalities or injuries.

Coils

Spring embolus coils are rarely used alone for the treatment of pelvic bleeding. They usually occlude too proximally to stop bleeding from small collateral vessels. Coils are permanent. Therefore, it is not possible to re-catheterize vessels in which they have been placed. They also create artifacts on magnetic resonance studies.

Occasionally, a large proximal branch of the internal iliac artery is lacerated. Gelfoam cubes may be swept through the laceration into the extravascular and consequently have no effect on the bleeding. In these situations, spring embolus coils should be used.

Optimally, coils are placed both distal and proximal to the bleeding site if the vessel has not been completely transected. Distal embolization will prevent retrograde bleeding from collaterals beyond the site of laceration.

Bleeding of large vessels can be slowed by inflation of an occlusion balloon catheter proximal to or at the bleeding site.

Coils are made of stainless steel or platinum and come in a wide variety of sizes. They may have Dacron fibers positioned at right angles to the long axis of the coil, or coatings such as hydrogel to increase surface area and thereby increase the rate and permanence of thrombosis (Fig. 3.9).

Coils rely on mechanical obstruction, platelet activation, and the patient's coagulation cascade to completely occlude vessels. Consequently, in the presence of thrombocytopenia and coagulopathy, the efficacy of embolization is compromised. It should be noted that all coils are permanent devices and should be used when permanent occlusion is desired. When larger nonterminal vessels are occluded with coils, collateral arteries form relatively rapidly and the distal vascular bed will still be perfused, albeit at a lower pressure than pre-embolization. Coil stability is essential to prevent untargeted embolization.

For embolization of large vessels, such as the ovarian veins in pelvic congestion syndrome, plugs can also be used. Vascular plugs are permanent occlusive devices that use nitinol mesh in a 3D disc geometry. The Amplatzer Plug product family (AGA Medical Corporation, Golden Valley, MN) consists of four devices. Devices I and II are available in the United States; the newer generations (III and IV) are available outside the United States. They have platinum bands as radiopaque markers, are attached to a delivery wire via a microsite, and must be deployed through a guide catheter or sheath (5 to 9 Fr). The maximum length of the delivery system is 100 cm for plugs I and II and 120 cm for plugs III. The Amplatzer Plug IV is available in sizes from 4 to 8 mm and can be implemented using a 0.038 in. guide wire compatible diagnostic catheter no longer than 125 cm. Caps should be oversized relative to the target vessel diameter by 30% to 50% as recommended by the manufacturer. The devices are deployed by unscrewing the block counterclockwise, so precise positioning and repositioning are possible.

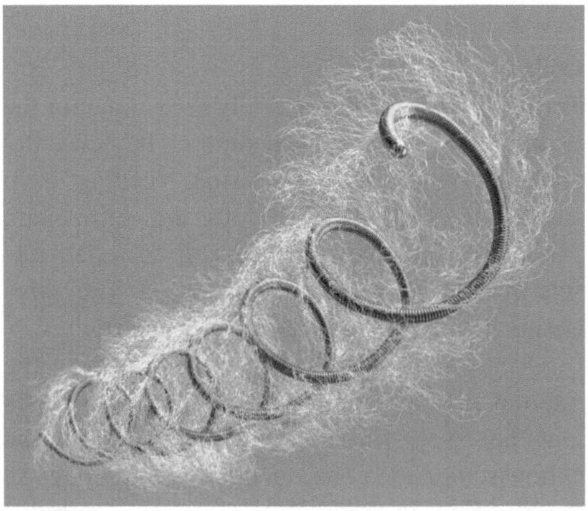

Fig. 3.9 Coil

In general, because of their compact design, relatively large surface area, and tight nitinol mesh structure, stoppers should be considered when single-pass occlusion of a larger vessel or branch is desired, or when an initial stopper is needed to act as a scaffold for subsequent additional embolization (e.g., with coils). In particular, plugs can be used to occlude internal iliac arteries before placement of aortoiliac stent grafts, exclusion of visceral arterial aneurysms, pseudoaneurysms of the ascending aorta, or emergency embolization of active bleeding.

3.1.2.5 Sclerosing Agents

Technically, all liquid embolic agents can be considered sclerosing agents; however, the term is usually applied to (mostly) low-viscosity agents used primarily in venous disease. Each has also been used with variable success in other types of embolization and cyst ablation. The properties of the most commonly used sclerosants will be described, but other agents such as hypertonic dextrose, bleomycin, acetic acid, triamcinolone, and methylmethacrylate have been or are being used, in some cases with spectacular results.

Polydocanol (Aethoxysklerol, Kreussler, Wiesbaden, Germany) is a nonionic surfactant sclerosant first developed as an anesthetic. It causes vascular injury through endothelial hyperhydration. The attractive anesthetic properties of the agent make it almost painless. Its use is primarily limited to venous disease [7, 8, 13, 33–36].

3.2 Complications

Overall complication rates for obstetric and gynecologic transcatheter embolization procedures are 6–9%.

3.2.1 Complications Related to Angiographic Procedure

Complications can be correlated to puncture site (hematoma) or to the vascular navigation (catheter-induced vessel dissection) or even to contrast medium administration (allergic phenomenon or nephrotoxic effect).

3.2.2 Complications Secondary to Embolization

A typical complication is the postembolization syndrome, characterized by pain, fever, nausea, and leukocytosis raised immediately after the procedure and lasting several days. This complication occurs in 50% of patients. Treatment includes analgesic and anti-inflammatory medications.

Other complications may include vaginal discharge and passage of fibroid tissue.

Severe complications such as uterine necrosis or rupture, sepsis, abscess, and ischemia of adjacent tissue also have been reported but they are rare. Embolization of nontargeted vessels may occur and typically cause bladder or rectal ischemic damages or sexual dysfunction.

Utero-ovarian anastomoses can cause unintended embolization of ovarian tissue causing premature ovarian failure and then amenorrhea. The reported rate of menopause within 1 year after uterine arterial embolization is approximately 15% for women aged 45 years or older [7, 17, 37–39] (Table 3.1).

Table 3.1 Embolic agents

Temporary embolic agents	Absorbable gelatin sponge (Gelfoam)
	Avitene
Permanent embolic agents	PVA
	Microsphere
	Liquid embolic agents
	Glue
	Liquid polymers
	Alcohol
	Metal coils and plugs
	Sclerosing agents

References

1. Varadharajan S, Ramalingaiah AH, Saini J, et al. Precipitating hydrophobic injectable liquid embolization of intracranial vascular shunts: initial experience and technical note. J Neurosurg. 2018;129:1217–22. https://doi.org/10.3171/2017.6.JNS16447.
2. Powerski M, Meyer-Wilmes P, Omari J, et al. Transcatheter arterial embolization of acute bleeding as 24/7 service: predictors of outcome and mortality. Br J Radiol. 2018;91:20180516. https://doi.org/10.1259/bjr.20180516.
3. Né R, Chevallier O, Falvo N, et al. Embolization with ethylene vinyl alcohol copolymer (onyx®) for peripheral hemostatic and non-hemostatic applications: a feasibility and safety study. Quant Imaging Med Surg. 2018;8:280–90. https://doi.org/10.21037/qims.2018.04.03.
4. Johnstone C, Rich SE. Bleeding in cancer patients and its treatment: a review. Ann Palliat Med. 2018;7:265–73. https://doi.org/10.21037/apm.2017.11.01.
5. Siskin GP, Englander M, Stainken BF, et al. Embolic agents used for uterine fibroid embolization. Am J Roentgenol. 2000;175:767–73. https://doi.org/10.2214/ajr.175.3.1750767.
6. Bakal CW, Silberzweig JE, Cynamon J, Sprayregen S. Vascular and interventional radiology principles and practice. New York: Thieme; 2002.
7. Katz MD, Sugay SB, Walker DK, et al. Beyond hemostasis: Spectrum of gynecologic and obstetric indications for transcatheter embolization. Radiographics. 2012;32:1713–31. https://doi.org/10.1148/rg.326125524.
8. Van Allan RJ, Pentecost MJ. Transcatheter control of hemorrhage in the cancer patient. Semin Intervent Radiol. 1992;9:38–44. https://doi.org/10.1055/s-2008-1074668.

9. Abada HT, Golzarian J. Gelatine sponge particles: handling characteristics for endovascular use. Tech Vasc Interv Radiol. 2007;10:257–60. https://doi.org/10.1053/j.tvir.2008.03.002.
10. Bensard DD, Beauchamp KM, Hurt RT, et al. Gelfoam. Encycl Intensive Care Med. 2012:977. https://doi.org/10.1007/978-3-642-00418-6_3122.
11. Scheurig-Muenkler C, Koesters C, Powerski MJ, et al. Clinical long-term outcome after uterine artery embolization: sustained symptom control and improvement of quality of life. J Vasc Interv Radiol. 2013;24:765–71. https://doi.org/10.1016/j.jvir.2013.02.018.
12. Marshburn PB, Matthews ML, Hurst BS. Uterine artery embolization as a treatment option for uterine myomas. Obstet Gynecol Clin N Am. 2006;33:125–44. https://doi.org/10.1016/j.ogc.2005.12.009.
13. Thabet A, Kalva SP, Liu B, et al. Interventional radiology in pregnancy complications: indications, technique, and methods for minimizing radiation exposure. Radiographics. 2012;32:255–74. https://doi.org/10.1148/rg.321115064.
14. El Shamy T, Amer SAK, Mohamed AA, et al. The impact of uterine artery embolization on ovarian reserve: a systematic review and meta-analysis. Acta Obstet Gynecol Scand. 2020;99:16–23. https://doi.org/10.1111/aogs.13698.
15. Laurent A. Microspheres and nonspherical particles for embolization. Tech Vasc Interv Radiol. 2007;10:248–56. https://doi.org/10.1053/j.tvir.2008.03.010.
16. Abramowitz SD, Israel GM, McCarthy SM, et al. Comparison of four embolic materials at uterine artery artery embolization by using postprocedural MR imaging enhancement. Radiology. 2009;250:482–7. https://doi.org/10.1148/radiol.2502080574.
17. Spies JB, Roth AR, Gonsalves SM, Murphy-Skrzyniarz KR. Ovarian function after uterine artery embolization for leiomyomata: assessment with use of serum follicle stimulating hormone assay. J Vasc Interv Radiol. 2001;12:437–42. https://doi.org/10.1016/s1051-0443(07)61881-8.
18. Lee KH, Liapi E, Ventura VP, et al. Evaluation of different calibrated spherical polyvinyl alcohol microspheres in transcatheter arterial chemoembolization: VX2 tumor model in rabbit liver. J Vasc Interv Radiol. 2008;19:1065–9. https://doi.org/10.1016/j.jvir.2008.02.023.
19. Howington JU, Kerber CW, Hopkins LN. Liquid embolic agents in the treatment of intracranial arteriovenous malformations. Neurosurg Clin N Am. 2005;16:355–63. https://doi.org/10.1016/j.nec.2004.08.013.
20. Capriotti K, Capriotti JA. Dimethyl sulfoxide: history, chemistry, and clinical utility in dermatology. J Clin Aesthet Dermatol. 2012;5:24–6.
21. Koçer N, Hanımoğlu H, Batur Ş, et al. Preliminary experience with precipitating hydrophobic injectable liquid in brain arteriovenous malformations. Diagn Interv Radiol. 2016;22:184–9. https://doi.org/10.5152/dir.2015.15283.
22. Müller-Wille R, Heiss P, Herold T, et al. Endovascular treatment of acute arterial hemorrhage in trauma patients using ethylene vinyl alcohol copolymer (onyx). Cardiovasc Intervent Radiol. 2012;35:65–75. https://doi.org/10.1007/s00270-011-0134-x.
23. Triano MJ, Lara-Reyna J, Schupper AJ, Yaeger KA. Embolic agents and microcatheters for endovascular treatment of cerebral arteriovenous malformations. World Neurosurg. 2020;141:383–8. https://doi.org/10.1016/j.wneu.2020.06.118.
24. Kurda D, Guduguntla G, Maingard J, et al. Precipitating hydrophobic injectable liquid (PHIL) embolic for the treatment of a uterine arteriovenous malformation: a technical report. CVIR Endovasc. 2019;2:17. https://doi.org/10.1186/s42155-019-0059-z.
25. Joseph S, Chadaga HC, Murali K. Endovascular treatment of cerebral AVM with onyx—initial experience. Interv Neuroradiol. 2005;11:171–8. https://doi.org/10.1177/15910199050110s121.
26. Vollherbst DF, Sommer CM, Ulfert C, et al. Liquid embolic agents for endovascular embolization: evaluation of an established (onyx) and a novel (PHIL) embolic agent in an in vitro AVM model. Am J Neuroradiol. 2017;38:1377–82. https://doi.org/10.3174/ajnr.A5203.
27. Lucatelli P, Corona M, Teodoli L, et al. Use of Phil embolic agent for bleeding in non-neurological interventions. J Clin Med. 2021;10:701. https://doi.org/10.3390/jcm10040701.
28. Vanninen RL, Manninen I. Onyx, a new liquid embolic material for peripheral interventions: preliminary experience in aneurysm, pseudoaneurysm, and pulmonary arteriovenous malformation embolization. Cardiovasc Intervent Radiol. 2007;30:196–200. https://doi.org/10.1007/s00270-006-0071-2.
29. Ayad M, Eskioglu E, Mericle RA. Onyx®: A unique neuroembolic agent. Expert Rev Med Devices. 2006;3:705–15. https://doi.org/10.1586/17434440.3.6.705.
30. Kolber MK, Shukla PA, Kumar A, Silberzweig JE. Ethylene vinyl alcohol copolymer (onyx) embolization for acute hemorrhage: a systematic review of peripheral applications. J Vasc Interv Radiol. 2015;26:809–15. https://doi.org/10.1016/j.jvir.2015.02.025.
31. Valek V, Husty J. Quality improvement guidelines for transcatheter embolization for acute gastrointestinal nonvariceal hemorrhage. Cardiovasc Intervent Radiol. 2013;36:608–12. https://doi.org/10.1007/s00270-012-0462-5.
32. Ginat DT, Saad WEA, Turba UC. Transcatheter renal artery embolization: clinical applications and techniques. Tech Vasc Interv Radiol. 2009;12:224–39. https://doi.org/10.1053/j.tvir.2009.09.007.

33. Bookwalter CA, Vanburen WM, Neisen MJ, Bjarnason H. Imaging appearance and nonsurgical management of pelvic venous congestion syndrome. Radiographics. 2019;39:596–608. https://doi.org/10.1148/rg.2019180159.
34. Laughlin-Tommaso S, Barnard EP, AbdElmagied AM, et al. FIRSTT study: randomized controlled trial of uterine artery embolization vs focused ultrasound surgery. Am J Obstet Gynecol. 2019;220:174.e1–174.e13. https://doi.org/10.1016/j.ajog.2018.10.032.
35. Andrews RT, Spies JB, Sacks D, et al. Patient care and uterine artery embolization for Leiomyomata. J Vasc Interv Radiol. 2004;15:115–20. https://doi.org/10.1097/01.RVI.0000109408.52762.35.
36. Pelage JP, Cazejust J, Pluot E, et al. Uterine fibroid vascularization and clinical relevance to uterine fibroid embolization. Radiographics. 2005;25:99–118. https://doi.org/10.1148/rg.25si055510.
37. Kitamura Y, Ascher SM, Cooper C, et al. Imaging manifestations of complications associated with uterine artery embolization. Radiographics. 2005;25:119–33. https://doi.org/10.1148/rg.25si055518.
38. Carrillo TC. Uterine artery embolization in the management of symptomatic uterine fibroids: an overview of complications and follow-up. Semin Intervent Radiol. 2008;25:378–86. https://doi.org/10.1055/s-0028-1102997.
39. Spies JB, Spector A, Roth AR, et al. Complications after uterine artery embolization for leiomyomas. Obstet Gynecol. 2002;100:873–80. https://doi.org/10.1097/00006250-200211000-00007.

Radioprotection

4

Marco Femia, Michela Lecchi, Ruggero Vercelli,
Michele Paternò, and Maurizio Cariati

4.1 Introduction

Until the second half of the twentieth century, the use of x-rays in medicine was limited to diagnosis, plain radiography and stratigraphy being the solely available methods. Subsequently, new x-ray-based technologies were introduced in daily clinical practice leading to a burst in the diagnostic power of radiologists and opening new scenarios in treatment options. Over the last three decades, image-guided interventions paved the way for new and minimally invasive management of many diseases, previously treated by more complex and invasive surgical interventions, with a constantly increasing number of people who benefited from such innovative procedures [1].

The vast majority of image-guided interventions are performed under real-time x-ray guidance (such as TIPS, artero-venous malformations, and prostate embolization), usually representing the most complex and long, whereas a minor part is supported by ultrasound imaging. In this setting, radiation safety measures are pivotal to gain a balance between benefits from minimally invasive image-guided interventions and potential future risks, due to ionizing radiation exposure. As interventional radiologists are a key figure to achieve this goal, they must acquire, during their training periods, a deep comprehension of the biological effects of ionizing radiations and the best strategies to minimize radiation dose in order to develop good work habits in their daily practice. However, despite the effort of minimizing radiation dose, there are some conditions which limit the impact of radiation protection measures. Obesity involves a raise in scatter radiation dose to the operator and a higher exposure to the patient undergoing the procedure while, for a fixed dose, pediatric patients have a higher risk of developing negative effects of ionizing radiations, compared to adults, due to their longer life expectancy and the higher sensitivity of developing tissues [2–4].

M. Femia (✉) · R. Vercelli · M. Cariati
Radiology Unit, ASST Santi Paolo e Carlo, Milan, Italy
e-mail: marco.femia@asst-santipaolocarlo.it; ruggero.vercelli@asst-santipaolocarlo.it; cariati.maurizio@sancarlo.mi.it

M. Paternò
Postgraduation School in Radiodiagnostics, Milan, Italy
e-mail: michele.paterno@unimi.it

M. Lecchi
Medical Physics, ASST Bergamo Ovest, Bergamo, Italy
e-mail: michela_lecchi@asst-bgovest.it

R. Niola et al. (eds.), *Diagnostic and Interventional Radiology in Gynecological and Obstetric Diseases*, https://doi.org/10.1007/978-3-031-11910-1_4

4.2 Damage Mechanisms of Ionizing Radiation

The harmful biological effect of ionizing radiations derives from cellular molecule damage. The damage mechanism of ionizing radiation can be either direct, due to the x-ray-induced ionization of DNA and/or other proteins and lipids, or indirect, secondary to the generation of free radicals mainly derived from x-ray interaction with O_2 and H_2O, the hydroxyl radical (OH) being mainly responsible [5, 6].

On a large scale, cellular death results in tissue damage named "tissue reaction" or the so-called deterministic effect. Deterministic effect is characterized by a threshold dose, below which the specific damage does not occur, while above the threshold, the probability of occurrence of a specific effect rises steeply to 100%. Moreover, above the threshold dose, deterministic effect is related to the dose: the higher the dose, the more severe the effect [7].

By contrast, stochastic effects follow a linear non-threshold (LNT) model, whereby no exposure is safe, and the risk increases with increased exposure [8]. This means that even at very low doses it is possible to induce cellular damage or death. The death of a few cells will not result in appreciable tissue damage, while genetic changes can lead to malignancies or heritable mutations if they occur in parental germ cells [9].

Unfortunately, it is not possible to accurately calculate the probability risk due to the inability to precisely quantify the radiation dose and variability in individual susceptibility.

4.3 The Dosimetric Quantities

The dosimetric quantities used in radiological protection are effective dose, equivalent dose [both with the unit of sievert (Sv)], and absorbed dose [with the unit of gray (Gy)].

Effective dose was introduced in the 1990 Recommendation of the International Commission on Radiological Protection (ICRP) [10] and now it is accepted internationally as the central radiological protection quantity, providing a risk-adjusted estimation of total body dose from external and internal sources in relation to risks of cancer and hereditary effects (i.e., mutations in germ cells that may affect future generations). It has proved to be a valuable and robust quantity for use in the optimization of protection for workers and members of the public, the setting of control criteria (constraints, reference levels, and limits), and the demonstration of compliance. Its use requires the assumption of the LNT dose response, the relationship between dose and risk at low doses or low dose rates, the equivalence of effect of acute and chronic low-level exposures, and the equivalence of effect of internal and external exposures. Effective dose will generally be used at doses below 100 mSv, but its use at acute doses in the range up to approximately 1 Sv is reasonable, noting the possibility of occurrence of tissue reactions, particularly from non-uniform distribution of dose.

Effective dose is used to compare patients' exposure doses from different medical procedures, informing judgments on justification, and establishing constraints for carers and volunteers in medical research.

While doses from the same technique are comparable, measurable quantities, characteristic of each modality (computed tomography, interventional procedures, etc.), are preferred.

Table 4.1 gives a scale linked to effective dose in the context of risks and benefits from medical imaging, with general terms to describe the dose linked to possible levels of cancer risk and examples of procedures within different dose ranges [11].

Organ/tissue equivalent dose is only an intermediate step in the calculation of effective dose that takes into account the differences between the radiation types (e.g., alpha particles and neutrons relative to gamma rays) in their effectiveness in relation to cancer induction.

Absorbed dose is the only measurable quantity for protection purposes and it is the primary scientific step from which effective dose is calculated for a "reference person," passing through

Table 4.1 Effective dose ranges and terminology for describing risks from different medical procedures for adult patients of average age (30–39) based on UK data

Effective dose (mSv)	Risk of cancer	Proposed term for dose level	Examples of medical radiation procedures within different dose categories
<0.1	Inferred $<10^{-5}$ on LNT model	Negligible	Radiographs of chest, femur, shoulder limbs, neck, and teeth
0.1–1	Inferred $<10^{-5}$–10^{-4} on LNT model	Minimal	Radiographs of spine, abdomen, pelvis, head, and cervical spine
1–10	Inferred $<10^{-4}$–10^{-3} on LNT model	Very low	CT scans of the head and combinations of chest, abdomen, and pelvis; barium enemas; cardiac angiography; interventional radiology
10–100	Risk $<10^{-3}$–10^{-2} based on LNT model and epidemiology[a]	Low	CT scans of chest, abdomen, and pelvis; double CT scans for contrast enhancement; interventional radiology (uterine fibroid embolization, embolization of ovarian veins)
			Renal/visceral angioplasty; iliac angioplasty; follow-up of endovascular aneurysm repair (35–100 mSv)
>100	$>10^{-2}$ based on epidemiology[a]	Moderate	Multiple procedures and follow-up studies

LNT linear non-threshold, *CT* computed tomography
[a]Risk bands are lifetime detriment-adjusted cancer incidence to nearest order of magnitude

Table 4.2 Dose thresholds for tissue reaction

Tissue or organ	Dose thresholds
Fetal abnormality	0.1–0.5 Gy
Cataracts	0.5 Gy
Sterility	2–3 Gy
Skin erythema	2–5 Gy
Hair loss	2–5 Gy
Lethality (whole body)	3–5 Gy
Irreversible skin damage	20–40 Gy

the intermediate level of organ/tissue equivalent dose estimation [11].

Absorbed dose is the quantity for use in setting limits on organ/tissue doses to prevent tissue reaction (Table 4.2).

4.4 Radiation Protection of Patients

Patients' radiation safety considerations differ from other situations in which radiation exposure is planned, as it is intentional and directed to a benefit. The justification and optimization principles represent the beacon in the difficult choice to expose a patient to ionizing radiations. The principle of dose limitation is not recommended as it could reduce the effectiveness of a diagnostic examination or a treatment, being more harmful than good [9, 12].

4.4.1 Radiation Protection in Diagnostic Imaging

The diagnosis of non-oncologic gynecological and obstetric pathologies is performed mainly with non-x-ray-based imaging. Indeed the most common imaging technique is transvaginal ultrasound (TV-US). However, a precise imaging mapping of vascular anatomy is sometimes suggested before the endovascular management of some gynecological pathologies, in order to ease the procedure and reduce its length. The best non-invasive imaging technique to depict vascular anatomy is contrast-enhanced computed tomography (CT). CT scan exposes patients to x-rays whose dose is not negligible. In many studies, the mean estimated effective dose for a standard abdominal CT examination is between 5 and 6 mSv [13–15].

This is why contrast-enhanced magnetic resonance imaging (MRI) may have a role as a preoperative examination, especially in young patients such as gynecological ones (e.g., women with pelvic congestion syndrome) [16].

4.4.2 Radiation Protection in Image-Guided Interventions

The first concept to be satisfied, in patients' radiation protection during interventional procedures, is the appropriateness of the indication. Taking it for granted, there are several tips and tricks which allow to reduce patient radiation exposure.

First of all, a careful evaluation of pre-procedural imaging is mandatory in order to plan the procedure accurately: clearly identify the target, choose the appropriate material, and define the best projections.

Commonly, operators take care of just fluoroscopy time; however, there are many other variables that can affect patient exposure such as x-ray tube output, x-ray beam geometry, image mode, and image sequence parameters. X-ray tube output can be modulated in both dose per single frame (low, normal, and high) and in the pulse rate reaching up to 30 frames per s. The low dose-low frame choice is not always the best, indeed low frame rate can lead to a retard in the image compared to the quick movement of the field of view resulting in a longer procedure. By contrast, a high dose-fast frame setting should be reserved for situations in which the best definition can prevent complications or allows to reach a more accurate result. Usually, fluoroscopy parameters are set at 7.5 frames/s with normal dose. Again, DSA runs frame rate strongly impacts radiation dose. It is usually set at 4 frames/s but it can be raised up to 7 frames/s depending on the necessity (e.g., artero-venous shunts in which high flows are involved).

Finally, x-ray beam geometry and image modality can significantly influence radiation dose to both patients and operators. Indeed, the lower the patient distance to the x-ray tube the higher the radiation dose; this is why for the best image quality and the lowest radiation dose, patients must be as far from the x-ray tube as possible and closest to the flat-panel receptor. The postero-anterior projection results in the lowest radiation dose, compared to other tube angulations, for both patient and operator. Indeed, an angulated x-ray beam crosses a thicker tract within the patient and there is a larger gap between the x-ray tube and the receptor. An oblique projection with the x-ray tube toward the operator results in a higher dose to the interventional radiologist, compared to the same contralateral grades, while it makes no difference to the patient. Although x-ray tube angulation globally results in a higher radiation dose to the patient, it may be a good strategy to reduce the peak skin dose by changing the entry point. Magnification tool limits the area of the exposed tissue but enhances the exposure of the remaining field of view thus increasing the risk of skin injury. However, the overall radiation dose to the patient remains unchanged [2].

4.4.3 Patient Shielding

Patient shielding was first introduced into U.S. Code of Federal Regulation in 1976, and it was justified as a matter of protection from hereditary risks (gonadal shielding only). However, 45 years later, no hereditary effects from radiation have yet been observed in humans (only in experimental animals) [17]. Moreover, the American College of Obstetricians and Gynecologists (ACOG) Guidelines, with endorsement from the American College of Radiology (ACR), states that "with few exceptions, radiation exposure through radiography, computed tomography scan, or nuclear medicine imaging techniques is at a dose much lower than the exposure associated with fetal harm" [18].

The current international position is to abandon the practice of gonadal and fetal shielding in radiology, as the associated risks are substantial (patient dose increment due to the need of exam repetition or the presence of shielding in the field of view of the automatic exposure control system), whereas the benefits are negligible or nonexistent [19].

4.5 Occupational Radiation Protection

The ICRP is the primary organization supervising the exposure to ionizing radiation and setting dose limits, which have been lowered over time.

In 2007, the Commission remarked an average effective dose limit of 20 mSv over 5 years (100 mSv in 5 years) and a maximum of 50 mSv in a single year for occupational exposure in planned situations [9, 12].

Interventional radiologists' activity requires the use of x-rays for most of the interventions, apart from US-guided procedures, leading to a daily exposure of the personnel for decades of career. Operators' exposure is mainly attributable to scatter from patient than to direct exposure.

The aim of every institution must be to provide the safest working environment which, in the fluoroscopy laboratories, means to reduce personnel radiation exposure to the minimum achievable. A modern angiographic suite should include ceiling-suspended clear acrylic shields, table-mounted flexible leaded strips, and eventually mobile barriers on wheels. Despite these environmental barriers, every interventional radiologist must be equipped with a lead equivalent apron, preferably custom made. Thyroid gland is the most radiation-sensitive organ unshielded with a classical apron, thus an adjunctive thyroid shield is usually employed. Additional shields can be used such as leaded caps, leaded goggles, and sterile radiation-resistant gloves. Radiation-resistant gloves deserve a special mention as their use may present a drawback in terms of radiation protection. Indeed, they may be useful when hands work outside the field of view, but they must be avoided in those procedures in which hands are directly hit by the x-ray beam as the raise in x-ray attenuation induces an automatic growth in x-ray tube output resulting in a greater exposure, both direct and scatter. In addition, leaded gloves reduce tactile sensation which may lengthen the procedure. Radiation protection of personnel can be divided into passive and active precautions. The first includes the above-mentioned protective equipment available in the angio suite, while the correct use of such protective tools as well as behaviors whose aim is to reduce exposure are part of active radiation protection. The acquisition of DSA runs from the control room or distant from the table and leads to a dramatic drop in radiation exposure, being among the most effective active radiation protection tools, according to the inverse square law. In addition, as previously mentioned, the operator's exposure is mainly due to scatter. As such, those behaviors aimed to lower patient dose also lead to a reduction in staff exposure; for this reason, they are considered part of active radiation protection.

4.6 Pregnant Patients and Personnel

Radiation exposure of patients and staff during pregnancy is a matter of concern. In these situations, exposure precautions must be further enhanced and dose monitoring is more careful. Radiation-related risk strongly depends on gestational age (sensitivity is the highest between 8 and 15 weeks of pregnancy) and the fetus' absorbed dose. The risk of abnormalities for fetal absorbed dose <100 mGy is small or probably absent [20]. Workers who declared their pregnant status should wear an additional dosimeter on the abdomen under the lead apron and be monitored monthly. Of course, this dosimeter overestimates the real dose to the embryo/fetus, as it registers the dose on the mother's abdomen without considering her tissue attenuation. Generally, the embryo/fetus dose can be considered as one half of the personal equivalent dose at 1 cm, Hp(10), for the additional dosimeter on the abdomen [20]. ICRP recommendations set the limit of an additional dose of 1 mSv during pregnancy [9], which would allow pregnant women to continue their working activity as long as they are strictly controlled. However, legislation differs between countries so that pregnant women often have to suspend their interventional activity. For example, in Italy, it is not possible for a woman who declared her pregnant state to be exposed to ionizing radiations for professional reasons.

The use of fluoroscopically guided procedures as well as diagnostic examinations involving ionizing radiations in pregnant women must be customized in order to reduce exposure to the minimum achievable (e.g., prophylactic occlusion balloon placement in internal iliac arteries). In such a setting, each measure needs to be care-

Table 4.3 Practical advices to minimize x-ray exposure in pregnant patients

Exclude the conceptus from direct x-ray beam when possible
Consider arm or wrist access
Keep beam-on time to the minimum
Keep the tube current as low as possible by keeping the tube potential (kVp) as high as possible
Keep the x-ray tube at maximal distance from the patient
Keep the flat-panel detector as close as possible to the patient
Do not overuse geometric magnification
Remove the grid when image intensifier cannot be placed close to the patient
Collimate as tightly as possible
Consider oblique projections for unexpectedly prolonged procedures (however, keep in mind that oblique projections could increase x-ray scatter to the conceptus)
Allow for posterior-anterior beam projections when possible
Use low-dose low-rate pulsed fluoroscopy (15 frame/s)
Use last image hold
Minimize DSA runs to the minimum enhancing the use of fluoroscopic loops

fully applied in order to reduce radiation dose to the minimum. This was matter of study by the Society of Interventional Radiology (SIR) and the Cardiovascular and Interventional Radiology Society of Europe (CIRSE) which produced a joint guideline document with the endorsement of the Canadian Interventional Radiology Association, whose main recommendations are summarized in Table 4.3 [21]. However, despite all the efforts to reduce radiation dose to the minimum, the most important feature to be evaluated in pregnant patients is the strict appropriateness of the indication of every x-ray-based diagnostic examination and interventional procedure, without which even extremely low doses are too much.

References

1. Marx MV. The radiation dose in interventional radiology study: knowledge brings responsibility. J Vasc Interv Radiol. 2003;14(8):947–51.
2. Schueler BA, Vrieze TJ, Bjarnason H, Stanson AW. An investigation of operator exposure in interventional radiology. Radiographics. 2006;26(5):1533–41; discussion 1541
3. ICRP. ICRP publication 121: radiological protection in paediatric diagnostic and interventional radiology. Ann ICRP. 2013;42(2):1–63.
4. Goodman TR, Mustafa A, Rowe E. Pediatric CT radiation exposure: where we were, and where we are now. Pediatr Radiol. 2019;49(4):469–78.
5. Wunderle K, Gill AS. Radiation-related injuries and their management: an update. Semin Intervent Radiol. 2015;32(2):156–62.
6. Rosen EM, Day R, Singh VK. New approaches to radiation protection. Front Oncol. 2015;4:381.
7. ICRP. ICRP publication 139: occupational radiological protection in interventional procedures. Ann ICRP. 2018;47(2):1–118.
8. Yu C. Don't be caught half-dressed when working with radiation. Cardiovasc Intervent Radiol. 2020;43(3):369–75.
9. ICRP. ICRP publication 103: the 2007 recommendations of the international commission on radiological protection. Ann ICRP. 2007;37(2–4):1–332.
10. ICRP. ICRP publication 60: 1990 recommendations of the international commission on radiological protection. Ann ICRP. 1991;21(1–3):1–201.
11. ICRP. ICRP publication 147: use of dose quantities in radiological protection. Ann ICRP. 2021;50(1):9–82.
12. ICRP. ICRP publication 73: radiological protection and safety in medicine. Ann ICRP. 1996;26(2):1–47.
13. Shrimpton PC, Hillier MC, Lewis MA, Dunn M. National survey of doses from CT in the UK: 2003. Br J Radiol. 2006;79(948):968–80.
14. Lahham A, ALMasri H. Estimation of radiation doses from abdominal computed tomography scans. Radiat Prot Dosim. 2018;182(2):235–40.
15. Matsunaga Y, Kawaguchi A, Kobayashi K, Kobayashi M, Asada Y, Minami K, et al. Effective radiation doses of CT examinations in Japan: a nationwide questionnaire-based study. Br J Radiol. 2016;89(1058):20150671.
16. Jens S, Koelemay MJ, Reekers JA, Bipat S. Diagnostic performance of computed tomography angiography and contrast-enhanced magnetic resonance angiography in patients with critical limb ischaemia and intermittent claudication: systematic review and meta-analysis. Eur Radiol. 2013;23(11):3104–14.
17. National Research Council. Health risks from exposure to low levels of ionizing radiation: BEIR VII—phase 2. Washington, DC: The National Academics Press; 2006.
18. Committee Opinion No. 723 summary: guidelines for diagnostic imaging during pregnancy and lactation. Obstet Gynecol. 2017;130(4):933–4.
19. Marsh RM, Silosky M. Patient shielding in diagnostic imaging: discontinuing a legacy practice. AJR Am J Roentgenol. 2019;212(4):755–7.
20. Dauer LT, Miller DL, Schueler B, Silberzweig J, Balter S, Bartal G, et al. Occupational radiation protection of pregnant or potentially pregnant workers in IR: a joint guideline of the Society of Interventional

Radiology and the Cardiovascular and Interventional Radiological Society of Europe. J Vasc Interv Radiol. 2015;26(2):171–81.

21. Dauer LT, Thornton RH, Miller DL, Damilakis J, Dixon RG, Marx MV, et al. Radiation management for interventions using fluoroscopic or computed tomographic guidance during pregnancy: a joint guideline of the Society of Interventional Radiology and the Cardiovascular and Interventional Radiological Society of Europe with Endorsement by the Canadian Interventional Radiology Association. J Vasc Interv Radiol. 2012;23(1):19–32.

5 Pharmaceutical Aspects: Pre-, Peri-, and Post-procedural

Aldo Victor Giordano, Sergio Carducci, and Marco Varrassi

5.1 Introduction

Over the years Interventional Radiology (IR) has developed many effective and less invasive procedures that continue to reshape the clinical management of patients in the obstetric-gynecological field.

As the number and types of interventions increase, interventional radiologists are increasingly involved in patient care. Their work includes the pre-intervention evaluation of the patient, the definition and modulation of an often sophisticated medical therapy, clinical/instrumental monitoring during interventions, regular visits during hospitalization, and complete follow-up management. Therefore, interventional radiologists are faced with a broad spectrum of both clinical and pharmacological issues.

Adjunctive medical therapy is expected to increase patient comfort, improve success rates, and further reduce the risks of the procedures. In order to fulfill our responsibility to patients, a thorough knowledge of certain drugs is essential.

In general, in the pre-, peri-, and post-procedural phases, the interventional radiologist must manage, from a pharmacological point of view, thrombotic/hemorrhagic problems, anxiety and pain, as well as possible procedural side effects (e.g., infections, nausea, vomiting, and arterial hypertension).

5.2 Peri-procedural Antithrombotic Management in Gynecological and Obstetric IR

Peri-procedural antithrombotic management for patients undergoing an interventional procedure is complex. The challenge derives from a continuous expansion of the procedures offered in terms of number and type as well as a simultaneous increase in the complexity of patients being treated with antithrombotic drugs, which are also increasingly numerous in terms of type and number.

A. V. Giordano (✉) · S. Carducci · M. Varrassi
Department of Interventional Radiology, San Salvatore Hospital, L'Aquila, Italy

R. Niola et al. (eds.), *Diagnostic and Interventional Radiology in Gynecological and Obstetric Diseases*, https://doi.org/10.1007/978-3-031-11910-1_5

There is a paucity of scientific evidence on peri-procedural management in IR for patients on antithrombotic drug therapy. Two opposing risks decide the peri-procedural management of patients receiving antithrombotic therapy: the risk of bleeding related to the procedure versus the risk of thromboembolic events resulting from the discontinuation of antithrombotic drugs. These risks vary according to various patient factors (e.g., age, comorbidities), the type of anticoagulation (rapid vs. slow offset and onset), the type of procedure (low or high bleeding risk), and the circumstances in which it occurs (election or emergency). Therefore, it is important, where possible, to discuss the perioperative anticoagulation plan with the patient and competent clinical teams (e.g., experts in hemostasis and thrombosis for patients with previous venous thromboembolism, or experts in cardiology or cardiothoracic surgery for patients with heart valves).

The risk of bleeding has been stratified by various publications in many ways often interchangeably, including: “no clinically important risk,” “low risk,” “moderate risk,” “intermediate risk,” and “high risk.” This was derived on the basis of post-procedure bleeding rates in predominantly non-randomized and uncontrolled studies and retrospective reports from databases.

Currently procedures with 2–4% major/clinically significant bleeding risk are considered moderate to high risk, while procedures with <2% major/clinically significant bleeding rates are considered low-risk procedures [1–4].

From a practical point of view, it is advisable to distinguish the procedures performed in urgency from those in election since the first, due to management complexity, require an additional figure, not involved in the execution of the procedure and an expert in the management of hemodynamically unstable patients.

The **IR emergency procedures** in the obstetric-gynecological field are essentially represented by uterine bleeding and in particular as a frequency by post-partum hemorrhages.

In these cases, the management of antithrombotic therapy may be particularly complex (with the use of antidotes, transfusions of blood, plasma, platelet jelly, fibrinogen, etc.) and associated with support measures for the circulation with careful monitoring of the patient’s vital parameters and should therefore be reserved to the anesthetist who must always be present in the room for these procedures.

Most of the **IR elective procedures** in the obstetric-gynecological setting are characterized by a low risk of bleeding (Table 5.1).

Vascular interventions in fact require an arterial or venous approach with introducers of caliber less than 7 F, in easily monitored and compressible access sites (common femoral artery/vein, radial artery/vein).

Low bleeding risk procedures involving venous access are performed safely with INR in the range of 2.0–3.0. For low bleeding risk procedures requiring arterial access, the recommended INR thresholds are <1.8 for femoral access and <2.2 for radial access. The platelet count must be >20,000/mm^3.

Table 5.1 Bleeding risk of the main obstetric-gynecological procedures

Low risk		High risk
Vascular	Extra-vascular	Extra-vascular
Uterine fibroid/adenomyosis embolization	MRgFUS uterine fibroids/adenomyosis	Drainage of tubo-ovarian abscess (percutaneous/transvaginals)
Congestion pelvic syndrome embolization	Fallopian tube recanalization	Biopsy (percutaneous/transvaginals)

Table 5.2 Guidance on when to stop and restart anticoagulation for procedures with low risk of bleeding

Procedures with low risk of bleeding			
	Discontinue	Hold duration prior to procedure	Restart time (h)[a]
Heparins			
Unfractionated heparin	Yes	4 h	6
LMWH (prophylactic)	Possible to continue	12 h	6
LMWH (therapeutic)	Yes	24 h	6–12
Vitamin K antagonists	Either continue and check INR 1 week before with VKA dose adjustment to ensure it is in range or hold prior to procedure at discretion of the physician undertaking the procedure. If warfarin is continued then check INR day of procedure to ensure it is within range and if warfarin is discontinued then check INR day of procedure to check it is <2		
Warfarin		3–5 days	12–24
Phenprocoumon		15–20 days	
Acenocoumarol		2–3 days	
Thrombin inhibitors			
Dabigatran	Either continue or omit the dose prior to procedure at discretion of physician undertaking procedure	1–2 days	6
Factor Xa inhibitors			
Apixaban	Either continue or omit the dose prior to procedure at discretion of physician undertaking procedure	1–2 days	6
Rivaroxaban		2 days (CrCl<50)	6
		2–4 days (CrCl<50)	
Edoxaban		1–2 days	6
Fondaparinux	Possible to continue	36 h	6–12
Fondaparinux (therapeutic)	Yes	48 h	6–12

[a]Restart time assumes post-procedure hemostasis has been achieved at the discretion of the physician undertaking the procedure

For extravascular procedures with a high risk of bleeding the desirable INR values are <1.8–1.5. The platelet count should be >50,000/mm^3 [5].

5.2.1 Anticoagulation Management Strategies for Elective Procedures

Current CIRSE Standards of Practice [6] on the management of perioperative anticoagulation during elective IR procedures include:

- For patients on anticoagulant treatment, without increased risk of thrombotic events/complications, who must undergo an elective low-risk bleeding IR procedure, consideration should be given to continuing anticoagulation or following the advice given in Table 5.2 regarding the suspension and restoration of anticoagulation.
- In patients treated with anticoagulants, with an increased risk of thromboembolic events/complications, who need to undergo an elective IR procedure with a low risk of bleeding, consider continuing anticoagulation therapy. However, the choice will depend on the specific procedure and on possible additional bleeding risk factors related to the patient's pathology.
- For patients on anticoagulants with increased risk of thromboembolic events/complications undergoing elective IR procedure with moderate/high bleeding risk, discontinuation of anticoagulation and bridging therapy (if applicable) should be considered (Table 5.3).

Table 5.3 Guidance on when to stop and restart anticoagulation for procedures with high risk of bleeding

Procedures with high risk of bleeding	Discontinue	Hold duration prior to procedure	Restart time (h)[a]
Heparins			
Unfractionated heparin	Yes	4 h	24
LMWH (prophylactic)	Yes	6–12 h	6–12
LMWH (therapeutic)	Yes	24 h	24–72
Vitamin K antagonists			
Warfarin	Discontinue VKA prior to procedure and on day of procedure check INR <1.5 prior to commencing procedure	3–5 days	12–24
Phenprocoumon		15–20 days	
Acenocoumarol		3 days	
Thrombin inhibitors			
Dabigatran	Yes	2–3 days (CrCl >50)	48–72
		3–5 days (CrCl <50)	
Factor Xa inhibitors			
Apixaban	Yes	1–2 days (CrCl >50)	48–72
Rivaroxaban	Yes	3–5 days (CrCl <50)	48–72
Edoxaban	Yes	3–4 days	48–72
Fondaparinux	Yes	36 h	6–12
Fondaparinux (therapeutic)	Yes	48 h	6–12

SC subcutaneous, *IV* intravenous, *CrCl* creatinine clearance, *LMWH* low molecular weight heparin

[a]Restart time assumes post-procedure hemostasis has been achieved at the discretion of the physician undertaking the procedure

5.2.2 Antiplatelet Management Strategies for Elective Procedures

- In procedures with low bleeding risk, it is not necessary to stop the antiplatelet therapy (single or double).
- In procedures with a high risk of bleeding, the current therapy with ASA can be continued (its suspension can be considered if the intake is for primary prevention). *Thienopyridine* therapy should be stopped 5 to 7 days before the procedure. However, it is necessary to verify the reasons for the prescribed therapy with particular attention, in the medical history, to the placement of coronary stents or intracranial stents.

The correct peri-procedural management of antithrombotic therapy will also be shared with other specialists possibly involved in the procedure. For example, the choice of the type of anesthesia may require different management of antithrombotic therapy. Specifically, during embolization of the uterine arteries double antiplatelet therapy is not a contraindication (low bleeding risk), but if it was decided to use epidural anesthesia, this approach is incompatible with the DAPT in the anesthetic guidelines.

5.3 Peri-procedural Sedation and Analgesia Management in Gynecological and Obstetric IR

The management of acute pain and anxiety associated with medical procedures remains one of the main health challenges, especially in the obstetric-gynecological field. Although minimally invasive diagnostic and therapeutic procedures are performed in IR, these procedures remain a potential source of anxiety and pain for patients.

Although anesthetists are better trained, they are not available to participate in all the IR procedures. Interventional radiologists therefore need to have a solid understanding of the basic principles and safety of anesthetic drugs as sedation can carry significant risks to the patient.

Sedation is the induction of a state of relaxation and calm by means of a drug. Sedation decreases perception and responsiveness to external stimuli, as well as reduces the patient's anxiety and irritability. Although sedation is a continuum, there are commonly four levels of sedation/analgesia, ranging from level 1 (minimal sedation or anxiolysis), in which there is a normal response to verbal stimulation with ventilation and cardiovascular function unaffected, up to level 4, in which the patient cannot be awakened even with painful stimuli and ventilation and cardiovascular function may be compromised.

Analgesia is defined as generalized pain relief without the intentional production of an altered mental state as in sedation. Pain signals are received, but drugs prevent/reduce the perception of pain. Sedation and analgesia are distinct processes: Some patients require mainly sedation, such as uncooperative patients, some mainly analgesia, and some both.

Sedation and analgesia protocols are highly variable between institutions and teams.

In IR moderate sedation/analgesia is often considered the ideal compromise by preserving patient cooperation, comfort, and procedural work, reducing drug levels and procedure duration compared to general anesthesia [7]. At this level of sedation, there is a depression of consciousness during which control of the patients' unwanted movements is obtained, who intentionally respond to verbal commands alone or accompanied by a light tactile stimulation. The perception of pain is also variously attenuated. Patent airways and spontaneous ventilation are maintained as well as cardiovascular function.

However, appropriate equipment and medications needed for cardiopulmonary resuscitation and airway support must be available in the area where sedation is performed.

Anesthesia is the pharmacological blocking of pain signal reception by the nervous system. Anesthesia can be general, regional, or local.

The European Society of Interventional and Cardiovascular Radiology (CIRSE) developed, in 2019, a document establishing the best therapeutic strategies to be followed for the safe administration of drugs for sedation and analgesia during IR procedures [8].

A general recommendation is that the operator administering the sedation should not be engaged in any other activity (e.g., performing the IR procedure). Properly trained staff and accredited teams should be able to safely deliver mild (anxiolytics) to moderate sedation/analgesia only. Deeper than moderate sedation levels or sedation in patients with ASA classification >2 (patient with severe systemic disease, whether life-threatening or not) should be performed by dedicated anesthetists, as functions and vital signs are likely (cardiovascular and/or respiratory) depressed and need support.

As a general principle, the choice of applying or not applying conscious or deep sedation, a loco-regional, sectorial, or general anesthesia depends on several factors which are: type and duration of the procedure, state of patient health evaluated with the ASA classification, and patient's anxiety state.

5.3.1 General Anesthesia

General anesthetics *Propofol* and *Ketamine* should be administered by an anesthetist. These two drugs do not guarantee the patient's immobility, so they must be combined with drugs such as curare, which in addition to assisted ventilation also require the monitoring of cardiovascular and respiratory parameters.

The selective μ-opioid agonist, *Propofol*, with rapid onset and very short duration is used in continuous infusion with a dosage of 3–12 mg/kg/h; as it can depress breathing and lead to loss of airway reflex, a respiratory and suction assist system must be available.

Ketamine gives dissociative general anesthesia, can be used iv or im, and must always be administered together with a *benzodiazepine* and *Atropine*: the im posology is 3–6 mg/kg, and the iv dose is 1 mg/kg, injected very slowly. *Ketamine* has a rapid onset and moderate duration of action.

5.3.2 Epidural Anesthesia

Epidural anesthesia involves the injection of drugs into the "epidural space." Because the drug has to cross the membrane (dura) that surrounds the spinal cord before reaching the targeted nerves, it usually takes about 10–15 min for pain relief to occur. The placement of a catheter during the insertion makes possible the continuous infusion of anesthetic drugs and, if necessary, painkillers for the whole duration of the procedure and especially in the following hours.

5.3.3 Spinal Anesthesia

Spinal anesthesia involves the injection of drugs into the fluid (cerebrospinal fluid or cerebrospinal fluid) that bathes the spinal cord. Spinal needles are much thinner than epidural needles and spinal doses are lower than epidural doses. However, the duration of pain relief is limited (approximately 1–2 h) because there is no catheter and therefore no continuous infusion.

5.3.4 Local Surface Anesthesia

Local anesthesia is the most used type in IR. Local anesthetics stabilize nerve membranes through a reversible link with sodium channels. Local anesthetics, injected into the subcutaneous skin, are divided into amides and esters; amides are more commonly used because they are, in general, more potent and have a longer duration of action. These include *Lidocaine*, *Mepivacaine*, *Bupivacaine*, and *Ropivacaine*.

In general, in gynecological/obstetric IR, "major" endovascular procedures, such as embolizations, require spinal or better epidural anesthesia, with subsequent pharmacological pain control in the immediate post-procedural phase by means of patient-controlled analgesia (PCA). "Minor" endovascular procedures, such as the treatment of Pelvic Congestion Syndrome, are performed under local anesthesia, possibly associated with mild sedation using Benzodiazepines. Immediately following the procedure the patient may experience mild to moderate discomfort for a few days and this typically responds quickly to common non-steroidal anti-inflammatory drugs. PCA is not normally required. Extravascular procedures (biopsies, drainages) are also conducted after local anesthesia of the access site with a possible association, depending on the case, with mild sedation. In these procedures, analgesic therapy is not normally necessary in the post-procedural continuation.

In adults, sedation and analgesia can be combined using a combination of different drugs.

5.3.4.1 Hypnotic Sedatives

Benzodiazepines: These are the most common type of sedatives used. They facilitate the actions of g-aminobutyric acid, the main inhibitory neurotransmitter of the central nervous system. They possess anxiolytic and amnesic properties. Most sedatives can be administered via a variety of routes, but the intravenous route is the most commonly used, before and during the procedure.

Among the BDZs, *Midazolam* is the most used. It has a fast onset time, a relatively short elimination half-life, and its antagonization is possible. It starts from 30 to 60 s and the maximum effect is reached after 13 min. The effects may be prolonged in elderly patients. Having no analgesic properties, it is typically combined with opioids for a synergistic action.

The initial dosage for sedation is: under the age of 60 a bolus of 2–2.5 mg iv; over the age of 60 or debilitated patients 0.5–1 mg iv.

Midazolam can be antagonized by *Flumazenil* at a dose of 0.2–0.5 mg in 15 s iv.

Dexmedetomidine: recently introduced alpha 2 adrenergic hypnotic sedative.

Its indication is for the sedation of adult patients not intubated before and/or during diagnostic or surgical procedures that require conscious procedural sedation.

Patients should be continuously monitored for early signs of hypotension, hypertension, bradycardia, respiratory depression, airway obstruction, apnea, dyspnea, and/or oxygen desaturation. The management of this drug by an anesthetist is therefore recommended.

5.3.4.2 Opioid Analgesics

Opioids are drugs that act on opioid receptors in the peripheral and central nervous system. They are powerful analgesics and are used to treat pain associated with injuries, surgery, and painful clinical conditions. They also have sedative, antitussive, and antirigor properties. Opioids are associated with unwanted side effects such as nausea, constipation, and depression of the central nervous and respiratory systems. Long-term opioid use can lead to tolerance and addiction. The action of opioids increases when they are administered with benzodiazepines. It is useful to use an iv anti-emetic drug (*Ondanserone*, *Dexamethasone*) in combination with opioids [9].

Opioids do not have a maximum dose and are titrated to effect.

Among the opioids, *Fentanyl* 50 mcg iv repeatable every 30–40 min, *Remifentanil* in continuous infusion with a dosage of 0.01–0.10 mcg/kg/min iv, *Sufentanil* 5 mcg iv repeatable every 40 min (0.1–0.3 mcg/kg), and *Morphine* 0.10–0.15 mg/kg iv as a bolus and with possible continuous infusion at 5–30 μg/kg/h.

The opioid antagonist is *Naloxone* 0.4 mg iv; its half-life is about 90 min.

Among the opiates analgesics *Tramadol* is used in acute and chronic pain, with a dosage of 50–100 mg iv every 4–6 h. The daily dose of 400 mg should not be exceeded. Since it is emetic, it should be combined with *Metoclopamide* 10 mg iv. It must not be combined with *Ondansetron* because they act on the same receptors and reduce their analgesic effect.

Patient-controlled analgesia is an important pain control modality. PCA allows the patient to self-administer small doses of opioid analgesic by controlled intravenous infusion. PCA pumps can be prescribed by both anesthetists and non-anesthetists. The PCA pump is programmable to control the dose delivered, the time between doses (lock-out interval), the total dose limit over a period of time (lock-out interval), and continuous background infusion. With PCA it is possible to relieve pain without the risk of overdose or long waiting times between doses. PCA increases patient satisfaction and reduces the total dose needed to control acute pain. It is most useful in patients with good neurological, lung, and kidney function [9].

5.3.4.3 Non-opioid Analgesics

Non-opioids are not typically used intra-procedurally and are usually reserved for outpatient use. The non-opioids in use are *Acetaminophen* and *NSAIDs*.

Acetaminophen can cause liver toxicity when taken in amounts greater than 4 g per day, but it does not damage the gastrointestinal tract or increase the risk of bleeding [9].

Its use is at a dose of 1000 mg iv in 15 min over 50 kg in weight, repeatable every 8 h.

NSAIDs have side effects that can potentially affect the cardiac, gastrointestinal, and renal systems in addition to interfering with normal platelets.

Among the NSAIDs, *Ketorolac* is used in adults: 10 mg iv up to a maximum of 90 mg/day and over 65 years maximum 60 mg/day iv to avoid reducing diuresis or *Ibuprofen* (400–600 mg per os). NSAIDs must always be combined with a gastro-protector.

5.4 Uterine Artery Embolization for Uterine Fibroids

The procedures for uterine fibroids, performed in IR, deserve a separate discussion because they numerically represent the most performed procedures in the gynecological/obstetric field and because they constitute an exciting challenge for the interventional radiologist in terms of peri-procedural pharmacological management.

Uterine artery embolization (UAE) represents a valid alternative to medical and surgical therapy of fibroids.

Some studies suggested the suspension of the Gn-RH analogs before the procedure, due to the effect that these drugs could have on the uterine vessels, deferring the operation for at least 3 months from the drug suspension; currently, the use of Gn-RH agonists is considered safe and does not compromise the efficacy of endovascular treatment.

It is important to perform pre- and postoperative antiemetic prophylaxis that can be carried out with *Droperidol* 0.5–1 mg iv or *Ondansetron* 8 mg iv plus *Dexamethasone* 4 mg iv or *Metoclopramide* 10 mg iv, repeatable up to 30 mg/day. Patients with known or suspected risk factors for cardiac arrhythmia or patients in whom the existence of a prolongation of the QT interval is suspected must be carefully examined before administration of *Droperidol*.

Necrotic material created during UAE can be contaminated by skin flora inoculated during arterial access or by direct invasion (submucosal lesions) of bacteria from the bladder or vagina, due to endocervical insufficiency. Serious infectious complications have been reported in about 2% of cases according to the data in the literature. However, the use of antibiotic prophylaxis continues to be debated [10].

In 2013, the Royal College of Obstetricians and Gynecologists recognized that a single dose of antibiotic agents targeted on skin flora was reasonable for UAE prophylaxis, extrapolating from data on prophylaxis used during a hysterectomy.

As antibiotic prophylaxis, it is common to administer 1 g of Cefazoline about 1 h before the procedure, but the choice of antibiotic administration is at the operator's discretion and also based on the patient's risk factors.

Embolization of the uterine arteries causes intense intraoperative and postoperative pain. Intraoperative pain usually begins during/after closure of the second uterine artery. It is mainly due to the ischemia of fibroids and the uterus (especially the endometrium and deeper layers of the myometrium). It can be of very strong intensity and alters the positive perception of UAE as a non-invasive procedure.

To counteract this type of pain there are three possibilities that can be associated:

- Use of opioids
- Epidural anesthesia
- Blockade of the superior hypogastric plexus

In many centers epidural anesthesia is the technique of choice.

The placement of the epidural catheter usually takes place at the level of the medullary segments between T10 and L1 associated or not associated with iv sedation.

For epidural anesthesia 15 mL of local anesthetic such as *Mepivacaine* 2% or *Levobupivacaine* 0.5% or *Ropivacaine* 0.5% can be used, in optional combination with opioids such as *Fentanyl* 50–100 mcg or *Sufentanil* 5–10 mcg.

The duration of this anesthesia is 3–4 h.

Postoperative analgesia is performed with an epidural infusion pump set with different protocols that can be modulated according to pain intensity:

1. Continuous infusion of 10 mL *Levobupivacaine* 0.12% or 0.15% + bolus on call of 5 mL with minimum interval (lock out) of 50 min
2. Periodic infusion every 60 min of 15 mL *Levobupivacaine* 0.12% or 0.15% + bolus on call of 5 mL with a minimum interval (lock out) of 60 min
3. Infusion at patient request after at least 50 min of 15 mL *Levobupivacaine* 0.12% or 0.15%

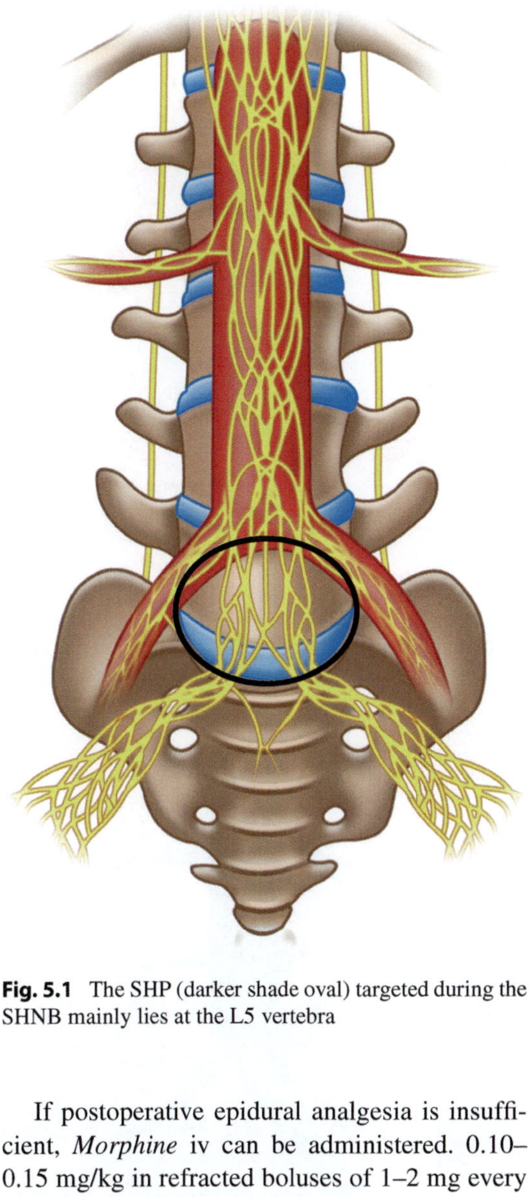

Fig. 5.1 The SHP (darker shade oval) targeted during the SHNB mainly lies at the L5 vertebra

If postoperative epidural analgesia is insufficient, *Morphine* iv can be administered. 0.10–0.15 mg/kg in refracted boluses of 1–2 mg every 10 min until the pain subsides.

A technique widely used for the treatment of intra- and postoperative pain in UAE is *blockage of the superior hypogastric plexus*.

The superior hypogastric plexus (SHP) is the part of the abdominal-pelvic sympathetic nervous system that conducts sympathetic-mediated pain pathways of the pelvic organs.

Topographically SHP is a retroperitoneal and median structure and is usually located anterior to the lower third of L5 and the upper third of S1 (Fig. 5.1) [11, 12]. Since UAE is performed in the fluoroscopy room with the patient supine, an anterior approach, guided by fluoroscopy, appears optimal. This reduces the chances of discitis from a posterior approach; however, the risk of vascular injury and intravascular injection remains.

Vascular structures closely related to the SHP target site at the level of the vertebral body L5 include the aortic bifurcation and the confluence of the inferior vena cava (IVC).

When performing uterine fibroid embolization (UFE) using a femoral approach it is easy to outline the aortic bifurcation after fluoroscopic evaluation of the catheter as it crosses over the aortic bifurcation. Several studies have shown that the aortic bifurcation is located between the vertebral levels L3 and L5 (Fig. 5.2a–c), most of it at the level of the L4 vertebra or the L4–L5 disc (63–80%) [11, 13].

The iliac-caval junction cannot be delineated with an angiogram and its anatomy is more subject to variations than the aorta. The iliac-caval junction is visible between the L4 and L5-S1 disc (Fig. 5.3a,b), particularly on the body of L5 in about 60–70% of cases. In relation to the aortic bifurcation, the iliac-caval junction is in most cases located approximately 19 mm below it [11, 14].

The typical target is the lower part of the L5 vertebral body in an attempt to remain distal to the aortic bifurcation. Under local anesthesia, a 21/22 G gauge Chiba needle is advanced to the anterior portion of the L5 vertebral body under fluoroscopic guidance. Once reached the bone plane, 2–5 mL of slightly diluted contrast medium is injected, with a typical triangular distribution in AP and a half-moon shape distribution in LL, without vascular opacification.

Typically, the onset of sensory block occurs within the first hour with a duration of up to 12 h after injection. After confirmation of a good needle tip position, a preliminary test dose of approximately 3 cc of *Ropivacaine* 0.5% is injected. If there is no change in heart rate or neurological status, the remainder of 17 cc of the total 20 cc (total of 60 mg of *Ropivacaine*) is slowly injected with intermittent aspiration [11].

Although the technical success has been high, technical problems can occur:

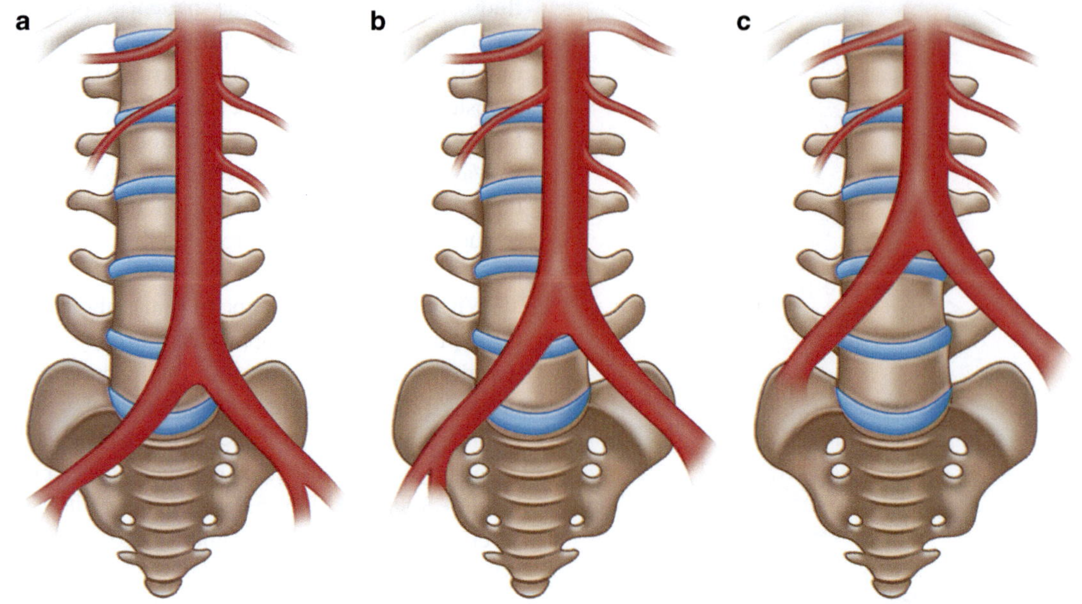

Fig. 5.2 Aortic bifurcation and relevant radiographic anatomy. In majority of cases (63–80%) the bifurcation is at the level of L4 vertebra or L4–5 disc (**b**). (**a** and **c**) represent the less commonly seen high and low bifurcations

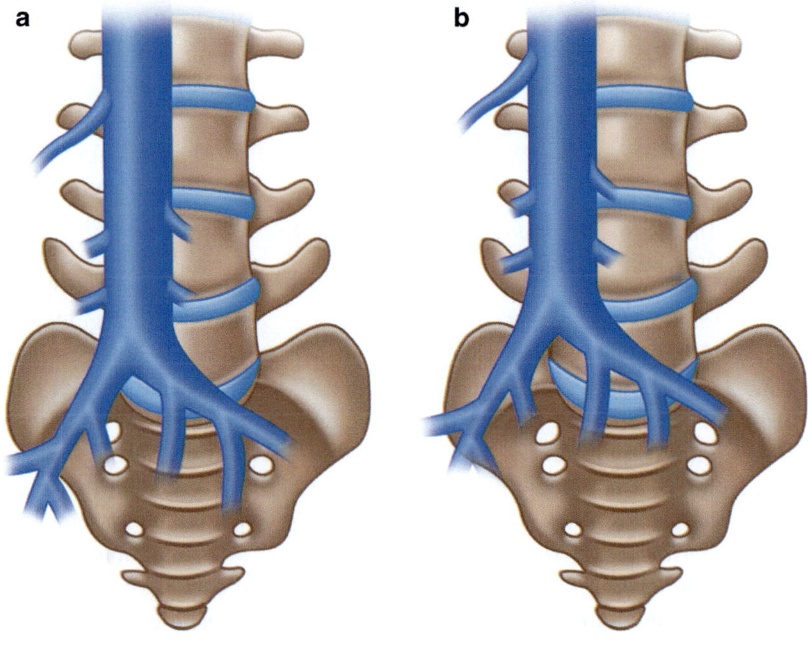

Fig. 5.3 Demonstration of iliocaval confluence and relevant radiographic anatomy. In 60–70% cases the iliocaval junction is seen between L4 and L5–S1 disc (**a**), specifically at the upper third and at right lateral third of the L5 vertebral body (**b**)

- *Crossing of a large uterine fibroid* in the percutaneous needle path toward the L5 vertebra. A 20 G and sometimes 18 G needle is preferred to a 21/22 G for better steerability and penetration, 15–20 cm length is often the best choice.
- *Vascular opacification:* If vascular opacification is observed it is important to reposi-

tion the needle before local anesthetic injection.

- *Systemic toxicity of local anesthetic (LAST)*: LAST can occur in the context of an unintended intravascular injection.

Several prospective or retrospective studies, single or multicenter, underline how the addition of the analgesic block of the superior hypogastric plexus increases pain control compared to conventional treatments. This technique takes less time to reduce pain and its use reduces the use of opioid and anti-emetic drugs.

The intra-arterial injection of diluted *Lidocaine* during the embolization phase, performed in order to reduce the pain, can cause a mild vasospasm of the afferent fibroid vessels with a potential increase in the percentage of incomplete fibroid necrosis cases due to a lower capacity of the particles to penetrate through the vessels within the fibroid.

Frequently, about 2/3 days after the UAE procedure, flu-like symptoms appear, such as increased body temperature, asthenia, and muscle and abdominal cramping pains (post-embolization syndrome). *Methilprednisolon* 40 mg iv before the procedure and *Ketorolac* 30 mg iv 6 h after the procedure can be given to prevent these symptoms.

The drugs used after discharge will be oral drugs. The therapy of choice is usually with *Ibuprofen* 600 mg 2–3 times a day after meals for 4–5 days, combining *Pantoprazole* 40 mg/day.

Acetaminophen up to 1000 mg × 3 or *Acetaminophen* with an opioid (often *Oxycodone* or *Hydrocodone*) can be associated for resistant pains.

The use of emollient laxatives twice a day can reduce the pain during evacuation.

The treatment of uterine fibroids/adenomyosis through the use of *MRI-guided focused ultrasound (MRgFUS)* requires much simpler pharmacological management.

In fact, the absence of treatment invasiveness does not require the use of local/regional anesthesia.

Intra- and postoperative pain management is also less complex as the treatment is aimed exclusively at the target fibroid without causing ischemic shock to the uterus as occurs in UAE.

Although the patient's discomfort is greater than in UAE (prone position, long duration of the procedure within the MR gantry, rectal probe, bladder catheter, etc.), patients undergoing MRgFUS are particularly motivated by the treatment and do not require particular sedation before the exam.

Generally, the following therapeutic scheme is performed:

- 100 mg *Diclofenac* sodium suppository.
- *Midazolam* 2 mg iv once the patient is positioned on the FUS table.
- *Pethidine* 50 mg and *Maxolon* 20 mg are administered just prior to performing sonications.

Administration of antibiotics remains at the discretion of the interventional radiologist.

Bibliography

1. Patel IJ, Davidson JC, Nikolic B, Salazar GM, Schwartzberg MS, Walker TG, et al. Consensus guidelines for periprocedural management of coagulation status and hemostasis risk in percutaneous image-guided interventions. J Vasc Interv Radiol. 2012;23:727–36.
2. Patel IJ, Rahim S, Davidson JC, Hanks SE, Tam AL, Gregory Walker T, et al. Society of interventional radiology consensus guidelines for the periprocedural management of thrombotic and bleeding risk in patients undergoing percutaneous image-guided interventions—part II: recommendations. J Vasc Interv Radiol. 2019;30(8):1168–1184.e1.
3. Spyropoulos AC, Douketis JD. How I treat anticoagulated patients undergoing an elective procedure or surgery. Blood. 2012;120(15):2954–62.
4. Atwell TD, Wennberg PW, McMenomy BP, Murthy NS, Anderson JR, Kriegshauser JS, et al. Periprocedural use of anticoagulants in radiology: an evidence-based review. Abdom Radiol (NY). 2017;42:1556–65.
5. Patel IJ, Rahim S, Davidson JC, Hanks SE, Tam AL, Walker TG, Wilkins LR, Sarode R, Weinberg

I. Society of interventional radiology consensus guidelines for the periprocedural management of thrombotic and bleeding risk in patients undergoing percutaneous image-guided interventions—part II: recommendations: endorsed by the Canadian Association for Interventional Radiology and the Cardiovascular and Interventional Radiological Society of Europe. J Vasc Interv Radiol. 2019;30(8):1168–1184.e1.
6. Hadi M, Walker C, Desborough M, Basile A, Tsetis D, Hunt B, Müller-Hüllsbeck S, Rand T, van Delden O, Uberoi R. CIRSE standards of practice on peri-operative anticoagulation management during interventional radiology procedures. Cardiovasc Intervent Radiol. 2021;44(4):523–36.
7. Cornelis FH, Monarda E, Moulina M-A, Vignauda E, Laveissierea F, Ben Ammara M, Nouri-Neuvillea M, Barral M, Lombart B. Sedation and analgesia in interventional radiology: where do we stand, where are we heading and why does it matter? Diagn Interv Imaging. 2019;100(12):753–62.
8. Romagnoli S, Fanelli F, Barbani F, Uberoi R, Esteban E, Lee MJ, Nielsen PT, Mahnken AH, Morgan R. CIRSE standards of practice on analgesia and sedation for interventional radiology in adults. Cardiovasc Intervent Radiol. 2020;43:1251–60.
9. Moran TC, Kaye AD, Mai AH, Bok LR. Sedation, analgesia, and local anesthesia: a review for general and interventional radiologists. Radiographics. 2013;33(2):E47–60.
10. Venkatesan AM, Kundu S, Sacks D, Wallace MJ, Wojak JC, Rose SC, Clark TWI, d'Othee BJ, Itkin M, Jones RS, Miller DL, Owens CA, Rajan DK, Stokes LAS, Swan TL, Towbin RB, Cardella JF. Practice guideline for adult antibiotic prophylaxis during vascular and interventional radiology procedures. J Vasc Interv Radiol. 2010;21:1611–30.
11. Pereira K, Morel-Ovalle LM, Taghipour M, Sherwani A, Parikh R, Kao J, Vaheesan K. Superior hypogastric nerve block (SHNB) for pain control after uterine fibroid embolization (UFE): technique and troubleshooting. CVIR Endovasc. 2020;3(1):50.
12. Benzon H, Rathmell JP, Wu CL, et al. Practical management of pain. Philadelphia: Elsevier Mosby; 2014.
13. Chithriki M, Jaibaji M, Steele RD. The anatomical relationship of the aortic bifurcation to the lumbar vertebrae: a MRI study. Surg Radiol Anat. 2002;24(5):308–12.
14. Appaji A, Kulkarni R, Balaji Pai S. Level of bifurcation of aorta and iliocaval confluence and its clinical relevance. IOSR J Dent Med Sci. 2014;13(7):2279–861.

Ethics and Safety

6

Antonio Pinto, Raffaella Capasso, Franco Guida, Claudia Rossi, Sabrina Segreto, and Daniela Vecchione

6.1 Introduction

Since its genesis in the 1960s when the first cases of transluminal angioplasty were reported [1], interventional radiology has developed considerably, with a growing number and variety of image-guided percutaneous procedures.

A wide range of imaging equipment is available for providing high-quality interventional radiology services, ranging from non-invasive imaging such as ultrasound, magnetic resonance, and computed tomography to dedicated digital angiographic suites equipped with flat panel detector technology for high-quality fluoroscopy with cone beam CT for 3D guidance. The requirements will vary with the needs of the unit and the type of intervention being carried out [2, 3].

Examples of treatments administered by interventional radiologists include angioplasty, biopsies, stenting, thrombolysis, embolization, and radiofrequency ablation [4–8].

Most of the interventional procedures are performed percutaneously with little associated patient discomfort and with conscious sedation instead of general anesthesia [9].

Through the improvement of new procedures and enhancement of standard techniques, the interventional radiologist can now offer many services to the obstetrician-gynecologist [10–15].

Interventional radiologists could receive consults for procedures that seem to have little to no chance of achieving meaningful benefit: understanding whether a request is potentially inappropriate or futile relies heavily on understanding the goals of care, the communicated goals between patient/surrogatedecision maker and treating physicians [16].

Unnecessary radiation, suffering, hazardous interventions, and any potential risk ofsevere consequence should all be avoided. Procedures with unjustified risks that are non-scientifically sound should be avoided [17–19].

Moreover, in interventional radiology, as in all medical disciplines, the need for improvements in patient safety is progressively being recognized [20–28]. Patient safety is the absence of preventable harm to a patient during the process of health care and reduction of risk of unnecessary harm associated with health care to an acceptable minimum [21].

6.2 Interventional Radiology and Ethical Issues

Performing an interventional procedure imposes a commitment on interventional radiologists to conduct the initial patient assessment, determine

A. Pinto (✉) · R. Capasso · F. Guida · C. Rossi
S. Segreto · D. Vecchione
Department of Support Health Services, Unit of Radiology, CTO Hospital, Azienda Ospedaliera dei Colli, Naples, Italy

R. Niola et al. (eds.), *Diagnostic and Interventional Radiology in Gynecological and Obstetric Diseases*, https://doi.org/10.1007/978-3-031-11910-1_6

the best course of therapy, and provide long-term care after the procedure is completed.

A key strength of interventional radiology is the dynamic equipoise interventional radiologists can strike, shifting the degree to which they are clinicians, radiologists, or surgeons from patient to patient. Very few, if any, specialties receive formal clinical, surgical, and radiologic training to the degree proposed by new interventional radiology residencies [29].

As interventional radiologists have adopted a more "clinical identity," they have assumed more responsibility in patient management. With this evolving role, interventional radiologists have an even greater obligation to understand the ethical challenges specific to their specialty.

The intersection of ethics and medicine becomes more apparent during a global pandemic when resources are limited and risks run high. Health-care leaders in all fields of medicine are faced with ethical dilemmas that they have never encountered before. They must decide whom to risk on the front lines, which patients are more emergent, and where to allocate resources [30].

Specifically, four ethical issues involving interventional radiology have emerged during the recent 2019 novel coronavirus disease (COVID-19) pandemic: duty to treat, futility, distributive justice, and tribalism [30].

6.3 The Interventional Radiology Suite

Interventional radiology is a medical specialty offering diagnostic and therapeutic minimally invasive procedures. In the oncologic field, the so-called interventional oncology allows to manage some issues related to cancer. The concept unifying all the interventional radiology procedures is the imaging guidance which means that an adequate environment is mandatory, that can be located outside operative rooms [31].

The COVID-19 pandemic has had a devastating impact on the economies and health-care systems across the world. It has highlighted the unpreparedness of virtually every health-care system in the world. Strict adherence to hand hygiene practices, proper use of appropriate personal protective equipment, and implementation of team segregation and social distancing emerged as the most relevant measures in preventing intra-hospital transmission and cross-infection of patients and operators. Other strategies to minimize cross-transmission include segregating patients of different infection risks, identifying and isolating COVID-19 patients early and minimizing their movements, and when necessary, performing procedures for COVID-19 patients at the bedside [32].

Interventional radiology services are delivered by a team consisting of different health-care professionals with different, but equally important roles. Ideally, these teams should include professional interventional radiologists, interventional radiology trainees, radiographers, nurse practitioners/physician assistants, nursing staff, and anesthetists. Clerical/cleaning staff and porters also play an important role. The scope of responsibility of each team member will vary depending on common practice within their institutions and/or the legal requirements of their country of practice [3].

Perhaps one of the most critical, yet often overlooked, aspects of performing interventional radiology procedures is organization: while each interventional radiologist will have his or her own preferred organization techniques, there are several important factors to consider when a specific strategy should be decided.

Modern interventional radiology suites should have one or two rooms built to operating room standards which include laminar air flow, mandatory air exchanges, a positive in-suite pressure with respect to the surrounding rooms and corridors, and appropriate flooring. Staffing is guided by patient safety and resource efficiencies. The anesthesiologist is available for procedures requiring general anesthesia or moderate-deep sedation in selected cases (transjugular intrahepatic portosystemic shunt, intracranial vascular procedures, hemorrhagic urgencies, and pediatric patients) [33, 34].

Guidelines stated that each procedure required three personnel in addition to the physician: one to be scrubbed into the procedure along with the physician, one to circulate, and one to monitor the patient. In certain situations, four nonphysician health-care practitioners may be needed per case [26].

A wedge is needed for pregnant patients. In emergencies, control of postpartum hemorrhage frequently involves the transfer of the post-natal woman to the interventional radiology suite for the insertion of catheters. In the elective situation, the site of the cesarean section after the procedure remains a topic of debate. If catheters are placed in the obstetric theatre, then an interventional radiology–compatible table is necessary, but the radiological imaging quality through a C-arm is inferior. If catheters are placed electively in the radiology suite with subsequent transfer of the woman to obstetric theatre for the cesarean section, then there is a risk of sheath and catheter displacement during transport [33].

Moreover, in the case of pregnant patients, it is of paramount importance to strictly follow the SIR and CIRSE guidelines for the use of radiation during pregnancy [35]. Several measures should be applied to achieve an appropriate balance between image quality and radiation dose to the fetus. These measures include low-dose rate pulsed fluoroscopy with the lowest pulse rate allowed by the equipment, no angiography exposure, use of the "last image hold" to record the study and plan techniques, no enlargement of the field of view, use of a half-dose filter, posteroanterior beam projection, x-ray tube at maximal distance from the patient, and tube current as low as possible by keeping the tube potential as high as possible. Finally, the fluoroscopy beam-on time is one of the primary factors that interventional radiologists have to control in order to reduce both patient and staff doses [36].

Another crucial topic related to patient safety is represented by hand hygiene and sterile technique [37]. The prominence of hand hygiene for reducing infection rates in health-care environments was first described by Semmelweis and Holmes in the mid-nineteenth century [38]. Since interventional radiologists perform so many procedures as part of daily practice, it is crucial to appreciate the current guidelines for both hand hygiene and sterile technique for procedures, especially central venous catheter placement. Hand hygiene, as defined by the 2002 Centers for Disease Control and Prevention Guideline for Hand Hygiene in Health-Care Settings [39], requires decontamination of hands by using either an alcohol-based hand rub (recommended as a first-line method) or hand washing with antimicrobial soap (preferred) or plain soap (acceptable) and water.

A good aseptic technique represents a serious step in reducing procedure-related infections. Skin sites can be disinfected by using 2% chlorhexidine-based agents (preferred), tincture of iodine, or 70% alcohol and should be allowed to dry completely before starting the procedure. For most procedures, it is also appropriate to use either clean or sterile gloves or a sterile drape.

For the placement or guidewire exchange of central venous catheters, the Centers for Disease Control and Prevention guidelines require the use of maximal sterile barrier precautions, which mandate an aseptic technique and the use of a cap, mask, sterile gown, sterile gloves, and sterile drape [40].

During the outbreak of COVID-19, there was the need for a correct selection of interventional radiology procedures, and a well-organized preparation of staff and interventional suite before the arrival of patients: execution of interventional radiology procedures in situations with suspected airborne infections needs particular precautions to reduce the risk of transmission to the health-care workers. As far as possible, procedures on patients with suspected or confirmed COVID-19 infection should be performed at a specially designed isolation facility [41].

6.4 Adverse Events and Errors in Interventional Radiology

Adverse events that occur during vascular and interventional radiology procedures are frequently related to poor pre-procedural planning and ineffective communication between health-care team members and operator or patient and operator [42]. An adverse event results in unintended harm to the patient by an act of commission or omission, rather than by the underlying disease or condition of the patient [43].

It has been estimated that 50% of all in-hospital adverse events are related to surgery and at least 50% of these could be avoided because they are caused by errors [44]. Error is defined as “the failure of a planned action to be completed as intended (i.e. error of execution) or the use of a wrong plan to achieve an aim (i.e. error of planning)” [25]. Errors are inevitable. We live in a universe that, at its most fundamental level, is governed by the laws of probability. As a result, eliminating errors is an unattainable goal. A realistic goal is to reduce the burden caused by errors [45].

Literature indicates that the majority of errors in interventional radiology are preventable [46]. Interventional radiology procedures place the team in circumstances comparable to those experienced in operating theatres (persistent stress, operator tiredness, and team inexperience) that can lead to mistakes: This explains the need to enhance patient safety measures through larger standardization of procedures and enlarged quality of care in interventional radiology procedures. Moreover, in addition to the most commonly recognized errors in medicine, some errors are specific to interventional radiology and can potentially occur at any time during the patient’s stay in the angiographic suite [47]. The American College of Radiology’s Task Force on Patient Safety recommends a list of preventable patient errors [48].

Factors leading to error rarely occur in isolation and reflect a combination of events, including judgment errors, vigilance/memory failure, lack of technical competence, and communication breakdown [49].

When errors occur, we must answer ethically what we owe patients and families, ourselves, and our colleagues. To some degree, the answers are similar: reflection, confession, and resolution. Truth-telling and trustworthiness have long been virtues of the medical profession. Patients trust that health-care professionals have their best interests in mind, and it is that trust that allows health-care providers to manipulate patients’ bodies in ways that would be considered assault and battery in any other context. Complications can weaken that trust, not only in that episode of care but in health care in general. This is why we owe it to our patients, selves, and colleagues to rebuild that trust by re-conveying truthfulness and trustworthiness [50].

6.5 Safety Checklist in Interventional Radiology

The increasing demand for interventional radiology services in a wide range of clinical scenarios has stretched the capabilities of many hospitals to provide high-quality, sustainable service, particularly on a 24/7 basis. Inequality of access to interventional radiology services has a detrimental effect on patient safety and care by denying access to life-saving minimally invasive treatments. It is imperative that sufficient interventional radiology posts are established and interventional radiologists trained to ensure equity of access [3].

Checklists are an important tool for achieving standardization. Checklists safeguard consistency and team communication, thereby overcoming limitations in human memory and attention span. Checklists ensure that procedural steps are performed in the correct order and that the procedure is complete [51]. A safety checklist should be utilized prior to any interventional radiology procedure and formally documented.

Starting in 2009, the World Health Organization developed its own Safety Surgical Checklist to standardize the surgical patient’s pathway and enhance safety. This checklist led to a significant reduction in clinical adverse events and in morbidity and mortality caused by human error on patients during their stay in the operating room [52]. Subsequently, the Cardiovascular and Interventional Radiological Society of Europe published its own safety checklist recommending its use in IR suites [53, 54].

Interventional radiology procedures have many aspects in common with surgery (complexity, fast patient turnover, urgency and emergency procedures, multilevel or diffuse diseases, and teamwork) and consequently carry a risk for potential error. Therefore, implementing the use of safety checklists in the interventional radiology suite could have the same usefulness in increasing patient safety as surgical safety checklists.

Safety checklists provide a verification tool to support the interventional radiologists' team, with the aim of facilitating adhesion to recommended patient safety standards and preventing avoidable adverse events [54].

A safety checklist can be used in different health-care environments because it includes the following three important safety goals: (1) improving accuracy in patient identification; (2) improving communication between health-care coworkers; and (3) eliminating all wrong-site, wrong-patient, and wrong-procedure interventions [53].

6.6 Safety Steps Related to Interventional Radiology Procedures

According to the Royal College of Radiologists, interventional radiology can be subdivided into three distinct disciplines: general and nonvascular interventions, vascular interventions, and interventional neuroradiology. Furthermore, the different types of procedures undertaken by interventional radiology can be considered under four broad headings: percutaneous procedures, arteriovenous interventions, ablation, and embolization, although each subdivision of interventional radiology has its own specific range of procedures [55].

Interventional radiologists should be encouraged to change their practice model to incorporate the clinical care of patients before, during, and after a procedure. There must be an improved emphasis on patient care, management of patients, setting up of clinic and office facilities, increasing the visibility and recognition of interventional radiologists, and working to establish interventional radiology as a well-defined independent clinical specialty providing complementary value to diagnostic radiology. Clinical practice must include reviewing patients in the outpatient clinical setting to determine suitability for a procedure; discussing benefits, risks, alternatives, and potential contraindications; taking informed consent; rounding on hospital inpatients; and being willing to manage procedure-related complications, which are all important parts of a successful interventional radiology practice [56].

After the patient's admission to the interventional radiology department, an interventional radiologist usually checks the blood tests ordered for the requested procedure and verifies that the patient has received all information regarding the interventional procedure. Coagulation parameters and pharmacological therapy should be clearly investigated before the procedure; the coagulation status of patients undergoing image-guided interventions should be assessed whenever the procedure involves direct entry into the arterial or venous system as an anticipated part of the procedure or whenever there is a possibility of inadvertent entry into the arterial or venous system with significant-sized interventional devices or tools [57].

Before the patient enters the interventional radiology suite (preprocedural period), it is mandatory to check the following items:

- Correct identification of patient's name and surname
- Patient's knowledge of the type and side of the procedure, crosschecking with the information in the patient list and informed consent form
- Informed consent form up to date and correctly filled
- Availability of peripheral venous access
- Knowledge of the risk of contrast-induced nephropathy and possible allergies
- The patient has discontinued anticoagulant/antiplatelet therapy (when required) [53].

The operating room model of anesthesia care is extended to procedures in the interventional radiology suite. The model of care includes:

- Adequate preprocedural assessment to determine the patient's need for anesthesia
- Care during the procedure
- Standardized monitoring and anesthesia equipment
- Clearly marked and easily accessible emergency equipment (code cart, defibrillator)
- Adequate backup in case of emergencies or difficulties
- Postoperative care in a postanesthesia care unit setting [58].

The practice of interventional radiology encompasses a wide range of procedures on many different organ systems. Approximately 70% of the procedures performed are booked less than 48 h in advance because of the relatively urgent or emergent nature of the bulk of interventional radiology procedures. Even though most of these procedures are done with a nurse providing moderate sedation and analgesia, there is a continual discussion between the anesthesia and interventional radiology staff about how best to provide for patient comfort and safety. An accurate and complete preprocedural assessment is key to having a patient comfortably tolerate a procedure (i.e., hold still, breathe, and experience no pain) [58].

When the patient is prepared for the procedure in the interventional radiology suite (on the operating table, asleep, sedated, or under locoregional anesthesia), with all of the team in the room, it is important to verify: (1) that all the team members are present and all the radiological images required for the procedure are ready (if necessary); (2) that the patient data displayed on the angiography system are correct and up to date and correspond to the patient submitted to the interventional procedure; (3) patient's identity, surgical site, and type and side (if required) of the procedure [53].

At the end of the procedure and before the patient leaves the angiography suite, a team member in the recovery room verifies that:

- The nursing assessment and radiological report have been completed and attached to the patient's clinical record
- The acquired images have been correctly uploaded and sent to the PACS
- The biopsy or biological sample containers have been correctly labeled and the requests and forms for the pathology laboratory have been correctly completed [53].

6.7 The Informed Consent

Health-care professionals and researchers have a legal and ethical responsibility to inform patients before carrying out diagnostic tests or treatment interventions [59].

Interventional radiologists should routinely attend or lead multidisciplinary team meetings to ensure patients get the most appropriate management for their particular condition. Interventional radiologists are best placed to discuss the treatments they offer and should have access to outpatient, inpatient, and day-care facilities to counsel and consent patients appropriately, review patients following interventional radiology treatments, and arrange further imaging and management as necessary [3].

Given that patient-centered decision-making has been increasingly viewed as an eminent quality of care indicator, assessment of the patient's desire for information about radiation exposure is imperative [60–62].

Physicians have the responsibility to obtain informed consent from patients, and this involves the health-care provider verbally explaining the risks and benefits of a procedure as well as alternative treatment options. Although the failure to do this properly is considered malpractice, and there is an extensive difference on informed consent regulations internationally and among states, the practice of formalizing the informed consent process with a signed document has been embraced worldwide [63, 64].

Topics to discuss during the informed consent process may include the purpose and nature of the procedure, the technique of performing the procedure, procedural risks and potential complications, the estimated benefits, the risks of not performing the procedure, reasonable alternatives and likely risks and benefits, and the right to refuse the procedure [38, 65, 66].

Since the patient must be able to fully understand the consent process, consent should be obtained before any sedation is administered. Finally, the necessary patient preparation for the treatment needs to be explained [64].

The interventional radiologist who performs the procedure (or a suitable delegate) should obtain the patient's consent, preferably on the evening before the procedure, unless there are remarkable circumstances and the patient should be allowed sufficient time to decide on or even to refuse the proposed interventional procedure.

During the consent process, the patient and the patient's family should understand that the site of skin entry and the site of treatment may be different [21].

Moreover, effective communication is fundamental to a successful patient-interventional radiologist relationship; shifting the communication model to be more patient-centered has been shown to improve both quality of care and patient satisfaction [67, 68].

In emergencies, the need for any immediate intervention must be documented in the patient's medical record, including situational details, the necessity for fast intervention, the magnitude of the situation, and the reason for not obtaining consent. If an intervention has a potential for higher levels of radiation, the risks of radiation-induced injuries should be included during the consent process: The medical record should note the estimated radiation dose received, and the patient should be advised of any potential radiation-related injuries with follow-up instructions [60, 69, 70].

6.8 Conclusion

Interventional radiology is an essential part of modern medicine, delivering minimally invasive patient-focused care, which has been proven to be safe and effective in both elective and emergency settings.

Over the years, numerous interventional radiology procedures have increasingly replaced open surgical techniques as they are less invasive, with reduced morbidity and mortality rates, and allow more rapid patient recovery and early hospital discharge. Today interventional radiology procedures are an excellent alternative to surgical interventions in the management of gynecological and obstetric diseases.

Proper organization and training are essential to any procedural specialty. While many aspects of interventional radiology are similar to that of surgery, most often, interventional radiologists are themselves required to set up equipment and organize the procedural table.

The need for more standardization to improve patient safety and quality of care is increasingly being recognized in interventional radiology. Preprocedural planning and intraprocedural organization are important for time management, and more importantly, for patient safety.

Of all the targeted and effective actions that can be undertaken to reduce adverse events, the use of safety checklists might have a prominent role.

The development of a safety culture will be the most important factor in determining the real success of safety checklists and their overall effects on patient safety. Developing a culture of safety can be a difficult process, but through safety education, dedicated teams, behavioral interventions, and executive support culture can begin to change.

As interventional radiologists have adopted a more "clinical identity," they have assumed more responsibility in patient management. With this evolving role, interventional radiologists have an even greater obligation to understand the ethical challenges specific to their specialty.

References

1. Cazzato RL, de Rubeis G, de Marini P, et al. Interventional radiology outpatient clinics (IROC): clinical impact and patient satisfaction. Cardiovasc Intervent Radiol. 2021;44:118–26. https://doi.org/10.1007/s00270-020-02677-1.
2. White SB. Value in interventional radiology: achieving high quality outcomes at a lower cost. Radiology. 2020;297:482–3. https://doi.org/10.1148/radiol.2020203407.
3. Tsetis D, Uberoi R, Fanelli F, et al. The provision of interventional radiology services in Europe: CIRSE recommendations. Cardiovasc Intervent Radiol. 2016;39:500–6. https://doi.org/10.1007/s00270-016-1299-0.
4. Baum RA, Baum S. Interventional radiology: a half century of innovation. Radiology. 2014;273(2 Suppl):S75–91. https://doi.org/10.1148/radiol.14140534.
5. Velling TE, Brennan FJ, Hall LD, et al. Role of the interventional radiologist in treating obstetric-gynecologic pathology. AJR Am J Roentgenol. 2000;175:1273–8. https://doi.org/10.2214/ajr.175.5.1751273.
6. Giurazza F, Corvino F, Cangiano G, et al. Transarterial embolization of peripheral high-flow arteriovenous malformation with ethylene vinyl alcohol copolymer (onyx®): single-center 10-year experience. Radiol Med. 2019;124:154–62. https://doi.org/10.1007/s11547-018-0948-6.
7. Coppola M, Pane F, Borzelli A, et al. Traumatic and spontaneous hemothorax due to intercostal arteries hemorrhage: what the interventional radiologist needs

to know. J Radiol Rev. 2020;7:300–6. https://doi.org/10.23736/S2723-9284.20.00050-X.
8. Giurazza F, Corvino F, Borzelli A, et al. Role of interventional radiology in managing gastrointestinal bleedings. J Radiol Rev. 2020;7:173–84. https://doi.org/10.23736/S2723-9284.20.00025-4.
9. Ganeshan A, Nazir SA, Hon LQ, et al. The role of interventional radiology in obstetric and gynaecology practice. Eur J Radiol. 2010;73:404–11. https://doi.org/10.1016/j.ejrad.2008.11.020.
10. Shanbhogue AK, Menias CO, Lalwani N, et al. Obstetric (nonfetal) complications. Radiol Clin N Am. 2013;51:983–1004. https://doi.org/10.1016/j.rcl.2013.07.012.
11. Niola R, Giurazza F, Torbica A, et al. Predelivery uterine arteries embolization in patients with placental implant anomalies: a cost-effective procedure. Radiol Med. 2017;122:77–9. https://doi.org/10.1007/s11547-016-0690-x.
12. Thabet A, Kalva SP, Liu B, et al. Interventional radiology in pregnancy complications: indications, technique, and methods for minimizing radiation exposure. Radiographics. 2012;32:255–74. https://doi.org/10.1148/rg.321115064.
13. Weston M, Soyer P, Barral M, et al. Role of interventional procedures in obstetrics and gynecology. Radiol Clin N Am. 2020;58:445–62. https://doi.org/10.1016/j.rcl.2019.11.006.
14. Giurazza F, Corvino F, Silvestre M, et al. Role of interventional radiology in obstetric and gynecological diseases. J Radiol Rev. 2020;7:26–38. https://doi.org/10.23736/S2723-9284.20.00253-3.
15. Di Stasi C, Cina A, Rosella F, et al. Uterine fibroid embolization efficacy and safety: 15 years experience in an elevated turnout rate center. Radiol Med. 2018;123:385–97. https://doi.org/10.1007/s11547-017-0843-6.
16. Silberstein S, Shnayder-Adams MM, Keller EJ, et al. Ethics in interventional radiology: a case-based primer. Cardiovasc Intervent Radiol. 2021;44:1510–7. https://doi.org/10.1007/s00270-021-02894-2.
17. Wong KK, Chu WC. Ethics policies and procedures in imaging and interventional radiology. Australas Phys Eng Sci Med. 2015;38:375–6. https://doi.org/10.1007/s13246-015-0346-5.
18. Bozorghadad S, Newton IG, Perez AW, et al. Research ethics in IR: the intersection between care and progress. J Vasc Interv Radiol. 2020;31:846–8. https://doi.org/10.1016/j.jvir.2020.02.014.
19. Kon AA, Shepard EK, Sederstrom NO, et al. Defining futile and potentially inappropriate interventions: a policy statement from the society of critical care medicine ethics committee. Crit Care Med. 2016;44:1769–74. https://doi.org/10.1097/CCM.0000000000001965.
20. Borgstede JP, Zinninger MD. Radiology and patient safety. Acad Radiol. 2004;11:322–32. https://doi.org/10.1016/s1076-6332(03)00720-7.
21. Angle JF, Nemcek AA Jr, Cohen AM, et al. Quality improvement guidelines for preventing wrong site, wrong procedure, and wrong person errors: application of the joint commission "universal protocol for preventing wrong site, wrong procedure, wrong person surgery" to the practice of interventional radiology. J Vasc Interv Radiol. 2009;20(7 Suppl):S256–62. https://doi.org/10.1016/j.jvir.2009.04.023.
22. Morbi AH, Hamady MS, Riga CV, et al. Reducing error and improving efficiency during vascular interventional radiology: implementation of a preprocedural team rehearsal. Radiology. 2012;264:473–83. https://doi.org/10.1148/radiol.12110530.
23. Koetser IC, de Vries EN, van Delden OM, et al. A checklist to improve patient safety in interventional radiology. Cardiovasc Intervent Radiol. 2013;36:312–9. https://doi.org/10.1007/s00270-012-0395-z.
24. Pressman BD, Roy LT. Developing a culture of safety in an imaging department. J Am Coll Radiol. 2015;12:198–200. https://doi.org/10.1016/j.jacr.2014.07.010.
25. Larson DB, Kruskal JB, Krecke KN, et al. Key concepts of patient safety in radiology. Radiographics. 2015;35:1677–93. https://doi.org/10.1148/rg.2015140277.
26. Baerlocher MO, Kennedy SA, Ward TJ, et al. Society of Interventional Radiology position statement: staffing guidelines for the interventional radiology suite. J Vasc Interv Radiol. 2016;27:618–22. https://doi.org/10.1016/j.jvir.2016.02.010.
27. du Pisanie JL, Dixon R. Building a culture of safety in interventional radiology. Tech Vasc Interv Radiol. 2018;21:198–204. https://doi.org/10.1053/j.tvir.2018.07.012.
28. Bibbolino C, Ferrante Z, Canitano S, et al. Working hypothesis for the drafting of ethical-deontological regulations in radiodiagnostics and interventional radiology. J Radiol Rev. 2020;7:165–72. https://doi.org/10.23736/S2723-9284.20.00013-2.
29. Keller EJ, Vogelzang RL. Who we are and what we can become: the anthropology of IR and challenges of forming a new specialty. J Vasc Interv Radiol. 2018;29:1703–1704.e2. https://doi.org/10.1016/j.jvir.2018.07.021.
30. Shnayder MM, Keller EJ, Makary MS. COVID-19 ethics: what interventional radiologists need to know. J Vasc Interv Radiol. 2020;31:1720–3. https://doi.org/10.1016/j.jvir.2020.07.003.
31. Cornelis FH, Monard E, Moulin MA, et al. Sedation and analgesia in interventional radiology: where do we stand, where are we heading and why does it matter? Diagn Interv Imaging. 2019;100:753–62. https://doi.org/10.1016/j.diii.2019.10.002.
32. Giurazza F, Corvino F, Borzelli A, et al. Interventional radiology in the COVID-19 era: management experience from a tertiary care center in the South of Italy. J Radiol Rev. 2021;8:181–5. https://doi.org/10.23736/S2723-9284.21.00133-0.
33. Dhansura T, Shaikh N. The parturient in the interventional radiology suite: new frontier in obstetric anaesthesia. Indian J Anaesth. 2017;61:289–94. https://doi.org/10.4103/ija.IJA_438_16.

34. Romagnoli S, Fanelli F, Barbani F, et al. CIRSE standards of practice on analgesia and sedation for interventional radiology in adults. Cardiovasc Intervent Radiol. 2020;43:1251–60. https://doi.org/10.1007/s00270-020-02536-z.
35. Dauer LT, Thornton RH, Miller DL, et al. Radiation management for interventions using fluoroscopic or computed tomographic guidance during pregnancy: a joint guideline of the Society of Interventional Radiology and the Cardiovascular and Interventional Radiological Society of Europe with Endorsement by the Canadian Interventional Radiology Association. J Vasc Interv Radiol. 2012;23:19–32. https://doi.org/10.1016/j.jvir.2011.09.007.
36. Niola R, Giurazza F, Nazzaro G, et al. Uterine artery embolization before delivery to prevent postpartum hemorrhage. J Vasc Interv Radiol. 2016;27:376–82. https://doi.org/10.1016/j.jvir.2015.12.006.
37. Bibbolino C, Pittalis S, Schininà V, et al. Hygiene precautions and the transmission of infections in radiology. Radiol Med. 2009;114:111–20. https://doi.org/10.1007/s11547-009-0363-0.
38. Kohi MP, Fidelman N, Behr S, et al. Periprocedural patient care. Radiographics. 2015;35:1766–78. https://doi.org/10.1148/rg.2015150038.
39. Guideline for hand hygiene in health-care settings. Centers for Disease Control and Prevention. http://www.cdc.gov/mmwr/preview/mmwrhtml/rr5116a1.htm.
40. Guidelines for the prevention of intravascular catheter-related infections, 2011. Centers for Disease Control and Prevention. 2011. http://www.cdc.gov/hicpac/pdf/guide lines/bsi-guidelines-2011.pdf.
41. Ierardi AM, Wood BJ, Gaudino C, et al. How to handle a COVID-19 patient in the angiographic suite. Cardiovasc Intervent Radiol. 2020;43:820–6. https://doi.org/10.1007/s00270-020-02476-8.
42. Taslakian B, Georges Sebaaly M, Al-Kutoubi A. Patient evaluation and preparation in vascular and interventional radiology: what every interventional radiologist should know (part 1: patient assessment and laboratory tests). Cardiovasc Intervent Radiol. 2016;39:325–33. https://doi.org/10.1007/s00270-015-1228-7.
43. Brook OR, Kruskal JB, Eisenberg RL, et al. Root cause analysis: learning from adverse safety events. Radiographics. 2015;35:1655–67. https://doi.org/10.1148/rg.2015150067.
44. de Vries EN, Ramrattan MA, Smorenburg SM, et al. The incidence and nature of in-hospital adverse events: a systematic review. Qual Saf Health Care. 2008;17:216–23. https://doi.org/10.1136/qshc.2007.023622.
45. Duncan JR. Strategies for improving safety and quality in interventional radiology. J Vasc Interv Radiol. 2008;19:3–7. https://doi.org/10.1016/j.jvir.2007.09.026.
46. Mafeld S, Musing E, Conway A, et al. Avoiding and managing error in interventional radiology practice: tips and tools. Can Assoc Radiol J. 2020;71:528–35. https://doi.org/10.1177/0846537119899215.
47. Pinto A, Brunese L, Pinto F, et al. The concept of error and malpractice in radiology. Semin Ultrasound CT MR. 2012;33:275–9. https://doi.org/10.1053/j.sult.2012.01.009.
48. Carrafiello G, Floridi C, Pellegrino C, et al. Errors and malpractice in interventional radiology. Semin Ultrasound CT MR. 2012;33:371–5. https://doi.org/10.1053/j.sult.2012.01.008.
49. Mafeld S, Oreopoulos G, Musing ELS, et al. Sources of error in interventional radiology: how, why, and when. Can Assoc Radiol J. 2020;71:518–27. https://doi.org/10.1177/0846537119899226.
50. Keller EJ. Reflect and remember: the ethics of complications in interventional radiology. Semin Intervent Radiol. 2019;36:104–7. https://doi.org/10.1055/s-0039-1688423.
51. Siewert B, Hochman MG. Improving safety through human factors engineering. Radiographics. 2015;35:1694–705. https://doi.org/10.1148/rg.2015150107.
52. Haynes AB, Weiser TG, Berry WR, et al. A surgical safety checklist to reduce morbidity and mortality in a global population. N Engl J Med. 2009;360:491–9. https://doi.org/10.1056/NEJMsa0810119.
53. Corso R, Vacirca F, Patelli C, et al. Use of "time-out" checklist in interventional radiology procedures as a tool to enhance patient safety. Radiol Med. 2014;119:828–34. https://doi.org/10.1007/s11547-014-0397-9.
54. Lee MJ, Fanelli F, Haage P, et al. Patient safety in interventional radiology: a CIRSE IR checklist. Cardiovasc Intervent Radiol. 2012;35:244–6. https://doi.org/10.1007/s00270-011-0289-5.
55. Cashman JN, Ng L. The management of peri- and postprocedural pain in interventional radiology: a narrative review. Pain Manag. 2017;7:523–35. https://doi.org/10.2217/pmt-2017-0024.
56. Maingard J, Kok HK, Ranatunga D, et al. The future of interventional and neurointerventional radiology: learning lessons from the past. Br J Radiol. 2017;90(1080):20170473. https://doi.org/10.1259/bjr.20170473.
57. Patel IJ, Davidson JC, Nikolic B, et al. Consensus guidelines for periprocedural management of coagulation status and hemostasis risk in percutaneous image-guided interventions. J Vasc Interv Radiol. 2012;23:727–36. https://doi.org/10.1016/j.jvir.2012.02.012.
58. Schenker MP, Martin R, Shyn PB, et al. Interventional radiology and anesthesia. Anesthesiol Clin. 2009;27:87–94. https://doi.org/10.1016/j.anclin.2008.10.012.
59. Kompanje EJO, van Dijck JTJM, Chalos V, et al. Informed consent procedures for emergency interventional research in patients with traumatic brain injury and ischaemic stroke. Lancet Neurol. 2020;19:1033–42. https://doi.org/10.1016/S1474-4422(20)30276-3.

60. Miller DL, Balter S, Wagner LK, et al. Quality improvement guidelines for recording patient radiation dose in the medical record. J Vasc Interv Radiol. 2009;20(7 Suppl):S200–7. https://doi.org/10.1016/j.jvir.2009.04.005.
61. Zener R, Johnson P, Wiseman D, et al. Informed consent for radiation in interventional radiology procedures. Can Assoc Radiol J. 2018;69:30–7. https://doi.org/10.1016/j.carj.2017.07.002.
62. Torresin A, Evans S, Lizio D, et al. Practical recommendations for the application of DE 59/2013. Radiol Med. 2019;124:721–7. https://doi.org/10.1007/s11547-019-01031-x.
63. Mavroforou A, Giannoukas A, Mavrophoros D, et al. Physicians' liability in interventional radiology and endovascular therapy. Eur J Radiol. 2003;46:240–3. https://doi.org/10.1016/s0720-048x(02)00192-4.
64. O'Dwyer HM, Lyon SM, Fotheringham T, et al. Informed consent for interventional radiology procedures: a survey detailing current European practice. Cardiovasc Intervent Radiol. 2003;26:428–33. https://doi.org/10.1007/s00270-003-0058-1.
65. Pomara C, Pascale N, Maglietta F, et al. Use of contrast media in diagnostic imaging: medico-legal considerations. Radiol Med. 2015;120:802–9. https://doi.org/10.1007/s11547-015-0549-6.
66. Peralta F, Wong CA. Interventional radiology in the pregnant patient for obstetric and nonobstetric indications: organizational, anesthetic, and procedural issues. Curr Opin Anaesthesiol. 2013;26:450–5. https://doi.org/10.1097/ACO.0b013e3283625e89.
67. Itri JN. Patient-centered radiology. Radiographics. 2015;35:1835–46. https://doi.org/10.1148/rg.2015150110.
68. Ripley BA, Tiffany D, Lehmann LS, et al. Improving the informed consent conversation: a standardized checklist that is patient centered, quality driven, and legally sound. J Vasc Interv Radiol. 2015;26:1639–46. https://doi.org/10.1016/j.jvir.2015.06.007.
69. Pinto A, Giurazza F, Califano T, et al. Interventional radiology in gynecology and obstetric practice: safety issues. Semin Ultrasound CT MR. 2021;42:104–12. https://doi.org/10.1053/j.sult.2020.09.004.
70. Hill GQ, Ryu RK. A primer to understanding the elements of medical malpractice. Semin Intervent Radiol. 2019;36:117–9. https://doi.org/10.1055/s-0039-1688425.

Part III

Gynecological Pathologies

Management of Fallopian Tube's Obstructions

7

Anna Paola Mancini, Rita Stefanucci, Valeria Mancuso, Giuseppina Pacella, and Bruno Beomonte Zobel

7.1 Introduction

Infertility is defined as the inability to get pregnant after 12 months, or more, of unprotected sexual intercourse; according to the World Health Organization, about 48 million couples and 186 million individuals live with infertility globally [1].

Female infertility is a widespread condition, and the Centres for Disease Control and Prevention estimate that about 10 out of 100 (6.1 million) women in the United States aged 15–44 have difficulty getting or staying pregnant. The pelvic causes of female infertility are numerous and, among them, fallopian tube abnormalities are the most common, accounting for 30–40% of cases [2].

Screening for tubal occlusion is part of the investigation of subfertile couples and is classically performed using hysterosalpingography (HSG) or laparoscopy with chromopertubation in conjunction with hysteroscopy (dye test), which is considered the gold standard [3, 4].

A. P. Mancini (✉) · R. Stefanucci · V. Mancuso
G. Pacella · B. Beomonte Zobel
Radiology Department, Fondazione Policlinico Universitario Campus Bio-Medico di Roma, Rome, Italy
e-mail: a.mancini@policlinicocampus.it; r.stefanucci@policlinicocampus.it; v.mancuso@unicampus.it; g.pacella@policlinicocampus.it; b.zobel@policlinicocampus.it

In the last years, HSG has become widely used especially in women without suspected comorbidities (such as pelvic inflammatory disease, previous ectopic pregnancy, or endometriosis); and conversely, laparoscopy, being a more expensive and invasive procedure, is usually reserved for the assessment or treatment of another pelvic pathology. More recently, hysterosalpingo contrast sonography (HyCoSy), an ultrasound-based technique using a non-toxic gel containing hydroxyethyl cellulose and glycerol for dilation of the uterine cavity, was proposed as another minimally invasive alternative to laparoscopy [5].

This chapter aims to present the evaluation of tubal patency, using mainly HSG, and the management of abnormal findings.

7.2 Aetiology

Tubal occlusion can arise from congenital abnormalities, pelvic inflammatory disease (PID), certain sexually transmitted infections (STIs), endometriosis, and previous pelvic surgery. In rare cases, tubal infertility can be considered idiopathic.

Fallopian tubes develop from the unpaired distal ends of the Mullerian ducts. Congenital abnormalities are rare and among them partial or complete absence of one or both fallopian tubes can cause tubal occlusion. The atresia can be

R. Niola et al. (eds.), *Diagnostic and Interventional Radiology in Gynecological and Obstetric Diseases*, https://doi.org/10.1007/978-3-031-11910-1_7

complete or segmental, and the latter mainly includes the proximal isthmic portion or the proximal ampullary segment.

PID can affect the fallopian tube, with or without abscess formation. The true prevalence of PID is unknown, due to the difficulty in accurately diagnosing pelvic infections. The rate of tubal infertility has been reported to be 12%, 23%, and 54% after one, two, and three episodes of PID, respectively.

Acute PID is often associated with *Neisseria gonorrhoea* and *Chlamydia trachomatis* infections. The *gonococcus* causes a direct inflammatory response and is one of the pathogens of fallopian tube epithelial cells. In contrast, intracellular *C. trachomatis* does not cause an acute inflammatory response, but persistent chlamydial antigens can trigger a delayed hypersensitivity reaction with later tissue injury, tubal scarring, and destruction. *C. trachomatis* serological positivity reduces the possibility of a physiological pregnancy and increases the risk of an ectopic pregnancy. Another frequently found pathogen is *Trichomonas vaginalis*. *Mycoplasma genitalium* can damage the female reproductive tract, although its pathogenesis is not fully understood. Most female carriers are asymptomatic, but in some studies, it has been linked to urethritis, cervicitis, PID, and tubal-factor infertility.

Chronic PID is generally associated with *Mycobacterium tuberculosis*. Especially in developing countries, genital tuberculosis may account for 3–5% of infertility cases. *M. tuberculosis* bacilli reach the genital tract typically by haematogenous spread from an extragenital primary infection.

In endometriosis, chronic inflammation and intraperitoneal bleeding can cause pelvic adhesions resulting in tubal obstruction or alteration of their course. Other factors appear to decrease fertility, such as increased peritoneal inflammatory factors, abnormalities in endometrial immunologic function, alterations in oocyte capture or possibly altering oocyte development, embryonic quality, or impaired implantation.

Salpingitis isthmica nodosa is an inflammatory disease of the fallopian tube, typically bilateral, characterized by isthmic portion nodular thickening, following the proliferation of smooth muscle and diverticula of tubal epithelium. This uncommon condition progressively leads to tubal occlusion and infertility.

A previous ectopic pregnancy could result in significant tubal damage [6–10].

7.3 Radiological Anatomy

The HSG allows to correctly evaluate the cervical canal, the internal uterine orifice, the region of the isthmus, the uterine body, and the fallopian tubes.

The uterine cavity has a roughly triangular shape with the fundus of the uterus forming the base of the triangle while the internal uterine orifice is the vertex. Usually, the uterus' fundus is straight, but a modest concavity or convexity is considered normal; however, the concavity must not be deeper than 1 cm.

The cervical canal may or may not be evaluated, depending on the position of the catheter used for contrast introduction; it has a variable appearance: very thinned, filiform, broad, and the morphology of the mucosa can vary depending on the period of the cycle in which the investigation is performed. The *arbor vitae*, mostly evident in the *nullipara*, is particularly represented in the periovulatory phase. The cervical canal must always be evaluated especially in patients with suspected anatomical alterations and with a history of repeated miscarriages.

The fallopian tubes are divided into five anatomic segments, that differ from each other in calibre and direction (from lateral to medial):

- *Fimbriae*: projections that drape over the ovary.
- *Infundibulum*: the fimbriae originate from it. It opens into the peritoneal cavity at the abdominal ostium.
- *Ampulla*: the widest and longest section.
- *Isthmus*: characterized by a sphincter ring not visible in HSG, during the procedure operative pressure often has to overcome its continence in order to allow the contrast progression in the *isthmus*.

- *Interstitial* or *intramural segment*: the section within the myometrium appearing as a triangular or oval-shaped bulge [11, 12].

7.4 Diagnostic Techniques

The most common techniques to study the patency of the fallopian tubes are [10, 13]:

- Hysterosalpingography (HSG)
- Laparoscopy with chromopertubation in conjunction with hysteroscopy
- Hysterosalpingo contrast sonography (HyCoSy)
- *C. Trachomatis* antibody test
- Endoscopic techniques
- Magnetic resonance (MR)

Among these, HSG is becoming the most widely used one, even if laparoscopy has been the gold standard, thanks to its advantages, such as ease of execution, lack of anaesthesia, uncommon complications, and potential therapeutic effects [4, 7, 14].

7.4.1 Hysterosalpingography

Hysterosalpingography is considered the first-level investigation to evaluate the fallopian tubes, through the injection into the uterine cavity, of a radiopaque contrast medium under a fluoroscopical guide, giving information about their patency and morphology. HSG may also have healing benefits, especially for proximal tubes blockade, in which a selective salpingography, that is, a direct opacification of a fallopian tube through a catheter placed in the tubal ostium, is recommended as the first therapeutic step by the American Society for Reproductive Medicine, also according to its simplicity and reasonable cost [10, 14].

Diagnosis using HSG is subject to some indications and contraindications, as summarized in Table 7.1 [14].

7.4.1.1 Technique

The examination is performed during days 7–12 of the menstrual cycle, as the endometrium is thin during the proliferative phase; you will have a simplified interpretation and ensure there is no existing pregnancy; furthermore, at this time the uterus is toned and the fallopian ostia are hypotonic, helping the contrast medium progression.

No specific patient preparation is necessary; it is not a routinely required prophylactic antibiotic treatment. In the case of a patient with a history of PID, antibiotics might be prescribed one day before and for a few days after. A nonsteroidal anti-inflammatory drug or Butylscopolamine 1 h before the procedure is suggested, to decrease discomfort, and enema a day before.

Before starting the procedure, some professionals would rather have the patient empty her bladder to obtain a more realistic uterus orientation and better comfort, whereas others suggest

Table 7.1 HSG's indications and contraindications

Indications	Contraindications
• Infertility;	• Possible pregnancy: To avoid the risk before the study, serum β-human chorionic gonadotropin (β-hCG) is also required;
• Recurrent spontaneous abortion;	• Active pelvic infection: Laboratory tests to exclude vaginal and cervical infections are required;
• Postoperative evaluation following tubal ligation or reversal of tubal ligation;	• Severe allergy to iodine-based contrast agents;
• Preoperative evaluation prior to myomectomy;	• Severe cardiac or renal deficiency;
• As a preliminary exam before in vitro fertilization;	• Recent uterine or tubal surgery;
• Congenital or anatomic abnormalities.	• Vaginal or uterine bleeding: Because of the risk of unrestrained bleeding.

examining with a full bladder to improve the uterine fundus profile evaluation.

The patient is placed supine in the gynaecologic examination position on the fluoroscopy table with her arms placed over the chest. The external genitals need to be cleaned with an antiseptic solution (e.g. Betadine) and covered with sterile towels. A sterile speculum is inserted into the vagina for correct visualization of the cervix, which is cleaned with a povidone-iodine solution once localized.

HSG is performed with a two-way 5 Fr catheter, equipped with a filled balloon, preventing backflow of contrast media, while improving accuracy in evaluating tubal patency. In our centre, the contrast agent used is *Iohexol*, a non-ionic low osmolarity contrast medium, with an iodine concentration of 350 mgI/mL (Fig. 7.1).

Before cannulating the cervical canal with 5 Fr catheter, it is good practice to remove the presence of air from the catheter by sending contrast medium: air could be mistaken for intrauterine defects. Once the catheter is located, the balloon is inflated to anchorage, and the patient is helped to move into a supine decubitus position.

The contrast is then slowly introduced under fluoroscopic guidance to evaluate the uterine cavity (i.e. any filling defects or contour abnormalities); after full distention of the uterus, contrast have to pass through the fallopian tubes—allowing their evaluation—and eventually into the peritoneum in case of tubal patency (Fig. 7.2). Oblique views of the fallopian tubes may be obtained for better visualization of the tubes or for displacing superimposed structures.

If the fallopian tubes' opacification fails, the catheter is advanced into the interstitial region and contrast material is injected again (Fig. 7.3); in case selective salpingography reveals a proximal fallopian tube obstruction, tubal cannulation can be performed (see next paragraph: proximal tubal obstructions management).

In the following 24 h after the exam, the patient may feel some abdominal and/or pelvic pain, spotting, fever and, in addition, is advised to abstain from sexual intercourse 3 days after HSG

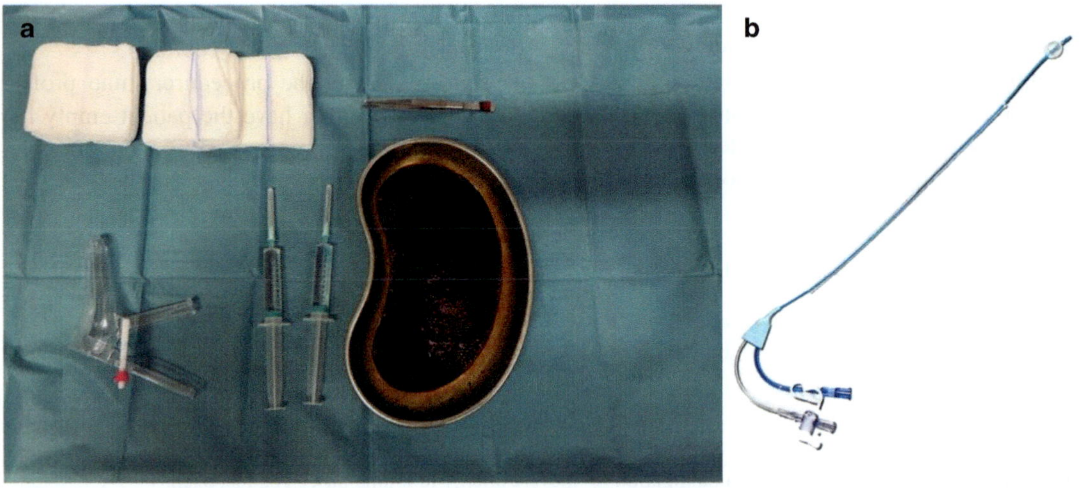

Fig. 7.1 HSG materials: (**a**) Speculum, contrast-filled syringes, povidone-iodine solution, forceps, and sterile gauzes. (**b**) 5 French catheter has two lower extremities: the right one is used to inflate contrast medium and the left one to inflate the balloon

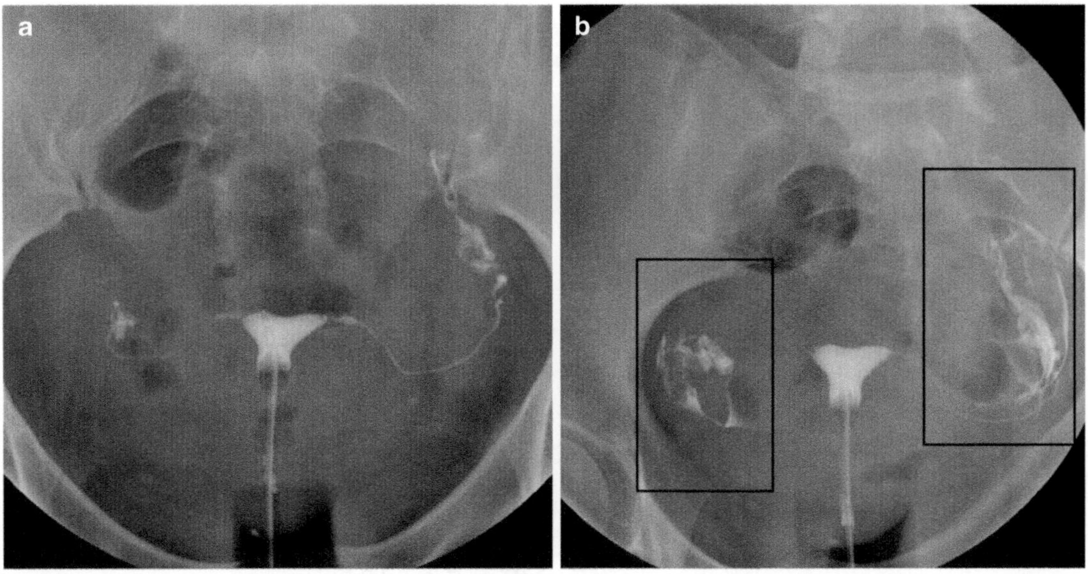

Fig. 7.2 Normal HSG: (**a**) the radiograph clearly shows portions of both fallopian tubes (infundibulum, ampulla, isthmus, and interstitial segment). (**b**) Contrast material flows into the peritoneal cavity (surrounded)

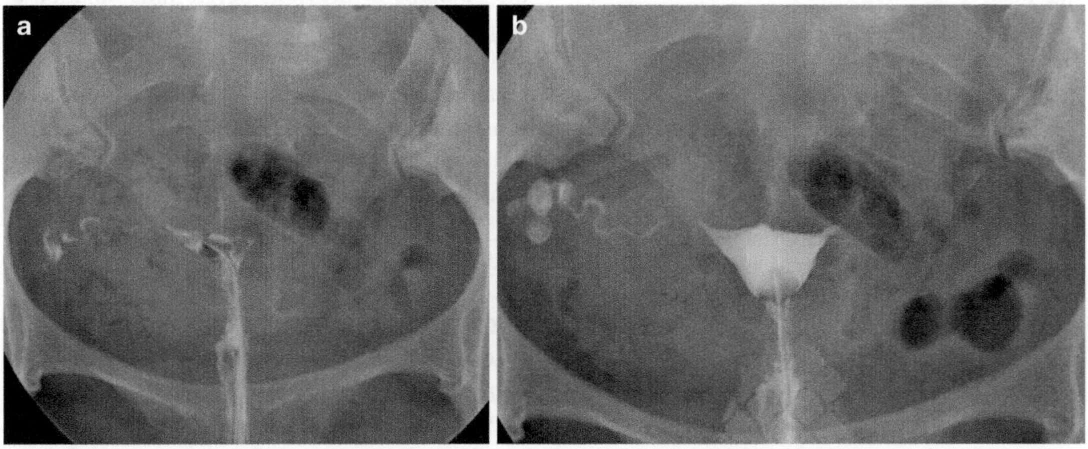

Fig. 7.3 Left tubal occlusion: (**a**) the radiograph shows the selective cannulation of the right tube. (**b**) The right tube is opacified by medium contrast visualized but there is no intraperitoneal spillage; only the interstitial segment of the left tube is visualized

and to have safe sex for 1 month after HSG to elude pregnancy [14, 15].

Some complications may occur during HSG, depending on the execution method of the examination or the contrast medium [14]. The most common ones are pain (Fig. 7.4), bleeding, and infection (Table 7.2) [14].

7.4.1.2 HSG Findings

Normal Findings

After the administration of contrast material, first, the uterine cavity with a roughly triangular shape is visualized. Second, fallopian tubes should appear as thin lines that widen in the

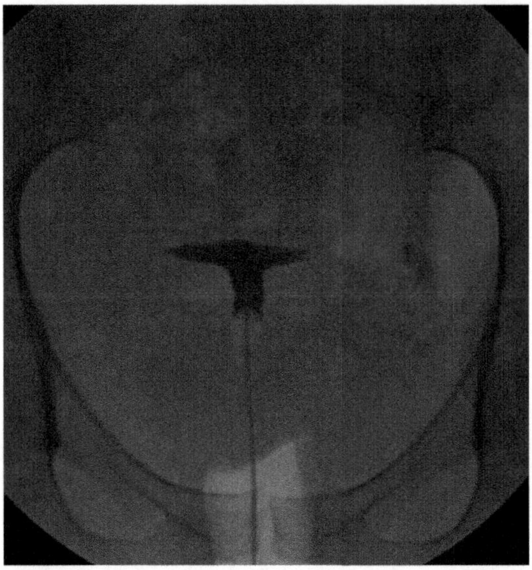

Fig. 7.4 Exam interrupted: one of the possible HSG side effects is patient fainting. In this case, the exam was interrupted due to a vasovagal reaction, spontaneously solved after 1 min

Table 7.2 Complications of HSG

HSG complications
Pain: Discomfort can be due to inflation of the catheter balloon in the endocervical canal or to contrast material distension of the uterine cavity or peritoneal irritation caused by contrast medium spillage.
Patients usually describe this pain as cramping, which is generally well tolerated; however, some may complain of severe pain, leading to an early end of HSG.
Bleeding: It is strongly recommended to advise patients about a light spotting after the procedure.
Infection: Being a sterile procedure, it minimizes the risk of infection. In our university hospital we suggest chloramphenicol ovules after HSG (250 mg × 6 days or 500 mg × 3 days).
Contrast material allergic reaction
Uterine perforation
Irradiation of an early and unsuspected pregnancy: Negative pregnancy test and appropriate timing of the examination minimize the risk.

ampullary segment and contrast should flow into the peritoneal cavity (Fig. 7.2) [14].

Pathological Findings

PID is the most common cause of tubal occlusion. Tubal occlusion appears as an abrupt cut-off of contrast material with failed opacification of the distal segments without contrast spillage into the peritoneal cavity (Figs. 7.5 and 7.6); it can be mono- or bi-lateral (Fig. 7.7) and can affect any portion of the tube.

The findings of cornual or proximal tubal blockage on HSG should be interpreted with caution: it can be functional, due to utero-tubal ostium spasm especially with elevated contrast injection pressure, or organic, due to a mucus plug or debris, or to fibrosis associated with *salpingitis isthmica nodosa* (SIN) resulting from endometriosis or infection.

PID can cause hydrosalpinx too; it is characterized by distal tubal occlusion (usually ampulla) with proximal segments dilatation and an absence of intraperitoneal spillover of contrast material (Figs. 7.8 and 7.9).

Peritubal adhesions (Fig. 7.10) are a significant cause of female infertility. Adhesions can be the outcome of previous pelvic inflammation or surgery: in the literature, the incidence of peritubal adhesions after salpingitis, at second-look laparoscopy, ranges from 38.5% to 54.6%. Even if laparoscopy remains the gold standard to make a diagnosis due to its direct view, HSG can be considered an accurate technique. In a practice a single or a combination of different radiographic findings have to be searched:

- Convoluted tubes: corkscrew tube appearance with regularly open tuba is a sign of modest *periviscеritis*.
- Vertical or horizontal tubes orientation.
- Halo effect: The contrast medium located along the tube's external surface produces a double-contour image of the fallopian tube, which allows for an assessment of the wall thickness.
- Hydro-/sacto-salpinx.
- Fixed latero-deviation of the uterus: is a sign of greater severity of *perivisceritis*, in which fibrosis causes the loss of uterus mobility.
- Irregular distribution of contrast in the peritoneal cavity: a round collection of contrast medium near the ampulla.
- Delayed progression of contrast in the fallopian tubes.

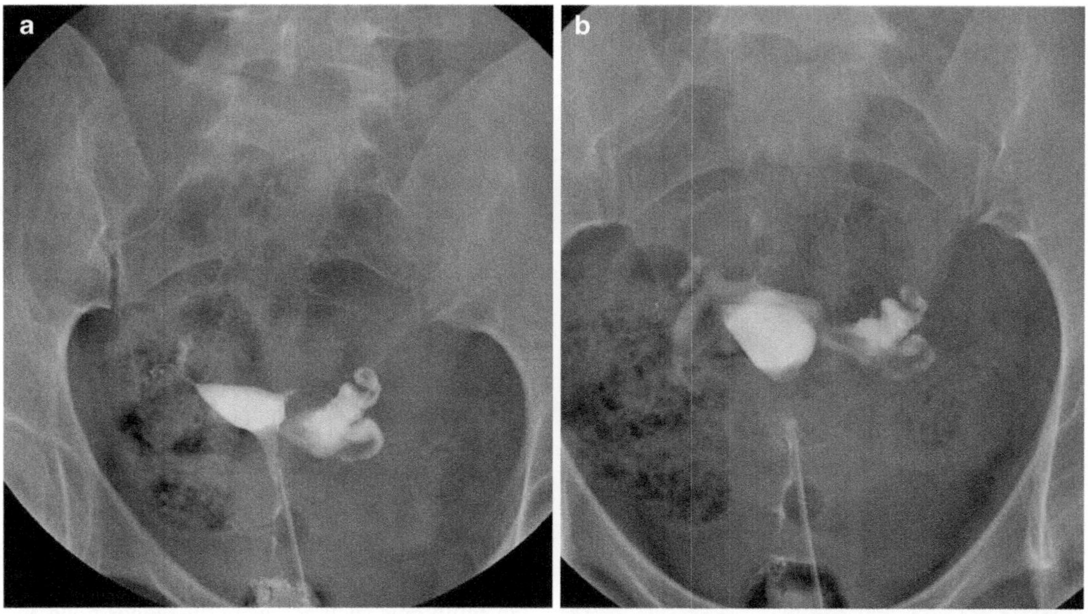

Fig. 7.5 Right tubal occlusion: (**a**) the right tube is highlighted by contrast until ampulla; the left tube is well opacified and presents contrast spillage into the peritoneal cavity. (**b**) Late radiograph shows the failed visualization of the right tube

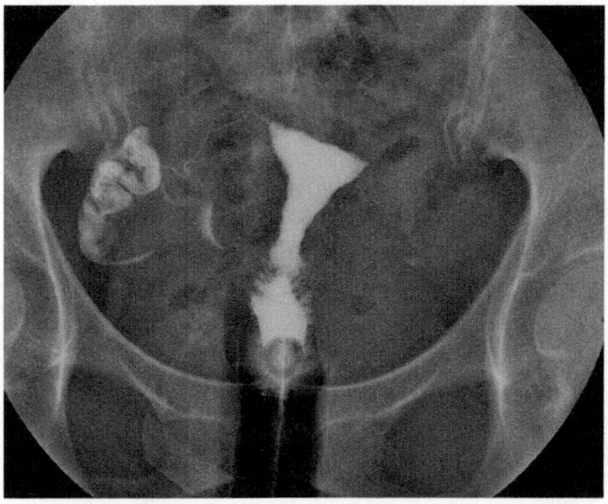

Fig. 7.6 Left tubal occlusion: the right tube is well opacified and presents contrast spillage into the peritoneal cavity, instead the left tube is highlighted by contrast until isthmus

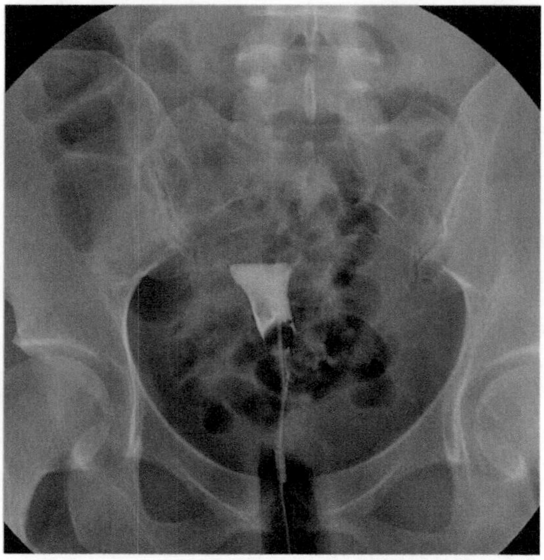

Fig. 7.7 Spot radiograph reveals a bilateral abrupt cut-off of the fallopian tubes, suggesting bilateral tubal occlusion

Tubal polyps are foci of ectopic endometrial tissue at the interstitial portion of the tube; they manifest as filling defects at the interstitial portion.

Post-operative assessment of tubal ligation is a common indication of HSG: successful treatment is seen as an abrupt termination of the tube at the surgical site or mild bulbous expansion of the tube with cut-off (Figs. 7.11 and 7.12). HSG can be performed to demonstrate tubal patency with no progression of contrast medium after the reversal of a ligation procedure.

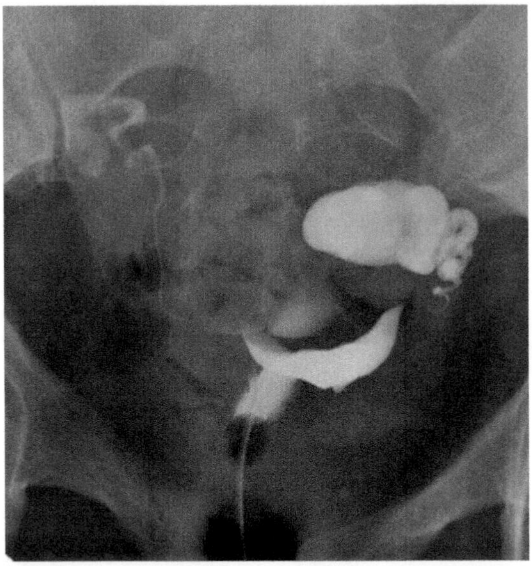

Fig. 7.8 Hydrosalpinx: the image shows dilatation of the ampullary portion of the left fallopian tube, with the loss of rugal folds. These findings are suggestive of hydrosalpinx. The right tube has normal calibre

SIN is a disease of unknown aetiology, presumably caused by pelvic inflammatory disease or endometriosis and it is associated with ectopic pregnancy and infertility; it appears at HSG as small outpouching or diverticula affecting one or both fallopian tubes [2, 12, 14, 16, 17].

7.4.2 Laparoscopy

Laparoscopy with chromopertubation in conjunction with hysteroscopy (dye test) is considered the "gold standard" for assessing tubal patency, and it is recommended in women who have an increased likelihood of pelvic pathology in presence of a history of PID, pelvic surgery, and significant pelvic symptoms such as severe dysmenorrhoea and dyspareunia. Laparoscopy offers the opportunity to treat coexisting pathologies. However, it could incur operative and anaesthesiological risks and increased operating costs [3, 10, 18].

7.4.3 Hysterosalpingo Contrast Sonography

Hysterosalpingo contrast sonography is considered a valid alternative to HSG to study tubal patency without the exposition to ionizing radiation and with a low incidence of side effects

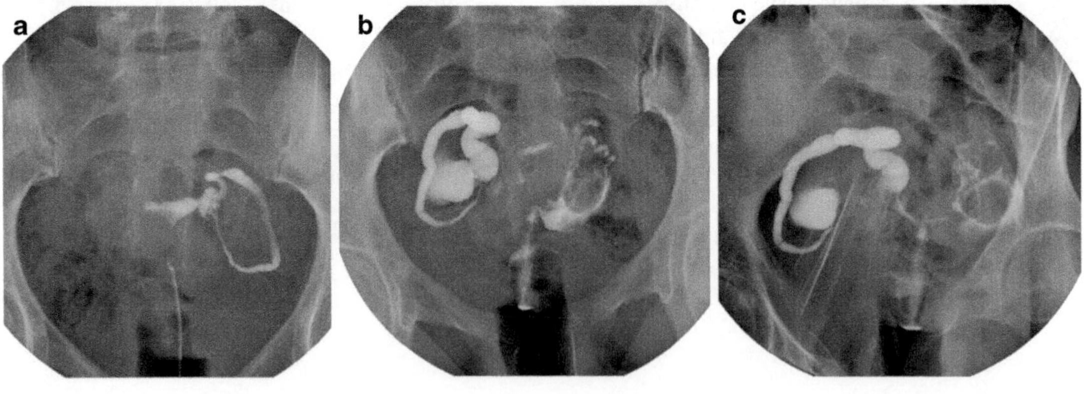

Fig. 7.9 Hydrosalpinx: (**a–c**) the images display dilatation of ampullary portion and of all proximal segments of the left fallopian tube, with the loss of rugal folds; these findings are suggestive of hydrosalpinx. The right tube has normal calibre, and intraperitoneal spillage of contrast medium is seen

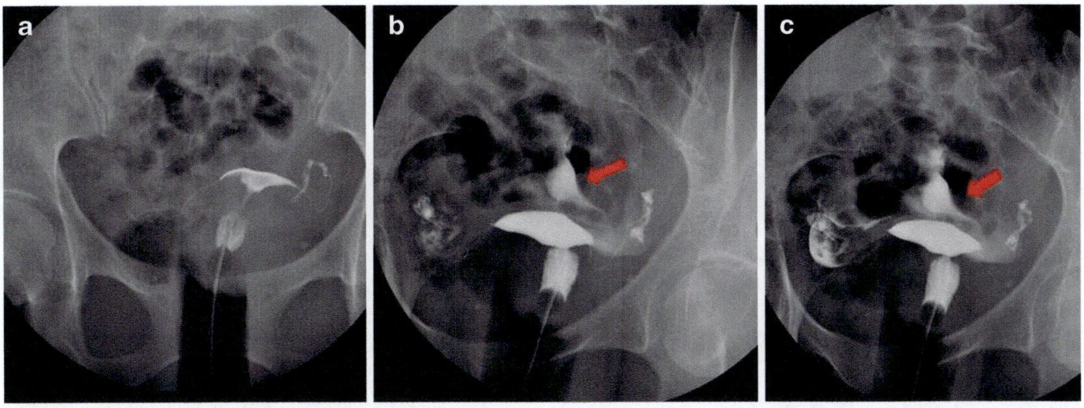

Fig. 7.10 Adhesions: (**a**) left dislocation of the uterus and the vertical position of the left tube are seen in the radiograph. (**b, c**) The radiographs show a well-demarcated collection of contrast material adjacent to the left tube (arrow). These three findings are strongly suggestive of peritubal adhesions

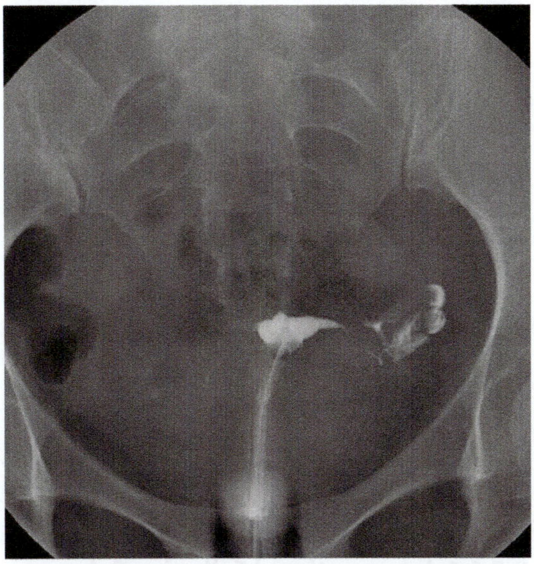

Fig. 7.11 Post tubal ligation findings: radiograph shows cut-off of contrast medium in the isthmic portion of the right tube due to surgical occlusion; the left tube is well opacified and presents contrast spillage into the peritoneal cavity

and complications. It consists of a transvaginal sonography in which a galactose solution, containing gas microbubbles, or an inexpensive mixture of air and saline solution, is injected into the uterine cavity by a cervical catheter. However, as the fallopian tubal course is not linear and lies on different planes, and rapid small movements of the probe are needed to visualize the fluid passage in the entire tube during infusion, recently a new non-toxic gel received the CE (European Conformity) approval for tubal patency evaluation. The gel, diluted and pushed into the uterine cavity and the fallopian tubes, produces a foam that is stable for several minutes.

HyCoSy could also be therapeutic for the subfertile female population; experts have linked this effect to the flushing effect of fluid through a partially occluded tube, but no statistically significant association between HyCoSy and the start of spontaneous pregnancy has been found.

Compared to HSG, HyCoSy has greater sensitivity and specificity for detecting intrauterine pathologies and enables concomitant visualization of the ovaries and the myometrium. The limits are that it is an operator-dependent technique and does not provide an image of the entire tube, but to exceed the latter, some infertility centres have recently introduced 3D HyCoSy [3, 10, 19–21].

7.4.4 *C. Trachomatis* Antibody Test

It is a non-invasive approach to evaluate fallopian tubes. The high presence of title of chlamydial antibodies is associated with tubal damage resulting from previous pelvic inflammatory disease.

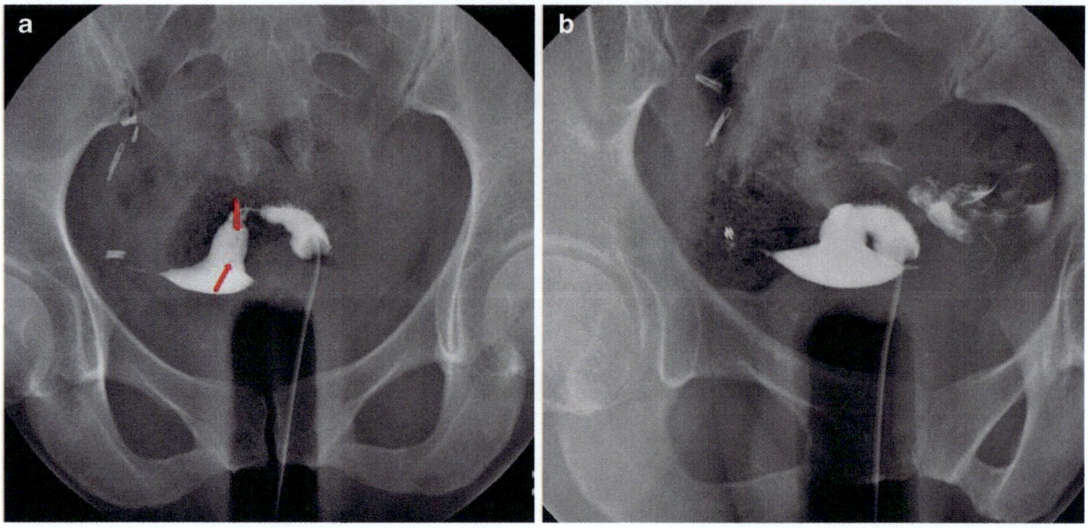

Fig. 7.12 Post tubal ligation findings: (**a**) retroverted uterus with some air bubbles into the cavity (arrow). Some metallic clips can be seen on the right side of the pelvic cavity as surgical operation sequela. (**b**) The image shows the outcomes of right tube surgical occlusion. No pathological findings are detected for the left tube

However, it cannot locate the site of damage and valuate the extension of tubal disease [3, 10, 18].

7.4.5 Endoscopic Techniques

A fallopian tube endoscopy by transvaginal (Falloscopy) or transabdominal (Salpingoscopy) approach diagnoses intraluminal tubal damage by a direct visualization of tubal epithelium. Being an expensive technique, it is rarely performed [3, 7].

7.4.6 Magnetic Resonance

In recent years, the role of 1.5 T MR-HSG has been emphasized due to its high contrast and spatial resolution which are helpful for accurately determining tubal patency and other pelvic causes of female infertility. Moreover, MR is typically used for problem solving when HyCoSy and/or HSG cannot provide definitive answers or show tubal occlusion due to endometriosis or contour abnormalities of the uterine cavity.

The MR advantages are being non-ionizing and non-operator dependent, but on the other hand, it is an expensive technique and the MR equipment is not commonly available for investigation of tube patency [22, 23].

7.5 Therapeutic Techniques

7.5.1 Proximal Tubal Occlusion

Proximal tubal blockage occurs in 10–25% of women with tubal disease [7].

7.5.1.1 Interventional Fallopian Tube Cannulation

If the tubal blockage cannot be overcome by the flushing action of the contrast medium, for fallopian tube access, a 5 Fr slightly curved polyethylene catheter is advanced over a 0.035-in. diameter (0.089 cm) guidewire to the uterine horn. The guidewire is removed and a full-strength contrast agent is injected through the 5 Fr catheter (selective salpingography) (Fig. 7.13). If the proximal tubal obstruction persists, a 0.015-in. diameter (0.038 cm) guidewire with a flexible platinum tip and 3 Fr Teflon catheter are inserted together into the fallopian tube and an attempt is made to recanalize the obstruction with gentle probing

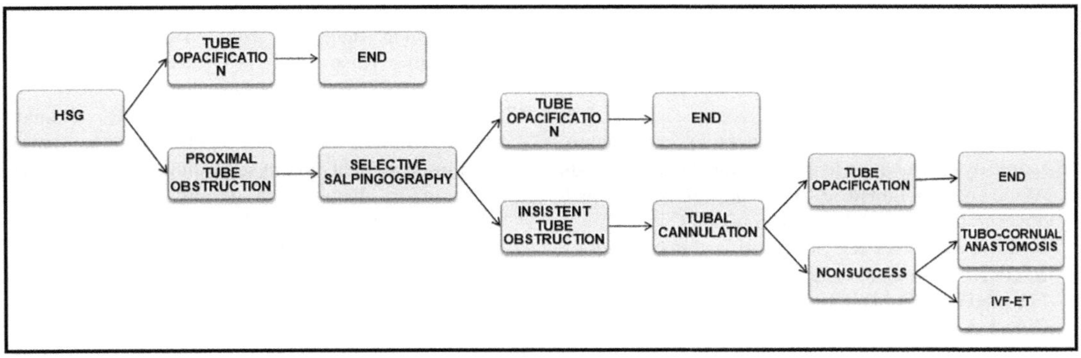

Fig. 7.13 Flow chart in proximal tubal obstruction management

movements of the guidewire. If there is an acute angulation in the tube at the site of the obstruction, or if the obstruction is in the isthmic portion of the tube, a softer tapered guidewire and catheter are used. The guidewire and catheter can be advanced as far as necessary to clear the obstruction, usually less than 4 cm from the tubal ostium. When the guidewire passes the obstruction, it is removed and the contrast agent is injected through the 3 Fr catheter. Once the recanalization is completed, the 3 Fr catheter is removed, and contrast agent is injected through the 5 Fr catheter still wedged in the tubal ostium to better delineate the tube and visualize the site of recanalization. A post-recanalization HSG can then be performed if desired.

Complications of the fallopian tube's recanalization are unusual and are of little clinical significance when they do occur: mild uterine cramping, vaginal bleeding, and tubal perforation (4%). The radiation dose to the ovaries during fluoroscopic catheterization has been documented to be less than 1 rad (10 Gy) [3, 7, 15, 24, 25].

7.5.1.2 Microsurgical Tubo-cornual Anastomosis

It could be considered after the failure of interventional tubal cannulation; it consists of the resection of the blocked cornual segment followed by a surgical anastomosis.

For microsurgical tubal reanastomosis in the setting of proximal tubal occlusion, the tubal isthmus is excised, the residual tube is axially incised along its antimesenteric border, and then reimplanted into a new uterotomy incision posterior to the horn.

Adverse prognostic factors for future fertility include a significant reduction of the residual length of the tube, evidence of pelvic inflammatory changes involving the other segment of the tube, and the presence of other infertility factors [3, 7].

7.5.2 Distal Tubal Occlusion

Distal tubal occlusions may be complete or incomplete and the most common causes are adhesive disease, tubo-ovarian abscess, hydrosalpinx, and ectopic pregnancy.

In this setting should be performed *salpingostomy* or *fimbrioplasty*. Salpingostomy consists of two phases, incision and eversion; the principle of fimbrioplasty is the lysis of fimbrial adhesions, separation of agglutination, or dilatation of fimbrial strictures [3, 10].

References

1. World Health Organization. International classification of diseases, 11th Revision (ICD-11). Geneva: WHO; 2018.
2. Steinkeler JA, Woodfield C, Lazarus E, Hillstrom MM. Female infertility: a systematic approach to radiologic imaging and diagnosis. RadioGraphics. 2009;29(5):1353–70. https://doi.org/10.1148/rg.295095047.
3. Kodaman PH, Arici A, Seli E. Evidence-based diagnosis and management of tubal factor infertility. Curr Opin Obstet Gynecol. 2004;16(3):221–9. https://doi.org/10.1097/00001703-200406000-00004.

4. National Institute for Health and Care Excellence London (UK). Fertility problems: assessment and treatment. 2017.
5. Exacoustos C, Zupi E, Carusotti C, Lanzi G, Marconi D, Arduini D. Hysterosalpingo-contrast sonography compared with hysterosalpingography and laparoscopic dye pertubation to evaluate tubal patency. J Am Assoc Gynecol Laparosc. 2003;10(3):367–72. https://doi.org/10.1016/S1074-3804(05)60264-2.
6. Barkwill D, Tobler KJ. Salpingitis Isthmica Nodosa. 2021 Jan 18. In: StatPearls [Internet]. Treasure Island, FL: StatPearls Publishing; 2021.
7. Gebeh AK, Metwally M. Surgical management of tubal disease and infertility. Obstet Gynaecol Reprod Med. 2017;27(11):346–51. https://doi.org/10.1016/j.ogrm.2017.08.002.
8. Hoffman BL. Williams gynecology. New York: McGraw-Hill; 2020.
9. Infertility workup for the women's health specialist: ACOG Committee Opinion, No. 781. Obstet Gynecol. 2019;133(6):e377–84. https://doi.org/10.1097/AOG.0000000000003271.
10. Sonal P, Sanja KP, Asim K. Donald School textbook of human reproductive & gynecological endocrinology. New Delhi: Jaypee Brothers; 2019.
11. La Fianza A. Isterosalpingografia attualità metodologiche, indicazioni cliniche e integrazioni diagnostiche. Idelson-Gnocchi; Naples, Italy; 2004.
12. Revzin MV, Moshiri M, Katz DS, Pellerito JS, Mankowski Gettle L, Menias CO. Imaging evaluation of fallopian tubes and related disease: a primer for radiologists. Radiographics. 2020;40(5):1473–501. https://doi.org/10.1148/rg.2020200051.
13. Imaoka I, Wada A, Matsuo M, Yoshida M, Kitagaki H, Sugimura K. MR imaging of disorders associated with female infertility: use in diagnosis, treatment, and management. Radiographics. 2003;23:1401–21. https://doi.org/10.1148/rg.236025115.
14. Simpson WL Jr, Beitia LG, Mester J. Hysterosalpingography: a reemerging study. Radiographics. 2006;26(2):419–31. https://doi.org/10.1148/rg.262055109.
15. Thurmond AS, Machan LS, Maubon AJ, Rouanet JP, Hovsepian DM, Moore A, Zagoria RJ, Dickey KW, Bass JC. A review of selective salpingography and fallopian tube catheterization. Radiographics. 2000;20(6):1759–68. https://doi.org/10.1148/radiographics.20.6.g00nv211759.
16. Karasick S, Goldfarb AF. Peritubal adhesions in infertile women: diagnosis with hysterosalpingography. AJR Am J Roentgenol. 1989;152(4):777–9. https://doi.org/10.2214/ajr.152.4.777.
17. Valentini AL, Muzii L, Marana R, Catalano GF, Summaria V, Felici F, Rossetti A, Destito C. Improvement of hysterosalpingographic accuracy in the diagnosis of peritubal adhesions. AJR Am J Roentgenol. 2000;175(4):1173–6. https://doi.org/10.2214/ajr.175.4.1751173.
18. Practice Committee of the American Society for Reproductive Medicine. Diagnostic evaluation of the infertile female: a committee opinion. Fertil Steril. 2015;103(6):e44–50. https://doi.org/10.1016/j.fertnstert.2015.03.019.
19. Graziano A, Lo Monte G, Soave I, Caserta D, Moscarini M, Marci R. Sonohysterosalpingography: a suitable choice in infertility workup. J Med Ultrason. 2013;40:225–9. https://doi.org/10.1007/s10396-012-0417-0.
20. Hajishafiha M, Zobairi T, Rasoli Zanjani V, Ghasemi-Rad M, Yekta Z, Mladkova N. Diagnostic value of sonohysterography in the determination of fallopian tube patency as an initial step of routine infertility assessment. J Ultrasound Med. 2009;28(12):1671–7. https://doi.org/10.7863/jum.2009.28.12.1671.
21. Luciano DE, Exacoustos C, Luciano AA. Contrast ultrasonography for tubal patency. J Minim Invasive Gynecol. 2014;21(6):994–8. https://doi.org/10.1016/j.jmig.2014.05.017.
22. Cipolla V, Guerrieri D, Pietrangeli D, Santucci D, Argirò R, de Felice C. Role of 3.0 tesla magnetic resonance hysterosalpingography in the diagnostic work-up of female infertility. Acta Radiol. 2016;57(9):1132–9. https://doi.org/10.1177/0284185115617351.
23. Jiugen R, Chunyan W, Changhua Z, Yao D, Qiuping T, Tao M. The imaging characteristics of magnetic resonance hysterosalpingography in infertile women. Int J Clin Exp Med. 2020;13(6):3955–62.
24. Badawy SZ, Singer S. Proximal tubal obstruction: pathogenesis and management. J Gynecol Surg. 2019;35(5):296–8. https://doi.org/10.1089/gyn.2019.0044.
25. Thurmond AS. Fallopian tube catheterization. Semin Intervent Radiol. 2013;30(4):381–7. https://doi.org/10.1055/s-0033-1359732.

8 Embolics and Sclerosis in Pelvic Congestion Syndrome

Giovanni Failla, Cecilia Gozzo, Francesco Vacirca, Serafino Santonocito, Daniele Falsaperla, Davide Castiglione, Stefano Palmucci, Domenico Patanè, and Antonio Basile

8.1 Introduction

Pelvic congestion syndrome (PCS) is characterized by chronic pelvic pain in female patients with gonadal vein dilatation and parauterine varices [1, 2].

Radiological examinations needed for PCS diagnosis include Doppler Ultrasound, CT scan, and MRI; transcatheter venography is considered the gold standard for diagnosis, but it is often performed after inconclusive noninvasive previous exams [3, 4]. Treatment of PCS includes medical, surgical, and endovascular treatments [5].

Transcatheter embolization for PCS consists of endovascular occlusion of uterine and pelvic refluxing veins with various embolizing materials and techniques [4].

The planning for PCS endovascular treatment is based on the choice of:

- Venous approach
- Target vessels to embolize
- Types of embolic agents
- Embolization technique

Our aim is to review all the embolic and sclerosis agents used for PCS treatment and their applications, clinical outcomes, and complications.

8.2 Patient Preparation

Detailed clinical assessment by a gynecologist is required for women with chronic pelvic pain, in order to exclude other causes of symptoms. Patients with lower extremities varicosities need clinical and duplex ultrasound assessment of venous reflux.

Patients should be evaluated in the interventional radiology unit prior to the procedures to explain to them the risks of the interventions. An informed consent specific to the procedure should be obtained by the interventional radiologist before the procedure [6]. It is important to know certain basic questions before starting: known allergies, medications, comorbidities, and symptoms: Post-coital ache (dyspareunia), menstrual disorders, bladder irritability, and functional GI symptoms must be noted.

Timing of the procedure in relation to the menstrual or pain cycle is unimportant [7].

The anatomical or pathological conditions of the access site (transfemoral, transbrachial,

G. Failla (✉) · S. Santonocito · D. Patanè
Department of Diagnostic and Interventional Radiology, Azienda Ospedaliera per l'Emergenza Cannizzaro, Catania, Italy

C. Gozzo · F. Vacirca · D. Falsaperla · D. Castiglione
S. Palmucci · A. Basile
Department of Medical and Surgical Sciences and Advanced Technologies-Radiodiagnostic and Radiotherapy Unit, University Hospital "Policlinico-Vittorio Emanuele", Catania, Italy
e-mail: S.palmucci@sirm.org

R. Niola et al. (eds.), *Diagnostic and Interventional Radiology in Gynecological and Obstetric Diseases*, https://doi.org/10.1007/978-3-031-11910-1_8

or transjugular) to perform the procedure should be evaluated before using an ultrasound machine.

8.2.1 Anesthesia and Pain Control

Intraprocedural sedoanalgesia with midazolam and Fentanyl and analgesics if necessary. Post-procedure for post-embolization syndrome (PES), nonsteroidal anti-inflammatory drugs are the mainstay of treatment.

8.3 Technique

8.3.1 Venous Approach

Percutaneous embolization for PCS can be performed through different venous approaches such as transjugular and transbrachial (i.e., transbasilic) venous approach [8–12].

The right internal jugular vein approach, along with the basilic vein one, affords an antegrade approach to the pelvic veins with higher material pushability [12, 13].

The transbrachial venous approach is preferred in the case of bilateral PCS [14] also because it increases patient compliance.

Standard materials for transbrachial access include:

1. 5F sheath and a 90-cm and 6F introducer sheath
2. 4 or 5F diagnostic catheters, typically with Multipurpose or Cobra configuration with 100 cm of length
3. 0.035″ standard and hydrophilic guidewires
4. PTA Dilatation catheters with diameters ranging from 6 to 20 mm
5. Various types of embolic agents (i.e., coils, plugs, and sclerotic agents)

8.3.2 Vessels to Embolize

In the literature, there is no consensus in terms of the number of vessels to embolize or embolic materials due to the lack of an adequate randomized controlled trial [5].

No statistically significant difference between unilateral and bilateral PCS embolization was seen [9, 15].

Therefore, the embolization can involve only refluxing veins (usually the left), both ovarian veins (OVs), and both OVs and internal iliac veins (IIVs) [16–18] (Fig. 8.1).

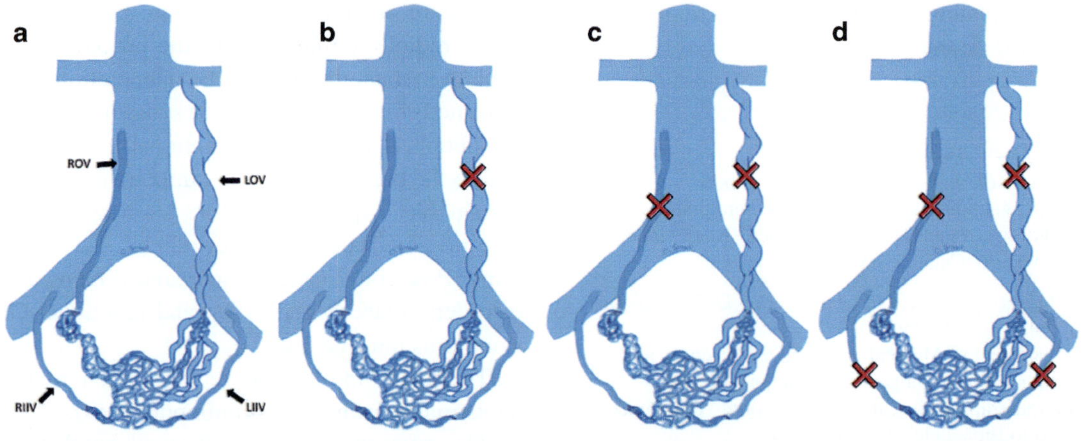

Fig. 8.1 Drawing illustrating left ovarian vein dilation (**a**); the different vessels that can be embolized are shown with a *red* "x": only LOV (**b**); both ovarian veins (OVs) (**c**); and both OVs and IIVs (**d**). LOV, left ovarian vein; OVs, ovarian veins; IIV, internal iliac veins; ROV, right ovarian vein; LOV, left ovarian vein; RIIV, right internal iliac vein; LIIV, left internal iliac vein

Bilateral OVs embolization, proposed by Edwards et al. in 1993, was first the chosen technique [17, 19, 20].

The persisting symptoms over a period of 3/6 months after PCS embolization or the documented communication with IIV can also require IIV embolization [16].

In the experience of Laborda et al., the PCS embolization of only one or two of them can result in hypertrophy of the remaining vessels, which might be due to their close connection; so they performed embolization of all four venous axes of the pelvis (both OVs and IIVs) using coils [21]. Also, Kim et al. usually performed the OVs embolization followed by IIV embolization in a subsequent procedure [18].

8.3.3 Embolic Agents

Embolic agents used for PCS embolization range from liquid to solid. Liquid embolic agents include sclerotic agents, that is, polidocanol, glue, or lipiodized oil [22–24].

As solid embolic agents, in addition to coils or plugs, Amplatzer Vascular Plug (AVP) can be used [15, 21, 25, 26]. Some authors suggest the use of temporary embolic agents such as gelatin foam (gelfoam) [18, 26, 27]. Different types of embolic agents are summarized in Table 8.1.

Table 8.1 Types of embolic agents and their constitution

Embolic agents	Mechanism of action	Materials
Coils:	Permanent mechanical occlusion	Platinum or stainless steel coated
Pushable or detachables	Platelets activation	With different materials like dacron, nylon, or silk fibers
Vascular plugs	Permanent mechanical	Disks of self-expanding nitinol mesh
Glue in combination with lipiodized oil	Polymerization in contact with blood	Enbucrylate plus lipiodized oil
	Damage to the vascular endothelium	
Sclerosing agents	Venous wall damage	Polidocanol
	Occlusion of the vessel	Sodium tetradecyl sulfate (STS) sodium morrhuate
		Ethanolamine oleate
Gelfoam plus sclerotic agent	Venous wall damage	Absorbable sterile gelatin compressed sponge and sodium morrhuate
	Occlusion of the vessel	

8.3.4 Embolization Techniques

Combined embolization of multiple embolic agents is preferred over single-agent embolization. Some groups perform PCS embolization with only coils [13, 17, 20, 21, 25]. Indeed, coils and plugs placement can be performed with the addition of sclerosant [22–28]. Among the other embolic agents added to coils, we find gelfoam [18, 27], glue, and lipiodized oil injection [23, 24]. Other authors promote sclerotherapy with 3% sodium tetradecyl sulfate [14, 29]. Technical success, defined as complete occlusion of refluxing vein, is achieved in all these techniques (98% to 100%) with few and minor complications [8]. Some authors propose the balloon-occluded technique which allows to determine when the pelvic varices are completely filled by the sclerosing agent and to avoid its systemic dispersion [5, 29]. Clinical improvement is similar among coil embolization, sclerotherapy, and combined use of embolic agents, whereas that of glue and lipiodized oil is relatively lower [9].

The choice of the embolic material is guided by the type of Insufficiency highlighted in the phlebographic study.

8.3.5 Phlebographic Study and Classification

The first step of every type of embolization is transcatheter venography which represents the gold standard for PCS diagnosis and allows classification (Fig. 8.2). Beard et al. proposed a scoring system based on three components:

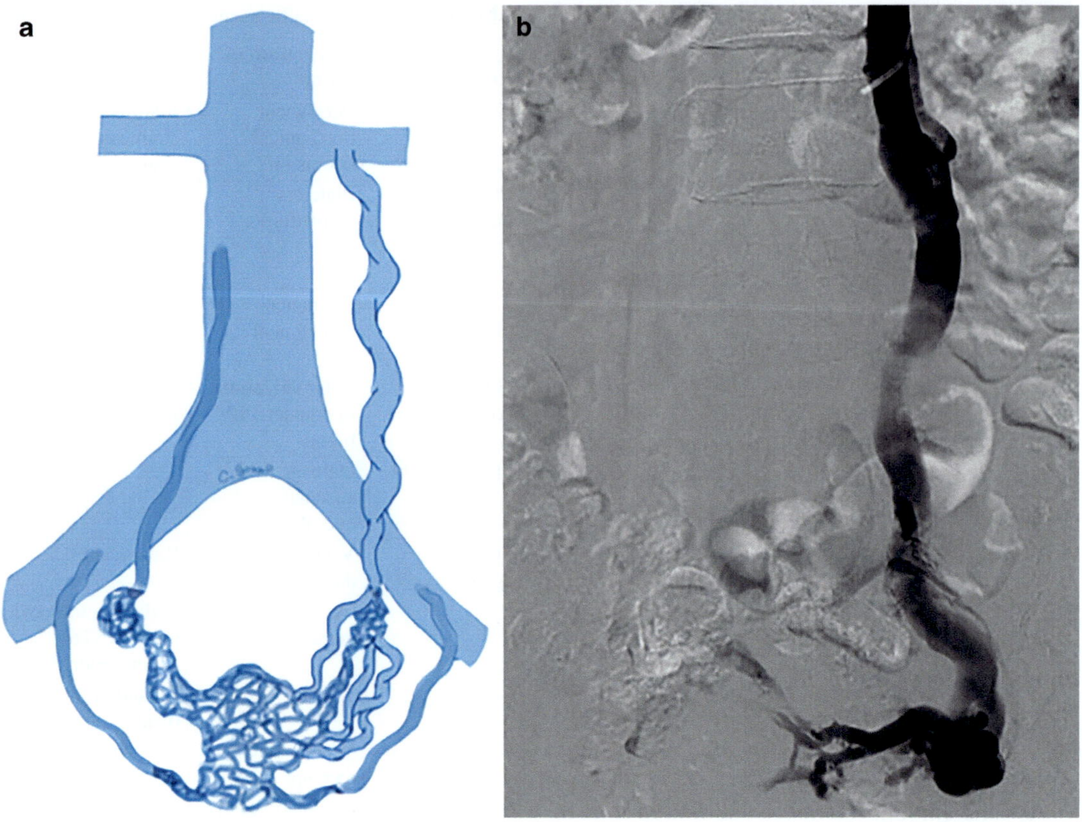

Fig. 8.2 Drawing (**a**) and phlebographic image (**b**) showing severe dilation of the left ovarian vein with uterine vein engorgement and initial partial filling of the contralateral vein

maximum diameter of the ovarian vein, time to disappearance of contrast material, and degree of congestion [30]. Each component is scored from 1 to 3 and a score of 5 or more is an objective measure of pelvic congestion. Ovarian vein diameter was considered normal between 1 and 4 mm; moderate, 5–8 mm; and severe, greater than 8 mm. Time to disappearance of contrast medium was scored on the basis of a time of 0, 20, or 40 s. Degree of congestion was considered normal if veins were small, straight, and easily seen; moderate when veins were tortuous with variable caliber; and severe if veins were highly tortuous, wide with great variation in caliber [30].

8.3.6 Embolization with Coils or Vascular Plugs

Transcatheter pelvic vein embolization with coils as the embolic agent (Fig. 8.3) was first reported in 1993 by Edwards et al. [19]. There are not enough clinical evidence or randomized studies to compare outcomes and recurrence using only coils or the combined treatment [21].

Initially, the coils used for PCS embolization include steel and platinum coils with a diameter ranging from 5 to 15 mm [13, 17]. More recently, 8–12 mm diameter coils 'fibered' with synthetic dacron rather than plain non-fibered coils have been proposed due to the more rapid occlusion

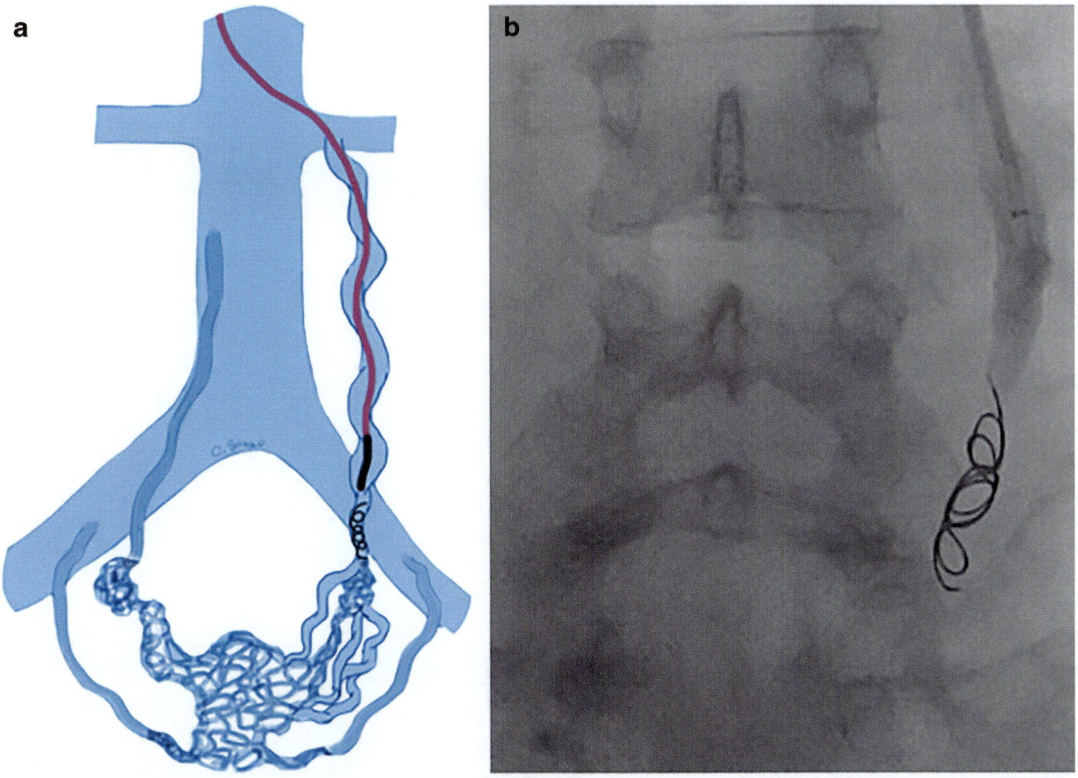

Fig. 8.3 Drawing (**a**) and fluoroscopic image (**b**) showing coils embolization of left ovarian vein. In detail, Retracta Detachable Embolization coils (Cook Medical, MWCER-35-7-8) were used

with fewer coils required and consequently lower procedural time [13].

In addition to their use alone, coils should be combined with other embolic materials such as sclerosant [22, 28], glue [23], and gelfoam [18, 27]. Clinical improvement following coil embolization ranges from about 82.1% to 100% even when combined with sclerosant agents [9].

In the case of medium-sized to large-sized venous vessels, in order to avoid the placement of multiple coils, AVPs (12–14 mm) in place of coils (Fig. 8.4) in combination with a sclerotic agent could be used [15, 31]. Although the number of devices was lower, the embolization with AVPs shows higher cost compared to the coils one [31]. The advantages of embolization with AVPs are short fluoroscopy time and lower radiation dose [31].

8.3.7 Embolization with a Mixture of Glue and Lipiodized Oil

Embolization with a mixture of glue (enbucrilate) and lipiodized oil showed a lower clinical improvement rate ranging from 68.3% to 73.7% [5, 9, 14, 24, 29, 32]. Other authors used enbucrilate/lipiodized oil mixture alone and also in combination with coils [23].

8.3.8 Embolization with Gelfoam

Gelfoam is a temporary absorbable embolic agent. The injection of gelfoam, used as a slurry made with a sclerotic agent (sodium morrhuate), is often followed by coil embolization [18, 27]. This combined technique has a clinical success rate of about 80–100% [9].

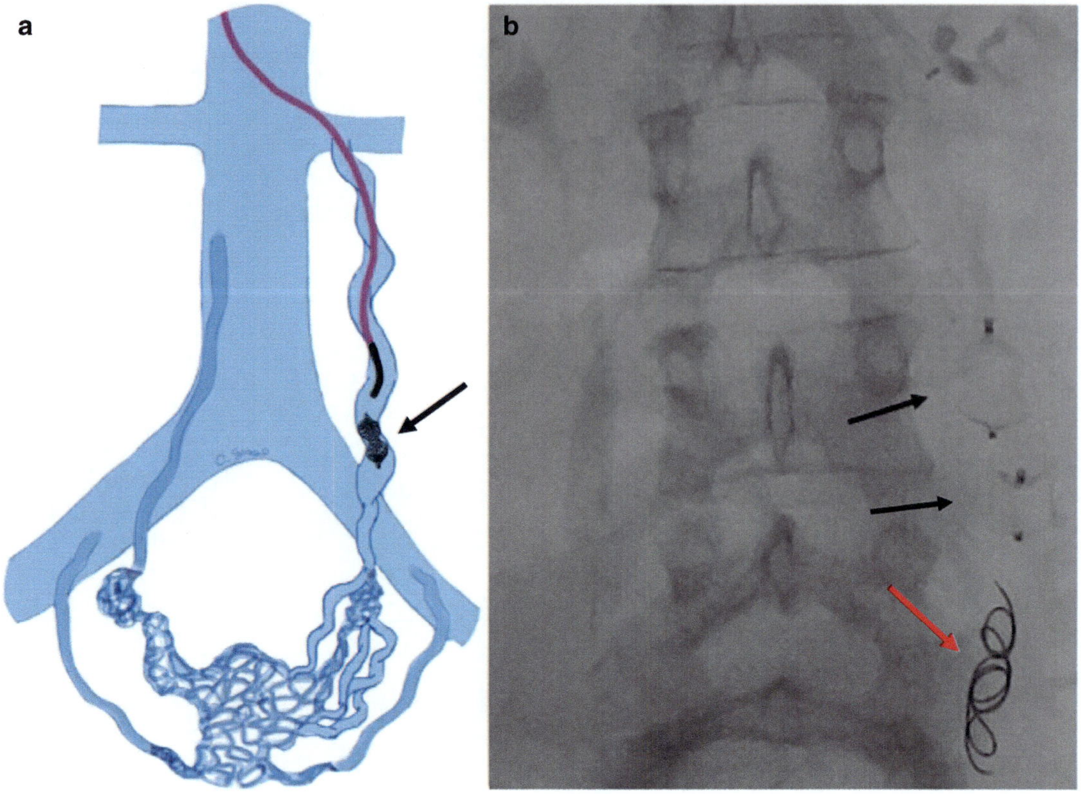

Fig. 8.4 Drawing (**a**) and fluoroscopic image (**b**) showing embolization of left ovarian vein with two AVPs type I (*black* arrows) and a coil (*red* arrow) released before in the ovarian vein

8.3.9 Sclerotherapy

Sclerotherapy is performed through the injection of sodium tetradecyl sulphate (STS) at 3% in foam form [14, 29]. The foam form allows increased contact with the endothelial surface and the use of smaller volumes of the sclerosing agent with reduced toxic effects [29]. This technique also requires the use of an occluding balloon catheter which is positioned at about the lower third of the sacroiliac joint (in the case of OVs embolization) and inflated during the STS foam injection [22, 29] (Fig. 8.5). Some groups performed coils placement after the STS injection [22]. Other authors performed embolization with polidocanol at 2% in foam form either alone for vessel segments not accessible to coil placement or in combination with coils in a 'sandwich' technique [28].

8.3.10 Balloon-Occluded Technique

The balloon-occluded retrograde transvenous embolization (B-RTO) was first described by Kanagawa et al. for the treatment of large gastric fundal varices [33]. Then a balloon-occluded retrograde transvenous embolization from the IIVs has been proposed as a completion of pelvic varicocele embolization with residual low-outflow collaterals that are tributaries to the hypogastric vein [18, 22, 27, 29]. For this purpose, a sub selective balloon-occlusion venography of the IIVs was performed to better visualize residual pelvic varices in the pelvic, vulvar, or thigh regions, in patients already treated with OVs embolization [18, 22, 27]. Therefore, in addition to the venography study, the occluding balloon catheter also plays a role in the embolization [18, 27, 29]. This technique consists of balloon infla-

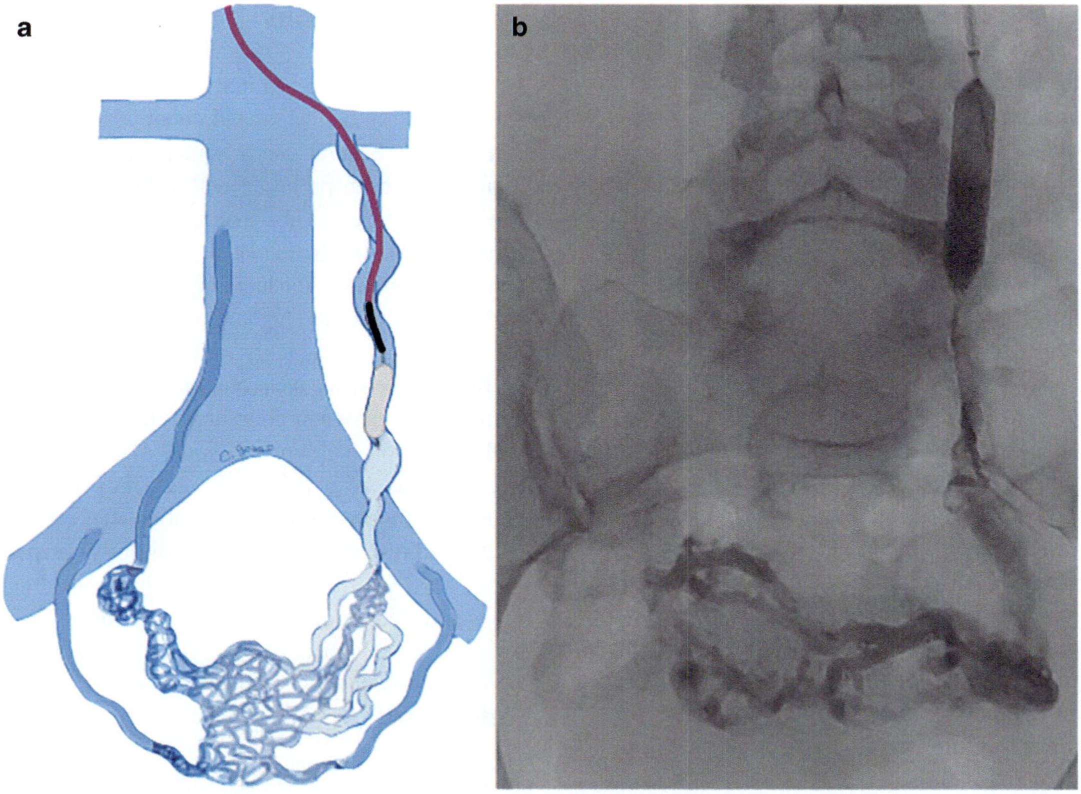

Fig. 8.5 Drawing (**a**) and fluoroscopic image (**b**) showing sclerotherapy with polidocanol at 3% of the left ovarian vein and uterine veins using the balloon-occluded technique

tion during sclerosant/gelfoam injection in order to determine when the pelvic varices are completely filled by the sclerosing agent, thus optimizing the quantity of the agent used and avoiding its systemic dispersion [29].

The occlusion balloon has to be positioned to the lower third of the sacroiliac joint (in the case of OVs embolization) or selectively to the incompetent vein (in case of IIVs embolization) [22].

8.4 Clinical Outcomes

In the last years, PCS treatment was reviewed by two important literature systematic reviews made by Brown et al. and Hansrani et al. [8, 9].

These reviews showed a similar clinical improvement rate (80–100%) between coil embolization, sclerotherapy, and combined use of these agents; a lower improvement rate (68.3–73.7%) was reported for embolization with glue and lipiodized oil [9, 27].

Regarding the territory to embolize, complete embolization (including ovarian, internal iliac, and additional variceal vessels) showed a range of clinical success lower than the limited one (ovarian and iliac interventions alone) [9].

In the literature, the recurrence rate is highly variable, ranging from 0% to 39% and providing worse results if only sclerosing agents are used [34].

8.5 Complications

Complications after PCS endovascular treatment are rare (0.85–10% rate) and often mild [9]. PCS complications can be immediate or delayed [13]. Immediate complications include access site related (i.e., hematoma, pneumothorax for venous catheterization via a neck vein); non-target embolization (i.e., coil misplacement, into the left external iliac or common femoral vein, or uncontrolled foam); and stroke (i.e., coil migration or uncontrolled foam) [9, 13, 35].

Delayed complications include enlarging pneumothorax and coil migration, for example, pulmonary embolization of coils [9, 13].

Another complication well recognized is PES, occurring in about 20% of patients undergoing endovascular coil embolization for PCS [36].

PES is characterized by gluteal and lumbar severe post-procedural pain (54%), hyperthermia (12.5%), and fatigue caused by an introduction of foreign bodies into the venous lumen and the development of inflammatory response in vessel walls [28, 36].

Cases of allergic reactions to nitinol coils implanted in the gonadal veins (as well as to contrast media) were reported [28].

Other reported complications are OV rupture and contrast extravasation without the need for reinterventions or glue migration in the pulmonary circulation.

Complications are summarized in Table 8.2.

Table 8.2 Summary of the types of complications distinguished between immediate and delayed

Complications	
Immediate	Delayed
Hematoma	Enlarging pneumothorax
Pneumothorax	Coil migration, for example, pulmonary embolization of coils
Non-target embolization (i.e., coil misplacement, into left external iliac or common femoral vein or uncontrolled foam)	PES
Stroke (i.e., coil migration or uncontrolled foam)	Allergic reactions to nitinol coils placed in ovarian veins
Allergic reactions to contrast media	
OV rupture and contrast extravasation	
Glue migration in the pulmonary circulation	

8.6 Conclusions

No consensus is achieved in the literature about the technique of embolization and about which vessels to embolize. Several endovascular treatment techniques have been proposed with different embolic agents, in some cases also in combination (i.e., sclerosant foam and coils, amplatzer plug, and sclerosant gents). According to the literature, clinical and technical success rates are high (about 80–100%) while the recurrence rate is highly variable.

In our experience we prefer embolization with a combination between coils and sclerosant agents with occlusion balloon technique, often performing bilateral OVs occlusion and IIVs only in patients with lower extremities varicosities.

Nowadays, interventional radiology is preferred for PCS treatment because it allows diagnosis and treatment in the same sessions.

References

1. Bookwalter CA, VanBuren WM, Neisen MJ, Bjarnason H. Imaging appearance and nonsurgical Management of Pelvic Venous Congestion Syndrome. Radiographics. 2019;39(2):596–608. https://doi.org/10.1148/rg.2019180159.
2. Jurga-Karwacka A, Karwacki GM, Schoetzau A, Zech CJ, Heinzelmann-Schwarz V, Schwab FD. A forgotten disease: pelvic congestion syndrome as a cause of chronic lower abdominal pain. PLoS One. 2019;14(4):e0213834.
3. Hiromura T, Nishioka T, Nishioka S, Ikeda H, Tomita K. Reflux in the left ovarian vein: analysis of MDCT findings in asymptomatic women. AJR Am J Roentgenol. 2004;183(5):1411–5.
4. Knuttinen MG, Xie K, Jani A, et al. Pelvic venous insufficiency: imaging diagnosis, treatment approaches, and therapeutic issues. AJR Am J Roentgenol. 2015;204:448–58.
5. Basile A, Failla G, Gozzo C. Pelvic congestion syndrome. Semin Ultrasound CT MR. 2021;42(1):3–12.
6. Kessel D, Ray CE. Transcatheter embolization and therapy. London: Springer-Verlag; 2010.
7. Kandarpa K, Machan L, Durham JD. Handbook of interventional radiologic procedures. Philadelphia: Lippincot Williams & Wilkins; 2016.
8. Hansrani V, Abbas A, Bhandari S, et al. Trans-venous occlusion of incompetent pelvic veins for chronic

pelvic pain in women: a systematic review. Eur J Obstet Gynecol Reprod Biol. 2015;185:156–63.
9. Brown CL, Rizer M, Alexander R, et al. Pelvic congestion syndrome: systematic review of treatment success. Semin Intervent Radiol. 2018;35:35–40.
10. Mongioì LM, Mammino L, Compagnone M, et al. Effects of varicocele treatment on sperm conventional parameters: surgical varicocelectomy versus sclerotherapy. Cardiovasc Intervent Radiol. 2019;42(3):396–404.
11. Di Silverio F, Gentile V, La Pera G, Minucci S, Morucci M. Transbrachial approach in spermatic phlebography. Br J Urol. 1991;68(1):108–9.
12. Pieri S, Agresti P, Morucci M, De'Medici L, Fiocca G, Calisti A. A transbranchial approach for the percutaneous therapy of pediatric varicocele. Radiol Med. 2003;106(3):221–31.
13. Lopez AJ. Female pelvic vein embolization: indications, techniques, and outcomes. Cardiovasc Intervent Radiol. 2015;38:806–20.
14. Pieri S, Agresti P, Morucci M, et al. Percutaneous treatment of pelvic congestion syndrome. Radiol Med. 2003;105:76–82.
15. Basile A, Marletta G, Tsetis D, et al. The Amplatzer vascular plug also for ovarian vein embolization. Cardiovasc Intervent Radiol. 2008;31:446–7.
16. Nicholson T, Basile A. Pelvic congestion syndrome, who should we treat and how? Tech Vasc Interv Radiol. 2006;9:19–23.
17. Kwon SH, Oh JH, Ko KR, et al. Transcatheter ovarian vein embolization using coils for the treatment of pelvic congestion syndrome. Cardiovasc Intervent Radiol. 2007;30:655–61.
18. Kim HS, Malhotra AD, Rowe PC, et al. Embolotherapy for pelvic congestion syndrome: long-term results. J Vasc Interv Radiol. 2006;17:289–97.
19. Edwards RD, Robertson IR, MacLean AB, et al. Case report: pelvic pain syndrome-successful treatment of a case by ovarian vein embolization. Clin Radiol. 1993;47:429–31.
20. Tarazov PG, Prozorovskij KV, Ryzhkov VK. Pelvic pain syndrome caused by ovarian varices: treatment by transcatheter embolization. Acta Radiol. 1997;38:1023–5.
21. Laborda A, Medrano J, de Blas I, et al. Endovascular treatment of pelvic congestion syndrome: visual analog scale (VAS) long-term follow-up clinical evaluation in 202 patients. Cardiovasc Intervent Radiol. 2013;36:1006–14.
22. Meneses L, Fava M, Diaz P, et al. Embolization of incompetent pelvic veins for the treatment of recurrent varicose veins in lower limbs and pelvic congestion syndrome. Cardiovasc Intervent Radiol. 2013;36:128–32.
23. Capasso P, Simons C, Trotteur G, et al. Treatment of symptomatic pelvic varices by ovarian vein embolization. Cardiovasc Intervent Radiol. 1997;2:107–11.
24. Maleux G, Stockx L, Wilms G, Marchal G. Ovarian vein embolization for the treatment of pelvic congestion syndrome: long-term technical and clinical results. J Vasc Interv Radiol. 2000;11(7):859–64.
25. Chung MH, Huh CY. Comparison of treatments for pelvic congestion syndrome. Tohoku J Exp Med. 2003;201:131–8.
26. Katz MD, Sugay SB, Walker DK, et al. Beyond hemostasis: spectrum of gynecologic and obstetric indications for transcatheter embolization. Radiographics. 2012;32:1713–31.
27. Venbrux AC, Chang AH, Kim HS, et al. Pelvic congestion syndrome (pelvic venous incompetence): impact of ovarian and internal iliac vein embolotherapy on menstrual cycle and chronic pelvic pain. J Vasc Interv Radiol. 2002;13:171–8.
28. Monedero JL, Zubicoa Ezpeleta S, Castro Castro J, et al. Embolization treatment of recurrent varices of pelvic origin. Phlebology. 2006;21:3–11.
29. Gandini R, Konda D, Abrignani S, et al. Treatment of symptomatic high-flow female varicoceles with stop-flow foam sclerotherapy. Cardiovasc Intervent Radiol. 2014;37:1259–67.
30. Beard RW, Highman JH, Pearce S, et al. Diagnosis of pelvic varicosities in women with chronic pelvic pain. Lancet. 1984;2:946–9.
31. Guirola JA, Sánchez-Ballestin M, Sierre S, Lahuerta C, Mayoral V, De Gregorio MA. A randomized trial of endovascular embolization treatment in pelvic congestion syndrome: fibered platinum coils versus vascular plugs with 1-year clinical outcomes. J Vasc Interv Radiol. 2018;29(1):45–53. https://doi.org/10.1016/j.jvir.2017.09.011.
32. Hansrani V, Abbas A, Bhandari S, Caress AL, Seif M, McCollum CN. Trans-venous occlusion of incompetent pelvic veins for chronic pelvic pain in women: a systematic review. Eur J Obstet Gynecol Reprod Biol. 2015;185:156–63.
33. Kanagawa H, Mima S, Kouyama H, et al. A successfully treated case of fundic varices by retrograde transvenous obliteration with balloon. Jpn J Gastroenterol. 1991;88:1459–62.
34. Tiralongo F, Distefano G, Palermo M, Granata A, Giurazza F, Vacirca F, Palmucci S, Venturini M, Basile A. Liquid and solid embolic agents in gonadal veins. J Clin Med. 2021;10:1596. https://doi.org/10.3390/jcm10081596.
35. Marsh P, Holdstock JM, Bacon JL, Lopez AJ, Whiteley MS, Price BA. Coil protruding into the common femoral vein following pelvic venous embolization. Cardiovasc Interv Radiol. 2008;31(2):435–8.
36. Gavrilov SG, Krasavin GV, Mishakina NY, Kirsanov KV. Post-embolization syndrome in endovascular interventions on the gonadal veins. J Vasc Surg Venous Lymphat Disord. 2021;9(3):697–702.

Endovascular Embolization of Uterine Myomas and Adenomyosis

9

Andrea Contegiacomo, Luigi Natale, Anna Rita Scrofani, Ernesto Punzi, Alessandro Cina, and Riccardo Manfredi

9.1 Introduction

Uterine fibroids and adenomyosis are common conditions that impair the quality of life of many women in their fertile age. Interventional treatment via endovascular embolization of both fibroids and adenomyosis has gained a central role in the management of these conditions during the last decades. This chapter focuses on the clinical and technical aspects of uterine fibroids and adenomyosis that interventionists need to know for a better approach to endovascular treatment.

9.2 Epidemiology and Clinical Features of Uterine Fibroids and Adenomyosis

9.2.1 Fibroids

Uterine fibroids, also known as leiomyomas and myomas, are the commonest gynecological tumors. In general, fibroids have a prevalence of 70–80% in women above the age of 50 [1, 2], showing a progressive increase with age, and peaking in women in their 40s [2, 3]. Fibroids are extremely heterogeneous in their pathophysiology, size, location, and clinical symptomatology [1]. The myometrium of the uterine corpus is involved in the majority of cases but myomas may also occur in the cervix in less than 5% of patients [4]. Leiomyomas are classified as submucosal, intramural, or subserosal according to anatomical location (Fig. 9.1). Submucosal leiomyomas are the less common type (approximately 5%), and they are commonly associated with dysmenorrhea, menorrhagia, or infertility, while intramural fibroids are the most common type of fibroids and are typically asymptomatic [4]. In some patients, myomas may cause significant morbidity including bulk symptoms (e.g., pelvic pressure/pain, obstructive symptoms); menstrual abnormalities (e.g., heavy, irregular, and prolonged uterine bleeding); anemia; and fertility disorders (lower pregnancy rates and a greater incidence of miscarriage in patients with submucosal fibroids, increase pregnancy risks) [5, 6], worsening quality of life as well as productivity [2]. Menorrhagia is the most common symptom and the primary indication for treatment, although bulk symptoms often occur and can be treated [5]. Submucosal fibroids are usually more symptomatic than subserosal or small intramural fibroids. Bulk symptoms are more

A. Contegiacomo (✉) · L. Natale · A. R. Scrofani
E. Punzi · A. Cina · R. Manfredi
Dipartimento di Diagnostica per Immagini, Radioterapia Oncologica ed Ematologia—Istituto di Radiologia, Fondazione Policlinico Universitario A. Gemelli IRCCS, Rome, Italy
e-mail: luigi.natale@policlinicogemelli.it; alessandro.cina@policlinicogemelli.it; riccardo.manfredi@policlinicogemelli.it

R. Niola et al. (eds.), *Diagnostic and Interventional Radiology in Gynecological and Obstetric Diseases*, https://doi.org/10.1007/978-3-031-11910-1_9

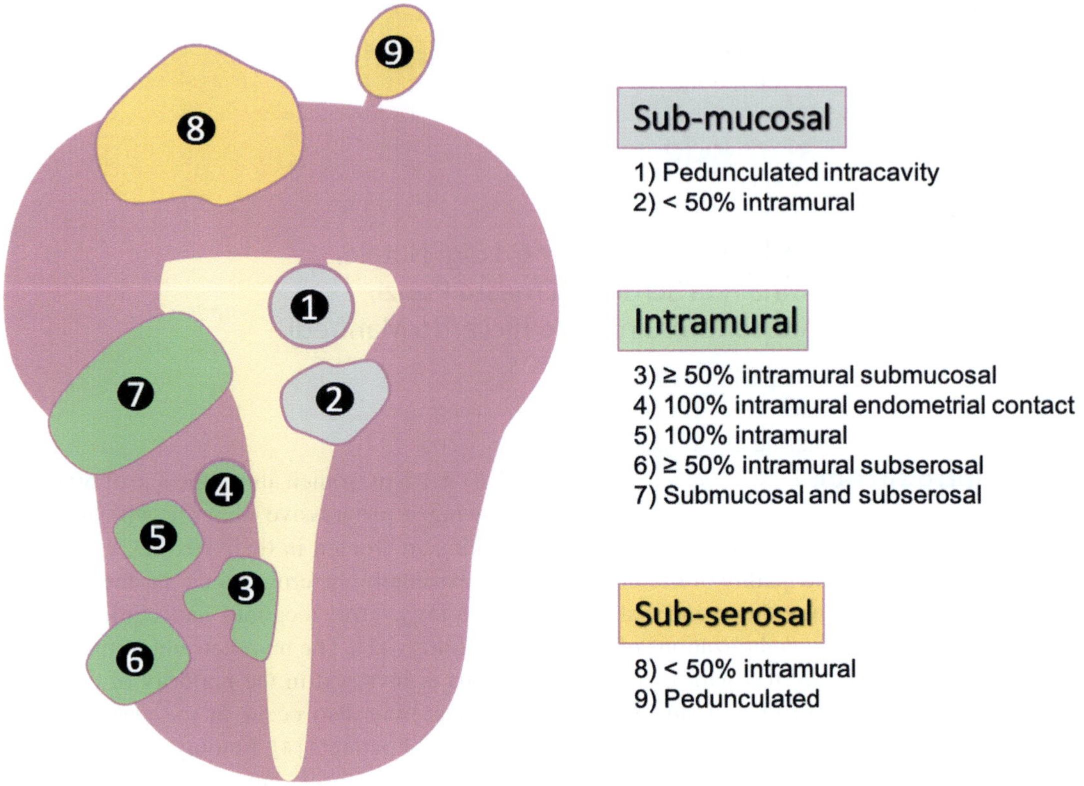

Fig. 9.1 Uterine fibroids classification

often seen with large intramural or subserosal fibroids due to their extra-compartimental development [6].

9.2.2 Adenomyosis

Adenomyosis is defined as the ectopic presence of endometrial glands and stroma within the myometrium with hypertrophy of the surrounding myometrial smooth muscle. Adenomyosis occurs in focal and diffuse forms, with the second one representing the most common type, predominantly located in the posterior uterine wall. Usually these elements are found at least 2.5 mm below the endometrial–myometrial junction. The prevalence of adenomyosis in tissues obtained from hysterectomy is reported to be between 8.8% and 31%. If broad criteria for the diagnosis of adenomyosis are used, some data suggest a prevalence as high as 70% in women between 40 and 50 years of age [4, 7]. Approximately one-third of women with adenomyosis are symptomatic [8] and the clinical manifestations of adenomyosis are similar to those occurring in fibroids [9], including abnormal menstrual bleeding, pain, bulk-related symptoms, and the coexistence with other pelvic diseases such as leiomyomas and endometriosis [10, 11].

9.3 Treatment Options and Clinical Indications to Uterine Artery Embolization

Multiple treatment options are available for uterine myomas and adenomyosis, ranging from surgery to medical therapy. The main indication for operative management is the presence of symptoms that reduce the patient's quality of life. Less frequently, the rapid growth of an asymptomatic myoma is an adequate indication for surgical removal because of the concern for malignancy [12].

In general, treatment options can be distinguished into medical, surgical, and mini-invasive. Medical treatment is focused on hormonal control of fibroids growth and includes progestins, gonadotropin-releasing hormone agonists and antagonists, progesterone receptor modulators, aromatase inhibitors, and hormone-containing intrauterine devices [13, 14].

Surgical management includes myomectomy via various routes including vaginal, hysteroscopic, laparoscopic (including robotics), and laparotomy. Hysterectomy remains the definitive treatment option, but it should be avoided in patients of childbearing age with a desire for offspring [15].

Other treatment options that enable uterine preservation include myolysis via freezing or hypothermia and thermal ablation via laser or radiofrequency electrical energy [16–18].

Mini-invasive treatment options include magnetic resonance imaging focused ultrasound (MRgFUS) and uterine artery embolization (UAE) or uterine fibroid embolization (UFE); these mini-invasive approaches offer the advantages of avoidance of surgical risks, potential preservation of fertility, and shorter hospitalization length [4]. Among mini-invasive treatments, recent meta-analysis and systematic reviews showed UFE superiority in respect of MRgFUS in terms of alleviation of symptoms, improvement in quality of life, postoperative reintervention rate, and pregnancy rate [19–21].

UAE is indicated for the treatment of symptomatic fibroids causing bleeding and/or mass-related symptoms (Table 9.1) and is considered an appropriate treatment from the American College of Radiology evidence-based 2018 guidelines in women affected by menometrorrhagia and with a desire for pregnancy [21].

Table 9.1 Classic indications to UAE

Menstrual	Disturbance menorrhagia
	Dysmenorrhea
	Pelvic pain
Mass-related symptoms	Urinary frequency
	Constipation

UAE uterine artery embolization

The success of UFE depends on appropriate patient selection [6]. In particular, patients with heavy menstrual bleeding or dysmenorrhea associated with intramural fibroids, premenopausal, and no desire for future pregnancy can be considered as optimal candidates for UFE [6, 22, 23]. Prospective cohort studies and randomized controlled trials of women who have undergone UFE have found a long-term improvement in bleeding symptoms as compared to bulk-related symptoms [24]. Moreover, a recent meta-analysis by Llewellyn et al. [25] attested that the treatment of giant fibroids (>10 cm) exposes women to a greater risk of reintervention and major complications compared to non-giant fibroids, suggesting that patients should be selected, counseled, and managed accordingly.

UAE was also investigated during the last two decades for the treatment of adenomyosis [26] mainly in women who do not respond to conservative treatment [27] and in whom hysterectomy was the only alternative treatment option.

Dueholm and Bruijn et al. reported up to 67% long-term (40 months) treatment success and up to 72% patient satisfaction rates, respectively [28].

Popovic et al. [7] proposed a review of the literature performed on 15 studies and 511 women with symptomatic adenomyosis showing an overall 75% symptom relief [7].

In a systematic review and meta-analysis by de Bruijn et al. [29], a short-term improvement was achieved in 89.6% of patients with only adenomyosis and 94.3% in patients with adenomyosis associated with uterine fibroids; the same study also established that long-term improvement was achieved in 74.0% of patients with pure adenomyosis and 84.5% of patients with adenomyosis and myomas [28].

An interesting prospective trial by Man Deuk Kin et al. proposed a new embolization technique for adenomyosis consisting of a progressive particles size range incrementation from 125–250 μm to 355–500 μm, obtaining an 82.5% complete necrosis of the adenomyosis, with complete symptoms relief in patients with complete

Table 9.2 Contraindications to UEA

Absolute	Ongoing pregnancy
	Active infection
	Suspected uterine, cervical, or adnexal malignancy
Relative	Coagulopathy
	Severe contrast medium allergy
	Renal impairment

UEA uterine artery embolization

necrosis at 18 months and absence of significant adverse events [30].

There is no definite agreement between absolute and relative contraindications to UAE (Table 9.2). Absolute contraindications to UFE are viable pregnancy; active infection without treatment; and suspected uterine, cervical, or adnexal malignancy (unless the procedure is being performed before the surgery). The relative contraindications to UAE include those typical of endovascular procedures such as coagulopathy, severe contrast medium allergy, and renal impairment [9, 31, 32].

9.4 Technical Aspects

UAE consists of the endovascular infusion of embolic agents into the uterine vascular district in order to reduce the blood supply to the fibroid, causing tumor infarction or volume reduction with subsequent symptom relief [33–35].

The procedure is usually performed under conscious sedation and local anesthesia, and general anesthesia is generally not required.

9.4.1 Type of Vascular Access

Arterial access is usually obtained through the right common femoral artery with a 21 G or 18 G cannula or metallic needle and Seldinger technique. A 5 French (Fr) introducer sheath is then placed in the common femoral artery [36]. Some authors proposed a transradial approach (TRA) for uterine artery embolization, comparing it to the trans-femoral approach (TFA) [37, 38]. These studies suggest that TRA is safe and feasible for UAE [39] with a safety profile comparable to TFA [38], similar technical and clinical outcomes, and lower rates of access site complications [40]. A recent study by Mortesens [41] compared the fluoro-time during UAE procedures performed with TRA versus TFA, suggesting that fluoro-time was similar for both approaches even though TRA requires a learning curve as it is a new technique.

9.4.2 Uterine Arteries Catheterization and Anatomy Evaluation

Whatever the access site, common and internal iliac arteries are usually engaged with a 4–5 Fr diagnostic catheter that is advanced into the uterine artery of each size distal to non-target branches (Fig. 9.2).

The internal iliac artery divides into an anterior and posterior branch in 57–77% of cases [42]. Uterine arteries usually arise from the anterior division of the internal iliac artery as the first (Fig. 9.3a) or the second/third branch (Fig. 9.3b) in 51% of cases [42]. Less frequently (15–40%), the internal iliac artery terminates in a trifurcation (uterine artery, inferior gluteal, and superior gluteal artery) (Fig. 9.3c), or the uterine arteries originate as the first branch of the internal iliac artery, above the level of gluteal arteries (6% of cases; Fig. 9.3d) [42, 43].

In patients with the most frequent bifurcation variants, the best angiographic projection is the contralateral anterior oblique with a 25°–40° angle [44]. The use of a micro-catheter is preferable in cases of complex anatomy or small uterine arteries in order to facilitate cannulation of the uterine arteries and may also reduce radiation exposure in fertile patients.

Uterine arteries show a typical U shape and are characterized by three segments: descending, transverse, and ascending. The descending segment has no side branches. A cervicovaginal branch typically arises from the mid- or distal portion of the transverse segment, and the vaginal artery can have a common trunk with the uterine artery. The ascending segment provides numer-

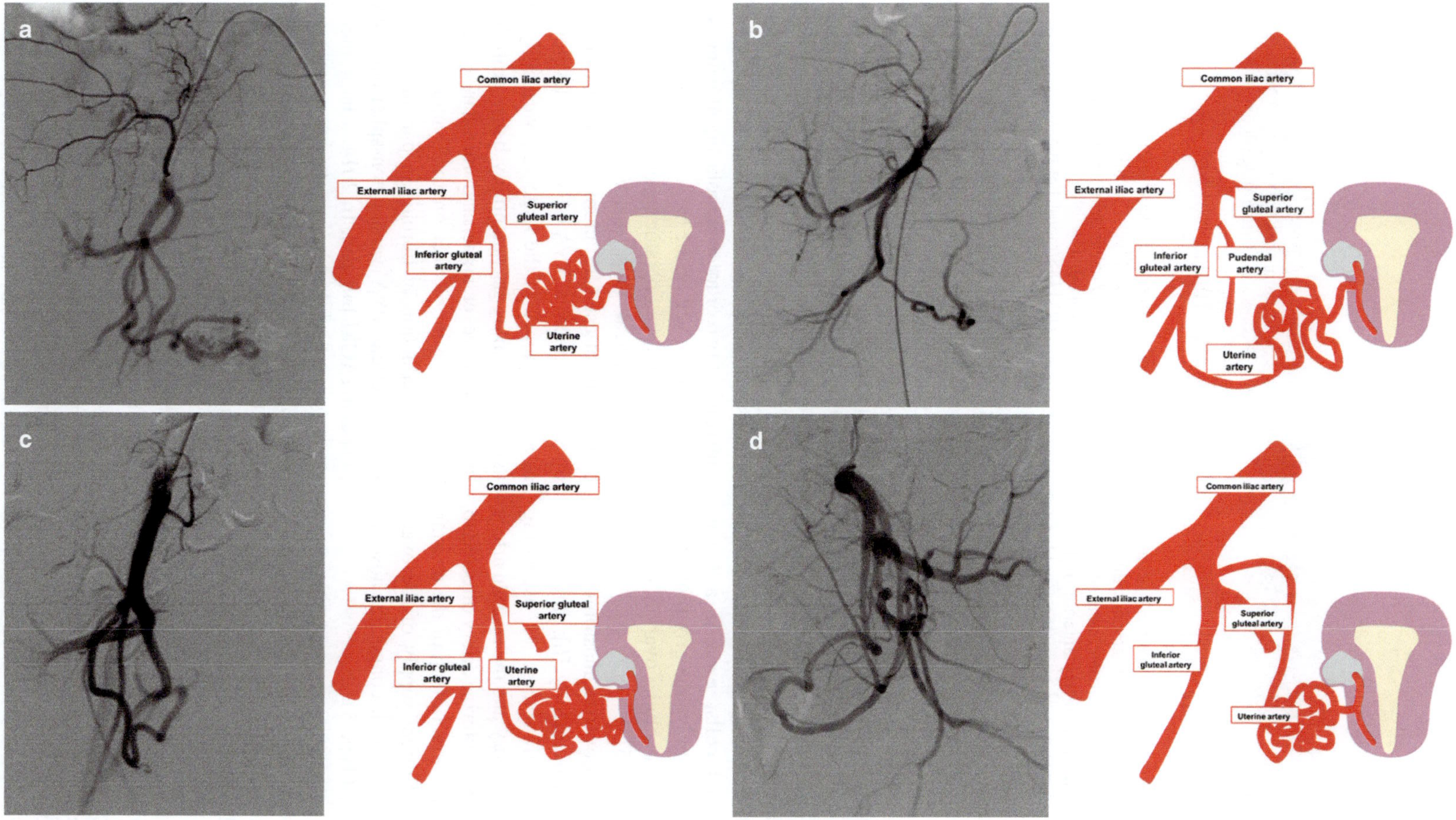

Fig. 9.2 Embolization steps: (**a**) Right internal iliac artery angiography; (**b–c**) The left (**b**) and right (**c**) uterine artery super selective angiographies with 2.7 F microcatheter show a large hypervascular fibroid; (**d**) Post-procedural complete embolization of right uterine artery

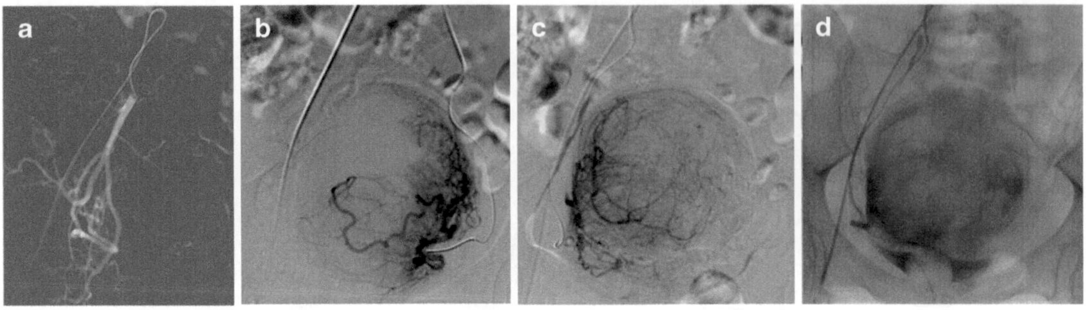

Fig. 9.3 (**a**) Type 1 anatomy: uterine artery arises as the first branch of the internal iliac artery anterior division. (**b**) Type 2 anatomy: uterine artery arises as the second or third branch of the internal iliac artery anterior division. (**c**) Type 3 anatomy: uterine artery arises at the same level of anterior and posterior division of the internal iliac artery (trifurcation). (**d**) Type 4 anatomy: uterine artery arises above the level of the anterior and posterior division of the internal iliac artery

ous branches coursing over the surface of the uterus sending numerous perforating arterioles.

After the uterine arteries have been cannulated, a diagnostic angiography should always be performed before embolization to rule out the presence of left-to-right and utero-ovarian anastomosis, which are present in about 50% of cases. The rationale for excluding these anastomoses is to prevent damage to the ovarian parenchyma and germinal cells, even if a recent meta-analysis carried out by the group of Tarek El Shamyl seems to exclude ovarian reserve reduction after UAE [45].

Three types of utero-ovarian anastomosis have been described most frequently [6]: direct connection between the transverse or ascending branch of the uterine artery and the ovarian artery (Type 1); a branch of the uterine artery directed to the fibroid connecting to a branch of the ovarian artery (Type 2); and direct supply of the ovary from the uterine artery with congenital absence of the ovarian artery (Type 3).

The congenital absence of both uterine arteries has also been described and is encountered in less than 1% of cases, with the ipsilateral ovarian artery replacing the uterine vascular supply.

9.4.3 Embolization Materials

Once the catheter is placed in the uterine artery and the presence of anastomoses has been excluded, embolization can be performed. Several embolic agents have been successfully used for UAE, such as polyvinyl alcohol (PVA), tris-acryl gelatin microsphere (TAGM), gelatin sponge, and microspheres. In the largest multicenter prospective voluntary registry of patients undergoing UFE (3160 patients enrolled at 72 contributing sites), calibrated microspheres were used in 73% of cases, PVA in 31% of cases, and gelatin sponge in 3% of cases with some cases of a mixture of two or more embolic agents suggesting that the choice of the embolic agent is probably based on the operator experience [46].

Non-spherical PVA (nsPVA) was the first embolic agent used for leiomyoma endovascular treatment. Spherical PVA (sPVA) was developed as a consequence of the large size variability of nsPVA, assuming its potentially better embolizing effect; however, some randomized trials demonstrated a minor effect on the symptoms and volume reduction of fibroids in patients treated with spherical PVA versus non-spherical PVA [47] and TAGM [48, 49]. In 2014, a large meta-analysis conducted on ten studies (five randomized controlled trials) compared the efficacy of five different embolic agents, nsPVA, sPVA, acrylamido PVA (aPVA), TAGM, and polyzene-F hydrogel microspheres, confirmed the inferiority of sPVA against TAGM, but did not show any difference in terms of procedural outcome among all the other embolic agents [50].

A more recent comparative meta-analysis between PVA and TAGM conducted on sixsix studies [51] confirmed the superiority of TAGM in terms of quality of life and procedural failure rate, in reducing symptom severity, and in reducing uterine volume; the authors also hypothesized that the lesser effect of PVA could be due to the size variability in particle preparations, the difficulty of injecting particulate PVA through a microcatheter, and the clumping of particles, which made the effective size of PVA larger than the actual size, leading to an embolic occlusion that was more proximal than intended as already reported [52–55]. Concerning acrylamido polyvinyl alcohol microspheres (a-PVAM), a hydrogel-based embolic agent, only a randomized trial compared its efficacy with TAGM showing no significant differences at 1 week, 3 and 6 months MR, in terms of leiomyoma perfusion, overall uterine volume, and dominant leiomyomas volume measured by contrast-enhanced magnetic resonance imaging, but with a slight superiority of TAGM in terms of overall quality of life at 3 months [56].

Also, gelatin sponge has been demonstrated to be an effective embolic agent in UAE [57]. This embolic agent is usually hand-prepared and cut from sheets of gelatin sponge to make a slurry. Therefore, the final composition can vary according to preparation, posing difficulties in quantitative comparison with other agents [50].

The only controlled randomized trial conducted by Yun Gyu Song [57] on uterine artery embolization performed with gelatin sponge particles versus non-spherical polyvinyl alcohol (nPVA) demonstrated a better outcome of gelatin sponge particles in terms of mean bleeding score improvement and volume reduction rate of dominant fibroid at 3 months follow-up after the procedure; in the same study, the infarction rate of dominant fibroid was similar across groups.

A multicentric phase I/II prospective Japanese study [58] conducted on 33 women demonstrated the safety of UAE performed with gelatin sponge and with an improvement of menorrhagia in 90% of patients, pelvic pain in 78%, and bulk-related symptoms in 97% with a 61% mean reduction in leiomyoma volume on MR imaging at 12 months, suggesting a comparable safety and efficacy of gelatin sponge in respect to other embolic agents. These results were confirmed by a comparative study by Tetsuya Katsumori et al. [59] conducted on 67 patients in which gelatin sponge was revealed to be as effective as TAGM in terms of tumor infarction on contrast-enhanced magnetic resonance imaging, symptom, and quality-of-life improvements in the early period (4 months).

Regarding particles size, the review by Jiang et al. [51] showed that the 500–700 μm size of TAGM was appropriate for leiomyoma embolization maybe because the target vessels for embolization were the vessels of the peri-leiomyoma vascular plexus; however, Bilhim et al. [60] compared the effect of 300 μm with 500 μm PVA particles in UAE without significant differences in the volume reduction rate of uterus and leiomyoma at 6 months.

9.5 Adverse Events

9.5.1 Procedural Complications

Overall, the reported complication rates for UAE remain low, with major complications occurring in <3% of patients [61]. The most common complications after UAE treatment are prolonged vaginal discharge and permanent amenorrhea (up to 10% of patients) [21] (Table 9.3). Less frequently prolonged or poorly controlled pain, infection (endometritis, pyomyoma, or tubo-ovarian abscess), vessel or nerve injury at the

Table 9.3 Complications of UEA

Complication	Reported rate (%)	Suggested threshold (%)
Permanent amenorrhea		
Age < 45	0–3	3
Age > 45	20–40	45
Prolonged vaginal discharge	2–17	20
Transcervical leiomyoma expulsion	3–15	15
Septicemia	1–3	3
DVT/pulmonary embolism	<1	
Nontarget embolization	<1	<1

UFE uterine fibroid embolization, *DVT* deep vein thrombosis access site, and urinary tract infection or urinary retention can occur. Rare major complications include sepsis or pulmonary embolism, inadvertent embolization of a leiomyosarcoma, uterine necrosis, buttock necrosis, labial necrosis, vesicouterine fistula formation, small-bowel volvulus, and acute renal failure [32]. Menstrual disturbances are most common in the case of nontarget embolization of the ovaries via uterine-to-ovarian arterial interconnections. Transient amenorrhea after UAE is usually limited to a few cycles and is not considered a major complication [62]. The authors of the Fibroid Registry for Outcomes Data (FIBROID) reported that permanent amenorrhea at 6 months and 3 years after UAE treatment has been correlated with the increasing age of the treated patients [46]. Permanent amenorrhea is classified as a major complication (permanent adverse sequelae), although some patients may not view it as such.

The risk for permanent amenorrhea appears to be age dependent. For women younger than 45 years of age, the risk is <3%, whereas it is up to 20% for those >45 years of age [63].

9.5.2 Impact on Pregnancy

There is no universal consensus about the role of UAE in women who wish to become pregnant, as it has been widely demonstrated that UAE does not preclude the possibility of obtaining conception and pregnancy at term [64]. Several studies compared UFE to myomectomy in fertility, but none of these produced definitive evidence [65]. For women who wish to conceive, an indication to UAE persists to be controversial on the increased risk of preterm delivery and malpresentation [66] or miscarriage [67, 68] after treatment. The systematic review by Homer H and Saridogan reported that UAE for fibroids is associated with an increased risk of miscarriage [67]. Conversely, two more recent systematic reviews [68] and meta-analysis [69] confirmed that a safe pregnancy after UAE is obviously possible resulting in a healthy and normal baby delivery.

In addition, pooled obstetrical complication rates, pregnancy rates and losses, preterm labor, and low birth rate seem to be mostly similar to the general population after age adjustment.

Regarding adverse events during UAE for adenomyosis, both the reviews by Popovic and de Brujin affirmed that postembolization syndrome and permanent amenorrhea were the most common complications, with a hysterectomy incidence in the long-term follow-up of 13.2% and 14.2%, respectively [7, 29].

9.6 Pain Management Protocols During Uterine Fibroid Embolization

Although uterine artery embolization is a minimally invasive procedure, there is usually significant post-procedural pain due to the embolization itself. There is no consensus about the most cost-effective analgesia protocols [70]. A review by Saibudden analyzed 26 studies with different analgesia protocols: opioids ± NSAIDs ± acetaminophen ($N = 17$), opioids ± NSAIDs ± acetaminophen + nerve block ($N = 4$), opioids ± NSAIDs ± acetaminophen + intrauterine arterial drug administration ($N = 3$), or opioids ± NSAIDs ± acetaminophen + other ($N = 2$). This study shows that despite opioids NSAIDs ± acetaminophen and intrauterine artery drug administration showing overall slightly better pain scores in comparison with the other treatment groups, this difference was not statistically significant. The use of intraarterial lidocaine may improve pain for the first 4 h post-procedure, without significant effect on the pain levels in the subsequent 7–24 h [70]. So there is no evidence to suggest the superiority of any pain protocol over others.

9.7 Imaging and Clinical Follow-Up

In patients who become asymptomatic, further imaging may not be necessary. Post-procedural MR is typically performed at 3–6 months following UFE, and at 12 or 24 months as clinically indicated [71].

However, MR imaging can be used to reassess for residual enhancement of leiomyomas in patients with continued symptoms, who possibly require re-embolization. Routine follow-up MR imaging will ideally show complete infarction of uterine leiomyomas, which is demonstrated on MR images as a lack of enhancement after contrast material administration [4].

Quantifying the volume reduction of the uterus and leiomyomata can be helpful in assessing treatment response. Typically, the majority of volume reduction occurs within the first 6 months following UFE, with further reduction occurring during the 6–12 month period [71].

Occasionally, a small amount of gas may be identified within a leiomyoma after embolization; this does not equate with a pyomyoma (is not a sign of superinfection).

9.8 Conclusions

UAE has gained great consideration for the management of symptomatic fibroids over the years and is also growing up as a valid therapeutic option for the management of women affected by adenomyosis that are not fit for medical therapies.

There are currently few randomized studies, systematic reviews, and meta-analysis on UAE; however, both the high clinical success and the low complication rate should expand the use of UAE to multiple clinical scenarios in the next few years, promoting the production of more evidence in the literature.

References

1. Stewart EA, Laughlin-Tommaso SK, Catherino WH, Lalitkumar S, Gupta D, Vollenhoven B. Uterine fibroids. Nat Rev Dis Prim. 2016;2:16043. https://doi.org/10.1038/nrdp.2016.43.
2. Vilos GA, Allaire C, Laberge PY, et al. The management of uterine leiomyomas. J Obstet Gynaecol Canada. 2015;37(2):157–78. https://doi.org/10.1016/S1701-2163(15)30338-8.
3. Baird DD, Dunson DB, Hill MC, Cousins D, Schectman JM. High cumulative incidence of uterine leiomyoma in black and white women: ultrasound evidence. Am J Obstet Gynecol. 2003;188(1):100–7. https://doi.org/10.1067/mob.2003.99.
4. Deshmukh SP, Gonsalves CF, Guglielmo FF, Mitchell DG. Role of MR imaging of uterine leiomyomas before and after embolization. Radiographics. 2012;32(6):E251–81. https://doi.org/10.1148/rg.326125517.
5. Silberzweig JE, Powell DK, Matsumoto AH, Spies JB. Management of uterine fibroids: a focus on uterine-sparing interventional techniques. Radiology. 2016;280(3):675–92. https://doi.org/10.1148/radiol.2016141693.
6. Young M, Coffey W, Mikhail LN. Uterine fibroid embolization. In: StatPearls [Internet]. Treasure Island, FL: StatPearls Publishing; 2021. https://www.ncbi.nlm.nih.gov/books/NBK519016/.
7. Popovic M, Puchner S, Berzaczy D, Lammer J, Bucek RA. Uterine artery embolization for the treatment of adenomyosis: a review. J Vasc Interv Radiol. 2011;22(7):901–9. https://doi.org/10.1016/j.jvir.2011.03.013.
8. Meredith SM, Sanchez-Ramos L, Kaunitz AM. Diagnostic accuracy of transvaginal sonography for the diagnosis of adenomyosis: systematic review and metaanalysis. Am J Obstet Gynecol. 2009;201(1):107.e1–6. https://doi.org/10.1016/j.ajog.2009.03.021.
9. Chen HT, Athreya S. Systematic review of uterine artery embolisation practice guidelines: are all the guidelines on the same page? Clin Radiol. 2018;73(5):507.e9–507.e15. https://doi.org/10.1016/j.crad.2017.12.005.
10. Habiba M, Benagiano G, Brosens I. The pathophysiology of adenomyosis. Uterine Adenomyosis. 2015;4(4):45–70. https://doi.org/10.1007/978-3-319-13012-5_3.
11. Bird CC, McElin TW, Manalo-Estrella P. The elusive adenomyosis of the uterus-revisited. Am J Obstet Gynecol. 1972;112(5):583–93. https://doi.org/10.1016/0002-9378(72)90781-8.
12. Parker WH, Fu YS, Berek JS. Uterine sarcoma in patients operated on for presumed leiomyoma and rapidly growing leiomyoma. Obstet Gynecol. 1994;83(3):414–8.
13. Engel JB, Audebert A, Frydman R, Zivny J, Diedrich K. Presurgical short term treatment of uterine fibroids with different doses of cetrorelix acetate: a double-blind, placebo-controlled multicenter study. Eur J Obstet Gynecol Reprod Biol. 2007;134(2):225–32. https://doi.org/10.1016/j.ejogrb.2006.07.018.
14. Sohn GS, Cho SH, Kim YM, Cho CH, Kim MR, Lee SR. Current medical treatment of uterine fibroids. Obstet Gynecol Sci. 2018;61(2):192–201. https://doi.org/10.5468/ogs.2018.61.2.192.
15. Munro MG. Uterine leiomyomas, current concepts: pathogenesis, impact on reproductive health, and medical, procedural, and surgical management. Obstet Gynecol Clin N Am. 2011;38(4):703–31. https://doi.org/10.1016/j.ogc.2011.09.006.

16. Fischer K, McDannold NJ, Tempany CM, Jolesz FA, Fennessy FM. Potential of minimally invasive procedures in the treatment of uterine fibroids: a focus on magnetic resonance-guided focused ultrasound therapy. Int J Women's Health. 2015;7:901–12. https://doi.org/10.2147/IJWH.S55564.
17. Shen SH, Fennessy F, McDannold N, Jolesz F, Tempany C. Image-guided thermal therapy of uterine fibroids. Semin Ultrasound CT MR. 2009;30(2):91–104. https://doi.org/10.1053/j.sult.2008.12.002.
18. Zreik TG, Rutherford TJ, Palter SF, et al. Cryomyolysis, a new procedure for the conservative treatment of uterine fibroids. J Am Assoc Gynecol Laparosc. 1998;5(1):33–8. https://doi.org/10.1016/S1074-3804(98)80008-X.
19. Liu L, Wang T, Lei B. Uterine artery embolization compared with high-intensity focused ultrasound ablation for the treatment of symptomatic uterine myomas: a systematic review and meta-analysis. J Minim Invasive Gynecol. 2021;28(2):218–27. https://doi.org/10.1016/j.jmig.2020.11.004.
20. Jeng CJ, Long CY, Chuang LT. Comparison of magnetic resonance-guided high-intensity focused ultrasound with uterine artery embolization for the treatment of uterine myoma: a systematic literature review and meta-analysis. Taiwan J Obstet Gynecol. 2020;59(5):691–7. https://doi.org/10.1016/j.tjog.2020.07.012.
21. Xu F, Deng L, Zhang L, Hu H, Shi Q. The comparison of myomectomy, UAE and MRgFUS in the treatment of uterine fibroids: a meta analysis. Int J Hyperthermia. 2021;38(2):24–9. https://doi.org/10.1080/02656736.2021.1933216.
22. Knuttinen MG, Stark G, Hohenwalter EJ, et al. ACR appropriateness criteria® radiologic management of uterine leiomyomas. J Am Coll Radiol. 2018;15(5):S160–70. https://doi.org/10.1016/j.jacr.2018.03.010.
23. Pérez-López FR, Ornat L, Ceausu I, et al. EMAS position statement: management of uterine fibroids. Maturitas. 2014;79(1):106–16. https://doi.org/10.1016/j.maturitas.2014.06.002.
24. Cooper S, Oceguera LM, Danes S. Uterine artery embolization: a vascular surgery procedure? One vascular surgery group's experience. Vascular. 2012;20(5):268–72. https://doi.org/10.1258/vasc.2011.oa0341.
25. Llewellyn O, Patel NR, Mallon D, Quinn SD, Hamady M. Uterine artery embolisation for women with giant versus non-giant uterine fibroids: a systematic review and meta-analysis. Cardiovasc Intervent Radiol. 2020;43(5):684–93. https://doi.org/10.1007/s00270-019-02359-7.
26. Dessouky R, Gamil SA, Nada MG, Mousa R, Libda Y. Management of uterine adenomyosis: current trends and uterine artery embolization as a potential alternative to hysterectomy. Insights Imaging. 2019;10(1):48. https://doi.org/10.1186/s13244-019-0732-8.
27. Ozdegirmenci O, Kayikcioglu F, Akgul MA, et al. Comparison of levonorgestrel intrauterine system versus hysterectomy on efficacy and quality of life in patients with adenomyosis. Fertil Steril. 2011;95(2):497–502. https://doi.org/10.1016/j.fertnstert.2010.10.009.
28. de Bruijn AM, Smink M, Lohle PNM, et al. Uterine artery embolization for the treatment of adenomyosis: a systematic review and meta-analysis. J Vasc Interv Radiol. 2017;28(12):1629–1642.e1. https://doi.org/10.1016/j.jvir.2017.07.034.
29. de Bruijn AM, Ankum WM, Reekers JA, et al. Uterine artery embolization vs hysterectomy in the treatment of symptomatic uterine fibroids: 10-year outcomes from the randomized EMMY trial. Am J Obstet Gynecol. 2016;215(6):745.e1–745.e12. https://doi.org/10.1016/j.ajog.2016.06.051.
30. Kim MD, Kim YM, Kim HC, et al. Uterine artery embolization for symptomatic adenomyosis: a new technical development of the 1-2-3 protocol and predictive factors of MR imaging affecting outcomes. J Vasc Interv Radiol. 2011;22(4):497–502. https://doi.org/10.1016/j.jvir.2011.01.426.
31. Das CJ, Rathinam D, Manchanda S, Srivastava DN. Endovascular uterine artery interventions. Indian J Radiol Imaging. 2017;27(4):488–95. https://doi.org/10.4103/ijri.IJRI_204_16.
32. Dariushnia SR, Nikolic B, Stokes LAS, Spies JB. Quality improvement guidelines for uterine artery embolization for symptomatic leiomyomata. J Vasc Interv Radiol. 2014;25(11):1737–47. https://doi.org/10.1016/j.jvir.2014.08.029.
33. McPherson K, Manyonda I, Lumsden MA, et al. A randomised trial of treating fibroids with either embolisation or myomectomy to measure the effect on quality of life among women wishing to avoid hysterectomy (the FEMME study): study protocol for a randomised controlled trial. Trials. 2014;15(1):468. https://doi.org/10.1186/1745-6215-15-468.
34. Scheurig-Muenkler C, Wagner M, Franiel T, Hamm B, Kroencke TJ. Effect of uterine artery embolization on uterine and leiomyoma perfusion: evidence of transient myometrial ischemia on magnetic resonance imaging. J Vasc Interv Radiol. 2010;21(9):1347–53. https://doi.org/10.1016/j.jvir.2010.05.008.
35. Ukybassova T, Terzic M, Dotlic J, et al. Evaluation of uterine artery embolization on myoma shrinkage: results from a large cohort analysis. Gynecol Minim Invasive Ther. 2019;8(4):165–71. https://doi.org/10.4103/GMIT.GMIT_50_19.
36. Contegiacomo A, Cina A, Di Stasi C, et al. Uterine myomas: endovascular treatment. Semin Ultrasound CT MR. 2021;42(1):13–24. https://doi.org/10.1053/j.sult.2020.07.002.
37. Resnick NJ, Kim E, Patel RS, Lookstein RA, Nowakowski FS, Fischman AM. Uterine artery embolization using a transradial approach: initial experience and technique. J Vasc Interv Radiol. 2014;25(3):443–7. https://doi.org/10.1016/j.jvir.2013.11.010.
38. Gjoreski A, Gjoreski J, Nancheva A. Uterine fibroid embolization via transradial versus transfemoral arte-

rial access: technical results. Open Access Maced J Med Sci. 2019;7(4):579–82. https://doi.org/10.3889/OAMJMS.2019.163.
39. Fischman AM, Horn CJ, Resnick NJ, et al. Uterine artery embolization using a transradial approach: initial experience and technique. J Vasc Interv Radiol. 2014;25(3):S67–8. https://doi.org/10.1016/j.jvir.2013.12.169.
40. Nakhaei M, Mojtahedi A, Faintuch S, Sarwar A, Brook OR. Transradial and transfemoral uterine fibroid embolization comparative study: technical and clinical outcomes. J Vasc Interv Radiol. 2020;31(1):123–9. https://doi.org/10.1016/j.jvir.2019.08.016.
41. Mortensen C, Chung J, Liu D, et al. Prospective study on total fluoroscopic time in patients undergoing uterine artery embolization: comparing transradial and transfemoral approaches. Cardiovasc Intervent Radiol. 2019;42(3):441–7. https://doi.org/10.1007/s00270-018-2100-3.
42. Pelage JP, Cazejust J, Pluot E, et al. Uterine fibroid vascularization and clinical relevance to uterine fibroid embolization. Radiographics. 2005;25(SPEC. ISS):99–118. https://doi.org/10.1148/rg.25si055510.
43. AbdElmagied AM, Vaughan LE, Weaver AL, et al. Uterine artery embolization for severe symptomatic fibroids: effects on fertility and symptoms. Cardiovasc Intervent Radiol. 2018;15(3):1–7. https://doi.org/10.1016/j.ajog.2016.04.001.
44. Pelage JP, Le Dref O, Soyer P, Jacob D, Kardache M, Dahan H, Lassau JP, Rymer R. Arterial anatomy of the female genital tract: variations and relevance to transcatheter embolization of the uterus. AJR Am J Roentgenol. 1999;172(4):989–94. https://doi.org/10.2214/ajr.172.4.10587133.
45. El Shamy T, Amer SAK, Mohamed AA, James C, Jayaprakasan K. The impact of uterine artery embolization on ovarian reserve: a systematic review and meta-analysis. Acta Obstet Gynecol Scand. 2020;99(1):16–23. https://doi.org/10.1111/aogs.13698.
46. Worthington-Kirsch R, Spies JB, Myers ER, et al. The fibroid registry for outcomes data (FIBROID) for uterine embolization: short-term outcomes. Obstet Gynecol. 2005;106(1):52–9. https://doi.org/10.1097/01.AOG.0000165828.68787.a9.
47. Rasuli P, Hammond I, Al-Mutairi B, et al. Spherical versus conventional polyvinyl alcohol particles for uterine artery embolization. J Vasc Interv Radiol. 2008;19(1):42–6. https://doi.org/10.1016/j.jvir.2007.08.016.
48. Spies JB. Current role of uterine artery embolization in the management of uterine fibroids. Clin Obstet Gynecol. 2016;59(1):93–102. https://doi.org/10.1097/GRF.0000000000000162.
49. Siskin GP, Beck A, Schuster M, Mandato K, Englander M, Herr A. Leiomyoma infarction after uterine artery embolization: a prospective randomized study comparing Trisacryl gelatin microspheres versus polyvinyl alcohol microspheres. J Vasc Interv Radiol. 2008;19(1):58–65. https://doi.org/10.1016/j.jvir.2007.08.034.
50. Das R, Champaneria R, Daniels JP, Belli AM. Comparison of embolic agents used in uterine artery embolisation: a systematic review and meta-analysis. Cardiovasc Intervent Radiol. 2014;37(5):1179–90. https://doi.org/10.1007/s00270-013-0790-0.
51. Jiang W, Shen Z, Luo H, Hu X, Zhu X. Comparison of polyvinyl alcohol and tris-acryl gelatin microsphere materials in embolization for symptomatic leiomyomas: a systematic review. Minim Invasive Ther Allied Technol. 2016;25(6):289–300. https://doi.org/10.1080/13645706.2016.1207667.
52. Siskin GP, Englander M, Stainken BF, Ahn J, Dowling K, Dolen EG. Embolic agents used for uterine fibroid embolization. Am J Roentgenol. 2000;175(3):767–73. https://doi.org/10.2214/ajr.175.3.1750767.
53. Beaujeux R, Laurent A, Wassef M, et al. Trisacryl gelatin microspheres for therapeutic embolization, II: preliminary clinical evaluation in tumors and arteriovenous malformations. Am J Neuroradiol. 1996;17(3):541–8.
54. Derdeyn CP, Graves VB, Salamat MS, Rappe A. Collagen-coated acrylic microspheres for embolotherapy: in vivo and in vitro characteristics. Am J Neuroradiol. 1997;18(4):647–53.
55. Choe DH, Han MH, Kang GH, Yeon KM, Han MC. An experimental study of embolic effect according to infusion rate and concentration of suspension in transarterial particulate embolization. Investig Radiol. 1997;32(5):260–7. https://doi.org/10.1097/00004424-199705000-00002.
56. Worthington-Kirsch RL, Siskin GP, Hegener P, Chesnick R. Comparison of the efficacy of the embolic agents acrylamido polyvinyl alcohol microspheres and tris-acryl gelatin microspheres for uterine artery embolization for leiomyomas: a prospective randomized controlled trial. Cardiovasc Intervent Radiol. 2011;34(3):493–501. https://doi.org/10.1007/s00270-010-0049-y.
57. Song YG, Jang H, Park KD, Kim MD, Kim CW. Non spherical polyvinyl alcohol versus gelatin sponge particles for uterine artery embolization for symptomatic fibroids. Minim Invasive Ther Allied Technol. 2013;22(6):364–71. https://doi.org/10.3109/13645706.2013.826674.
58. Sone M, Arai Y, Shimizu T, et al. Phase I/II multiinstitutional study of uterine artery embolization with gelatin sponge for symptomatic uterine leiomyomata: Japan interventional radiology in oncology study group study. J Vasc Interv Radiol. 2010;21(11):1665–71. https://doi.org/10.1016/j.jvir.2010.07.017.
59. Katsumori T, Miura H, Arima H, et al. Trisacryl gelatin microspheres versus gelatin sponge particles in uterine artery embolization for leiomyoma. Acta Radiol. 2017;58(7):834–41. https://doi.org/10.1177/0284185116674499.

60. Bilhim T, Pisco JM, Duarte M, Oliveira AG. Polyvinyl alcohol particle size for uterine artery embolization: a prospective randomized study of initial use of 350–500 μm particles versus initial use of 500–700 μm particles. J Vasc Interv Radiol. 2011;22(1):21–7. https://doi.org/10.1016/j.jvir.2010.09.018.
61. Spies JB, Spector A, Roth AR, Baker CM, Mauro L, Murphy-Skrynarz K. Complications after uterine artery embolization for leiomyomas. Obstet Gynecol. 2002;100(5):873–80. https://doi.org/10.1097/00006250-200211000-00007.
62. Pelage JP, Le Dref O, Jacob D, Soyer P, Rossignol M, Truc J, Payen D, Rymer R. Embolisation Utérine. Anatomie, technique, indications, résultats et complications [Uterine artery embolization: anatomical and technical considerations, indications, results, and complications]. J Radiol. 2000;81(12 Suppl):1863–72. French
63. Katsumori T, Kasahara T, Tsuchida Y, Nozaki T. Amenorrhea and resumption of menstruation after uterine artery embolization for fibroids. Int J Gynecol Obstet. 2008;103(3):217–21. https://doi.org/10.1016/j.ijgo.2008.07.010.
64. Pisco JM, Duarte M, Bilhim T, Cirurgião F, Oliveira AG. Pregnancy after uterine fibroid embolization. Fertil Steril. 2011;95(3):1121.e5–8. https://doi.org/10.1016/j.fertnstert.2010.08.032.
65. Gupta JK, Sinha A, Lumsden MA, Hickey M. Uterine artery embolization for symptomatic uterine fibroids. Cochrane Database Syst Rev. 2014;2014(12):CD005073. https://doi.org/10.1002/14651858.CD005073.pub4.
66. Goldberg J, Pereira L, Berghella V, et al. Pregnancy outcomes after treatment for fibromyomata: uterine artery embolization versus laparoscopic myomectomy. Am J Obstet Gynecol. 2004;191(1):18–21. https://doi.org/10.1016/j.ajog.2004.01.046.
67. Homer H, Saridogan E. Uterine artery embolization for fibroids is associated with an increased risk of miscarriage. Fertil Steril. 2010;94(1):324–30. https://doi.org/10.1016/j.fertnstert.2009.02.069.
68. Mohan PP, Hamblin MH, Vogelzang RL. Uterine artery embolization and its effect on fertility. J Vasc Interv Radiol. 2013;24(7):925–30. https://doi.org/10.1016/j.jvir.2013.03.014.
69. Ghanaati H, Sanaati M, Shakiba M, et al. Pregnancy and its outcomes in patients after uterine fibroid embolization: a systematic review and meta-analysis. Cardiovasc Intervent Radiol. 2020;43(8):1122–33. https://doi.org/10.1007/s00270-020-02521-6.
70. Saibudeen A, Makris GC, Elzein A, Wigham A, Patel R, Husainy MA, Anthony S, Uberoi R. Pain management protocols during uterine fibroid embolisation: a systematic review of the evidence. Cardiovasc Intervent Radiol. 2019;42(12):1663–77. https://doi.org/10.1007/s00270-019-02327-1.
71. Siddiqui N, Nikolaidis P, Hammond N, Miller FH. Uterine artery embolization: pre- and post-procedural evaluation using magnetic resonance imaging. Abdom Imaging. 2013;38(5):1161–77. https://doi.org/10.1007/s00261-013-9990-y.

Percutaneous Ablation of Uterine Myomas

10

Letizia Di Meglio, Anna Maria Ierardi, Giovanni Maria Rodà, Antonio Arrichiello, Pierpaolo Biondetti, Umberto G. Rossi, and Gianpaolo Carrafiello

10.1 Introduction

Uterine fibroids represent the most frequent benign tumor in women, in fact, literature data demonstrates the presence of fibroids in up to 77% of women. Uterine fibroids can be classified with the FIGO classification system in accordance with the position between the layers of the uterus. The classification includes the submucosal type 0–2, intramural type 3–5, and the subserosal type 6–7. An additional subtype is the 8 and it classifies the fibroids that are not located within the myometrium like the cervical ones [1, 2].

Fibroids can be found in an asymptomatic setting, while in other cases they can be related with clinical symptoms such as bleeding, infertility, pelvic pain, or compression manifestations on the bladder or bowel [3, 4].

There are several therapeutic options going from medical to surgical treatments.

The preferred therapy is chosen on the basis of the symptoms, the desire of pregnancy, and the type of fibroid.

Medical treatments are the first-line choice for bleeding manifestations with a variable success rate. Surgical myomectomy represents the standard approach for women with a desire to preserve fertility.

It is not free of adverse events, such as uterine rupture, implant abnormalities, and pre-term delivery.

Hysterectomy represents the first-line treatment for patients with multiple fibroids, with compression manifestations without a desire for preservation of fertility.

In the last years, non-surgical treatments have become available, such as uterine artery embolization (UAE) and fibroid ablation. The ablation can be performed using Microwave (MW), Radiofrequency (RF), High-focus Ultrasound (HIFU), or Cryotherapy (CRYO). These treatments are less invasive than surgical ones and have the advantage of preservation of the uterus;

L. Di Meglio · G. M. Rodà · A. Arrichiello
Postgraduation School in Radiodiagnostics, Università degli Studi di Milano, Milan, Italy

A. M. Ierardi (✉) · P. Biondetti
Operative Unit of Radiology, Fondazione IRCCS Ca' Granda Ospedale Maggiore Policlinico, Milan, Italy

U. G. Rossi
Department of Diagnostic Imaging, Interventional Radiology Unit, Ente Ospedaliero Galliera Hospital, Mura delle Cappuccine, Genoa, Italy
e-mail: umberto.rossi@galliera.it

G. Carrafiello
Operative Unit of Radiology, Fondazione IRCCS Ca' Granda Ospedale Maggiore Policlinico, Milan, Italy

Department of Diagnostic Imaging, Interventional Radiology Unit, Ente Ospedaliero Galliera Hospital, Mura delle Cappuccine, Genoa, Italy

Department of Health Sciences, Università degli Studi di Milano, Milan, Italy
e-mail: gianpaolo.carrafiello@unimi.it

R. Niola et al. (eds.), *Diagnostic and Interventional Radiology in Gynecological and Obstetric Diseases*, https://doi.org/10.1007/978-3-031-11910-1_10

however, the fibroids are not removed from the uterus and there is a shortage of data regarding the effect on future pregnancies.

Data regarding feasibility, technical success, clinical success, and safety have been analyzed.

The term safety was used for the evaluation of the immediate or delayed complications, categorized with the classification of the Socety of Interventional Radiology [5].

In literature the evaluation of the reduction of the symptoms was assessed with questionnaires, such as the Uterine Fibroids Symptom and Quality of Life (UFS-QoL) questionnaire and the Symptom Severity Score [3, 6, 7].

Clinical success is intended as the reduction of fibroids dimension and improvement of symptoms.

10.2 Percutaneous Techniques

10.2.1 Microwave Ablation

Percutaneous microwave ablation of fibroids is performed normally under conscious sedation and local anesthesia. The procedures may be performed via percutaneous, transvaginal, and transcervical approaches [3].

Literature data indicates the use of antennas ranging from 13 to 16 G with length ranging between 15 and 20 cm. Moreover, if the diameter of the fibroid is <5 cm a single antenna is used, meanwhile, if the target fibroid is >5 cm double antennas may be positioned within the fibroid 1 cm from the other, or the same antenna is positioned in two different areas (Fig. 10.1) [8].

Microwave ablation uses an antenna probe that emits microwaves (2.45 GHz) into the fibroid tissue, and the ablation can be performed in both continuous and pulsed microwave modes. Energy power ranges from 50 W to 100 W in literature, applied from 300 s up to 600 s.

The mean duration of the procedure described in literature is about 34.48 min [7].

10.2.2 Radiofrequency Ablation

RF ablation represents another alternative treatment for fibroids, and it is considered a minimally invasive and safe approach. The RF ablation can be performed both laparoscopically and percutaneously, with a transcervical, transabdominal, or transvaginal approach. The thermal ablation occurs using a monopolar radiofrequency electrode, inserted within the fibroid. The technique varies between different operators, and the ablation can be performed with low voltage (60 W) and high frequency (45–500 kHz) alternating current, or as reported in other works with higher voltages (100–150 W). The ablation is performed by inducing thermal damage inside the fibroid. The heat produces a coagulative necrosis of the cells, the formation of thrombosis in the vessels of the fibroid, and finally the inactivation of hormonal receptors within the myoma (Fig. 10.2) [9, 10].

A pre-procedural fibroid evaluation is necessary to establish the size of the fibroid and estimate the ablation diameter.

The mean during the RF ablation procedure in literature is around 49 min [7].

10.2.3 Cryotherapy Ablation

CRYO ablation is a technique that works by inducing cellular damage through the application of low temperatures. Generally, the procedure is executed with a percutaneous approach; the applicator is inserted into the target lesion and it is performed under MRI guidance with the patient in a supine or oblique position. Multiplanar T2-weighted images are used to locate the target

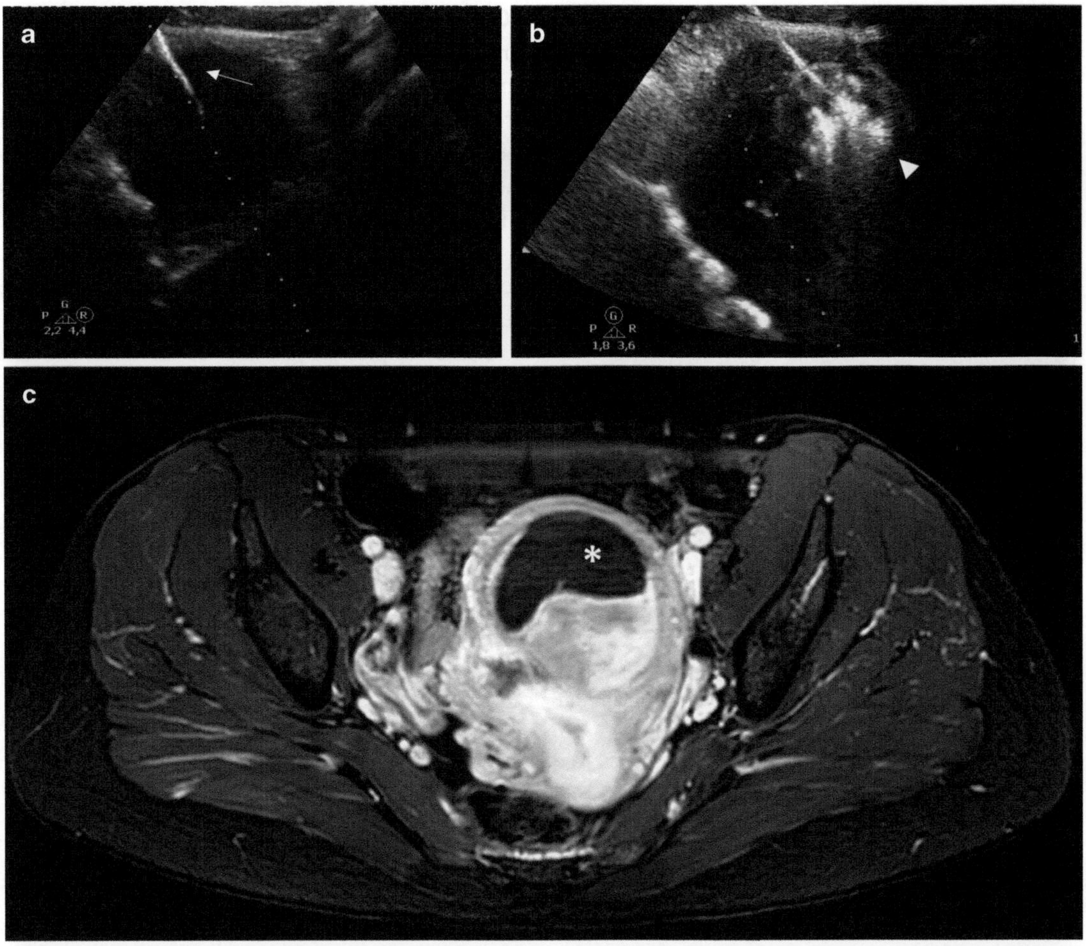

Fig. 10.1 MWA of a uterine fibroid with transabdominal US guide. (**a**) The antenna (arrow) is inserted within the fibroid. (**b**) US image during the ablation showing a hyperechoic area (point of arrow) inside the fibroid, as a result of the procedure. (**c**) Two months follow-up contrast-enhanced MRI, T1w images, showing an area of no enhancement inside the treated fibroid (asterisk)

lesion. Currently available systems work based on the Joule-Thomson effect. Real gases undergo a change in temperature after fast expansion. The used gases are argon and helium; the first one reaches low temperatures after expansion (up to −185 °C), meanwhile the second one reaches high ones. The gases are conveyed through cryoprobes (with a diameter between 2 and 3 mm) within the target lesion; at the tip of the probe there is an expansion chamber that allows the execution of the Joule-Thompson effect and the creation of the ice ball. Once the target is correctly reached, the ablation is performed and the ice ball is formed. Under MRI guidance the ice ball can be visualized three-dimensionally, and it is measured in terms of length, width, and depth and is calculated based on the volume of the target fibroid.

CRYO ablation can also be performed with a laparoscopic approach [11, 12].

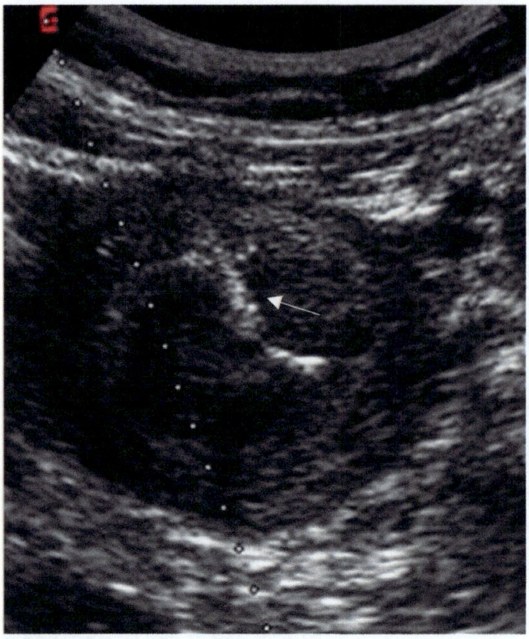

Fig. 10.2 RFA of a uterine fibroid with transabdominal US guide. The needle (arrow) is inserted within the fibroid

10.3 Outcomes

10.3.1 Percutaneous Microwave Ablation

10.3.1.1 Clinical and Technical Success

In literature, the shrinkage of the fibroids is reported to range between 15.6% and 94%; it can be assessed with MRI, in particular with T2-weighted sequences, or with CEUS [3, 13, 14].

Literature data report an increment of 72% from baseline scores of UFS-QoL questionaries after 12 months [13].

10.3.1.2 Complications

No serious complications were observed. Among the minor complications, the most frequent were abdominal pain, post-ablation syndrome, and vaginal discharge; however, these are considered to be normal phenomena probably due to endometrial inflammation caused by necrotizing liquefaction after ablation. Overall, percutaneous MWA may be considered a safe procedure [15, 16].

10.3.1.3 Fertility

The effect of microwave ablation on fertility has not been revealed. Given the novel nature of the procedure, it cannot be used to study its effect on fertility in patients who have reproductive requirement, and therefore, trials were restricted to patients with no desire for fertility in the future [17].

In literature unplanned pregnancies that occurred after treatment of uterine fibroids are described [18].

For example, Bing-Song et al. observed ten unplanned pregnancies in nine women in a follow-up study on 169 women. Six patients interrupted the pregnancy and three gave birth to a healthy term infant delivered by cesarean section [17].

10.3.2 Radiofrequency Ablation

10.3.2.1 Clinical and Technical Success

Literature data concerning the technical success reports a reduction rate from 80% up to 90.3%.

Data regarding the reduction of the symptoms report an increment from the baseline of quality-of-life scores between 66.7 and 82.7% [15].

Literature reports a rate of 11% of retreatments [19].

10.3.2.2 Complications

RF is considered a safe technique; however, there is a lack of data about the most common adverse effects. In literatures iatrogenic injury to the major abdominal organs or major bleedings are considered major complications. No cases of death have been reported in literature [20].

Data from the analysis of 1216 patients treated with RF by Yin et al. report three cases of bowel perforation related to the procedure. All cases occurred in the first 24 h in patients with multiple myomas [15].

10.3.2.3 Fertility

A review published in 2017 reports 20 cases of pregnancies following RF ablation, seven of them were undesired and asked for elective interruption. Among the others, there was one spontaneous abortion and 12 full-term live births (75% delivered by cesarian section) [18].

The only complication reported was a delivery complicated by the expulsion of a necrotic fibroid and a post-partum hemorrhage [21].

10.3.3 Cryotherapy Ablation

10.3.3.1 Clinical and Technical Success

CRYO ablation, like the previous techniques, has demonstrated to have promising results.

Cowan et al. report a case series of nine women with large symptomatic uterine fibroids, treated with CRYO ablation under MRI guidance [22]. Among the nine patients, only eight were available for follow-up until 12 months. All patients reported an improvement in the bleeding and bulk symptoms.

The mean shrinkage of the fibroid ranged between 58% and 72%. Sakuhara et al. reported a small series of six patients treated with CRYO ablation. All the patients completed a 12-month follow-up, and between them, only one did not report any benefit after the procedure. The reason was attributed to the presence of seven fibroids [23]. The mean reduction of fibroids dimensions at 12 months follow-up was estimated to be 79.4% [23]. The score of UFS-QoL questionaries demonstrated an increment of 55.8% from baseline value at 12 months after treatment [11].

10.3.3.2 Complications

Three of the nine treated patients reported in the work of Cowan et al. presented major complications: one had a laceration of a vessel that required laparotomy and surgical myomectomy, another had a peroneal nerve lesion associated that self-resolved after 4 months, and the last one had severe nausea that required hospitalization. Among the remaining six patients no major complications occurred [24].

Sakuhara et al. described two cases of major complications: one hepatic damage self-controlled and an abscess of the abdominal wall.

10.3.3.3 Fertility

Literature data evidence that all the patients who underwent CRYO ablation were evaluated by the institutional review board of each hospital and didn't have desire of prole [23].

The only work reporting pregnancy cases after CRYO ablation is that published by Ciavattini et al., regarding cases treated with a laparoscopic approach. Nine of the 64 women reported in the study presented unexpected pregnancies, among them two miscarried, meanwhile of the remaining seven, four delivered vaginally and the others by cesarean section. No complications were reported [11].

10.4 Technical Comparison

Recently, several new treatment options have become available for symptomatic uterine fibroids.

There are no randomized control trials available in literature, that compare the results of the different techniques, so it is not possibile to evaluate the better approach. As evidenced above, there are no guidelines to help with the selection of the best treatment among the different therapeutic options. The choice is generally based on the type of fibroid, the desire of pregnancy, and the expertise of the center [11, 22, 25, 26].

As evidenced above there is no significant difference in terms of technical success between the different approaches. All the approaches determine a reduction of the symptomatology related to fibroids. However, the mean reduction rate of the symptoms and the increment of UFS-QoL scores appear to be high for RF, MW, and CRYO [6, 7, 9, 27, 28].

Data from a metanalysis comparing MW ablation with other thermal ablation approaches evidence that MW is a safe, time-saving, and effective technique, in particular for the possibility to ablate larger ablation volumes compared with the other techniques [6, 7, 20].

None of the above-mentioned techniques is free of adverse events; however, literature data evidence that there is no significative difference

Table 10.1 Summary of the possible different approaches

Technique	Technical success	Clinical success	Fertility	Complications
MW	Mean shrinkage between 15.6% and 94%	Increment of 72% of UFS-QoL questionaries	Ten cases	Minor complications
RF	Mean shrinkage between 80% and 90.3%	Increment of 66.7–82.7% of UFS-QoL questionaries	20 cases	Minor and major complications
CRYO	Mean shrinkage between 58% and 72%	Increment of 55.8% of UFS-QoL questionaries	Nine cases	Minor and major complications

in terms of safety between the different approaches. A big leak in this field has been apprised since there are no data regarding the incidence of major and minor complications [1]. No cases of death related to the procedures have been reported (Table 10.1).

Until now all the above-mentioned treatments are not recommended for women with a desire of pregnancy, and all data regarding pregnancies refers mostly to unexpected pregnancies, some of which were interrupted. Therefore, it is not possible to determine which technique could be considered safe with no impact on future pregnancies. In addition, since literature data only includes treatments performed on menopausal women, it is not possible to estimate the incidence of pregnancies in treated women. Additionally, it is not possible to establish which one should be preferred for childbearing women with symptomatic fibroids [17, 18, 21, 29, 30].

10.5 Conclusion

This work aims to give a brief view of the possible different percutaneous approaches for uterine fibroids treatment. Few studies have been published comparing one technique over another, and there is no data regarding the superiority of a technique, making the development of additional randomized clinical studies highly requested, in order to create evidence-based guidelines. Moreover, future studies should be focused on pregnancy outcomes in treated patients, in order to establish the safest and more reliable option for childbearing women [4].

Finally, these treatments provide an alternative option, with preservation of the uterus, to invasive interventions, but until now there are only a few data reporting a lower rate of adverse events, a shorter recovery stay, and reduced postoperative complications. Further studies should be conducted [11, 25].

References

1. Lethaby A, Vollenhoven B. Fibroids (uterine myomatosis, leiomyomas). BMJ Clin Evid. 2011;2011:0814.
2. Munro MG, Critchley HOD, Broder MS, Fraser IS. FIGO classification system (PALM-COEIN) for causes of abnormal uterine bleeding in nongravid women of reproductive age. Int J Gynecol Obstet. 2011;113(1):3–13. https://doi.org/10.1016/j.ijgo.2010.11.011.
3. Ierardi AM, Savasi V, Angileri SA, Petrillo M, Sbaraini S, Pinto A, et al. Percutaneous high frequency microwave ablation of uterine fibroids: systematic review. Biomed Res Int. 2018;2018:2360107.
4. Havryliuk Y, Setton R, Carlow JJ, Shaktman BD. Symptomatic fibroid management: systematic review of the literature. JSLS. 2017;21(3):e2017.00041.
5. Khalilzadeh O, Baerlocher MO, Shyn PB, Connolly BL, Devane AM, Morris CS, et al. Proposal of a new adverse event classification by the Society of Interventional Radiology Standards of Practice Committee. J Vasc Interv Radiol. 2017;28(10):1432–1437.e3.
6. Zhao WP, Han ZY, Zhang J, Liang P. A retrospective comparison of microwave ablation and high intensity focused ultrasound for treating symptomatic uterine fibroids. Eur J Radiol. 2015;84(3):413–7. https://doi.org/10.1016/j.ejrad.2014.11.041.
7. Liu L, Wang T, Lei B. Ultrasound-guided microwave ablation in the management of symptomatic uterine myomas: a systematic review and meta-analysis. J Minim Invasive Gynecol. 2021;28(12):1982–92. https://doi.org/10.1016/j.jmig.2021.06.020.

8. Yang Y, Zhang J, Han Z-y, Yu M-a, Ma X, Zhou H-y, et al. Ultrasound-guided percutaneous microwave ablation for submucosal uterine fibroids. J Minim Invasive Gynecol. 2014;21(3):436–41. https://doi.org/10.1016/j.jmig.2013.11.012.
9. Fasciani A, Turtulici G, Siri G, Ferrero S, Sirito R. A prospective intervention trial on tailored radiofrequency ablation of uterine myomas. Medicina (Kaunas). 2020;56(3):1–11.
10. Yin G, Chen M, Yang S, Li J, Zhu T, Zhao X. Treatment of uterine myomas by radiofrequency thermal ablation: a 10-year retrospective cohort study. Reprod Sci. 2015;22(5):609–14. https://doi.org/10.1177/1933719114556481.
11. Patel A, Malik M, Britten J, Cox J, Catherino WH. Alternative therapies in management of leiomyomas. Fertil Steril. 2014;102(3):649–55. https://doi.org/10.1016/j.fertnstert.2014.07.008.
12. Mahnken AH, König AM, Figiel JH. Current technique and application of percutaneous cryotherapy. RoFo. 2018;190(9):836–46.
13. Liu H, Zhang J, Han ZY, Zhang BS, Zhang W, Qi CS, et al. Effectiveness of ultrasound-guided percutaneous microwave ablation for symptomatic uterine fibroids: a multicentre study in China. Int J Hyperth. 2016;32(8):876–80.
14. Lei F, Jing Z, Bo W, Dongmei H, Zhencai L, Xue J, et al. Uterine myomas treated with microwave ablation: the agreement between ablation volumes obtained from contrast-enhanced sonography and enhanced MRI. Int J Hyperth. 2014;30(1):11–8.
15. Ierardi AM, Carnevale A, Pellegrino F, Di Stefano G, Bonelli C, Renzulli M, et al. Uterine myomas: extravascular treatment. Semin Ultrasound CT MR. 2021;42(1):56–74.
16. Ierardi AM, Petrillo M, Fumarola EM, Coppola A, Angileri SA, Garanzini E, et al. Percutaneous microwave ablation of uterine fibroids: correlation between shrinkage and trend symptoms. Minim Invasive Ther Allied Technol. 2021;30(1):33–9. https://doi.org/10.1080/13645706.2019.1668417.
17. Bing-Song Z, Jing Z, Zhi-Yu H, Chang-Tao X, Rui-Fang X, Xiu-Mei L, et al. Unplanned pregnancy after ultrasound-guided percutaneous microwave ablation of uterine fibroids: a follow-up study. Sci Rep. 2016;6:1–5.
18. Keltz J, Levie M, Chudnoff S. Pregnancy outcomes after direct uterine myoma thermal ablation: review of the literature. J Minim Invasive Gynecol. 2017;24(4):538–45.
19. Lukes A, Green MA. Three-year results of the SONATA pivotal trial of transcervical fibroid ablation for symptomatic uterine myomata. J Gynecol Surg. 2020;36(5):228–33.
20. Bradley LD, Pasic RP, Miller LE. Clinical performance of radiofrequency ablation for treatment of uterine fibroids: systematic review and meta-analysis of prospective studies. J Laparoendosc Adv Surg Tech A. 2019;29(12):1507–17.
21. Berman JM, Bolnick JM, Pemueller RR, Garza Leal JG. Reproductive outcomes in women following radiofrequency volumetric thermal ablation of symptomatic fibroids. a retrospective case series analysis. J Reprod Med. 2015;60(5–6):194–8.
22. Cowan BD. Myomectomy and MRI-directed cryotherapy. Semin Reprod Med. 2004;22(2):143–8.
23. Sakuhara Y, Shimizu T, Kodama Y, Sawada A, Endo H, Abo D, et al. Magnetic resonance-guided percutaneous cryoablation of uterine fibroids: early clinical experiences. Cardiovasc Intervent Radiol. 2006;29(4):552–8.
24. Cowan BD, Sewell PE, Howard JC, Arriola RM, Robinette LG. Interventional magnetic resonance imaging cryotherapy of uterine fibroid tumors: preliminary observation. Am J Obstet Gynecol. 2002;186(6):1183–7.
25. Stovall DW. Alternatives to hysterectomy: focus on global endometrial ablation, uterine fibroid embolization, and magnetic resonance-guided focused ultrasound. Menopause. 2011;18(4):437–44.
26. Donnez J, Dolmans MM. Uterine fibroid management: from the present to the future. Hum Reprod Update. 2016;22(6):665–86.
27. Cheung VYT. High-intensity focused ultrasound therapy. Best Pract Res Clin Obstet Gynaecol. 2018;46:74–83. https://doi.org/10.1016/j.bpobgyn.2017.09.002.
28. Luo X, Rong SS, Ma XF, Shuai HL. The research of feasibility and efficacy of radiofrequency ablation in treating uterine fibroids. Medicine (Baltimore). 2015;94(47):e1956.
29. Qin J, Chen J-Y, Zhao W-P, Hu L, Chen W-Z, Wang Z-B. Outcome of unintended pregnancy after ultrasound-guided high-intensity focused ultrasound ablation of uterine fibroids. Int J Gynecol Obstet. 2012;117(3):273–7. https://doi.org/10.1016/j.ijgo.2012.01.011.
30. Rabinovici J, David M, Fukunishi H, Morita Y, Gostout BS, Stewart EA. Pregnancy outcome after magnetic resonance-guided focused ultrasound surgery (MRgFUS) for conservative treatment of uterine fibroids. Fertil Steril. 2010;93(1):199–209. https://doi.org/10.1016/j.fertnstert.2008.10.001.

High-Intensity Focused Ultrasound Surgery of Uterine Myomas

11

Giulia Alfieri, Monica Mattone, Lucia Manganaro, Francesco Pecorini, Carlo Catalano, and Alessandro Napoli

11.1 Introduction

Uterine fibroids (UFs), or leiomyomas, are the most common benign tumor of the genital tract in women of reproductive age, as they occur in about 70% of the female population [1]. About 30–50% of women with uterine fibroids have significant symptoms requiring therapy. Symptoms of myomas can be classified into three distinct categories: abnormal uterine bleeding, pelvic pressure and pain, and reproductive dysfunction [2].

Several treatment strategies are available for the management of UFs. Hysterectomy and laparoscopic and hysteroscopic myomectomy are the most widely used surgical interventions for myomas. However, surgery is burdened by a non-negligible risk of complications and adverse events, such as infection, venous thromboembolism, genitourinary and gastrointestinal tract injuries, and bleeding. Moreover, a hysterectomy causes total deprivation of fertility [3].

Alternatives to surgical intervention include uterine artery embolization (UAE) and high-intensity focused ultrasound surgery (HIFU) [4].

Focused ultrasound surgery (FUS) is a noninvasive technique that has the potential to ablate tumor lesions precisely [5], relying on the combination of HIFU and an imaging method for procedure guidance.

There have been nearly 375,000 patients treated with focused ultrasound; among these, 64% have been for prostate diseases and uterine fibroids [6]. The FDA has approved the use of FUS also for the treatment of essential tremor, Parkinson's disease, painful bone metastases, and osteoid osteoma [7]. Promising results were achieved in managing other neoplastic diseases, including liver, kidney, and breast, and neuropsychiatric disorders [7–10].

G. Alfieri · M. Mattone (✉) · L. Manganaro
C. Catalano
Department of Radiological, Oncological and Pathological Sciences, Policlinico Umberto I—Sapienza University of Rome, Rome, Italy
e-mail: giulia.alfieri@uniroma1.it; lucia.manganaro@uniroma1.it; carlo.catalano@uniroma1.it

F. Pecorini
Department of Gynecology, Obstetrics and Urology, Policlinico Umberto I —Sapienza University of Rome, Rome, Italy
e-mail: francesco.pecorini@uniroma1.it

A. Napoli
Department of Radiological, Oncological and Pathological Sciences, Policlinico Umberto I—Sapienza University of Rome, Rome, Italy

Spine Unit, Centro SaNa Servizi Sanitari Privati, Aprilia, Italy
e-mail: alessandro.napoli@uniroma1.it

11.2 Physical Principle and Biological Effects

The principle behind FUS is that a high-intensity ultrasound beam brought to a tight focus may kill cells lying within the focal volume while all other tissues in the ultrasound beam path are spared [11].

FUS is performed using a piezoelectric transducer that generates acoustic pressure waves

R. Niola et al. (eds.), *Diagnostic and Interventional Radiology in Gynecological and Obstetric Diseases*, https://doi.org/10.1007/978-3-031-11910-1_11

when an alternating electric current is applied [12], with frequencies of around 1 MHz and intensity of 102–104 W/cm^2 [13]. Ultrasounds can be focused with lens or reflector or, more recently, with phased-array transducers [12]. The incident ultrasound beam is absorbed and converted into heat at the focal point, resulting in local temperature elevation. At a microscopic level, the mechanical energy of ultrasounds causes pressure fluctuations that produce a vibratory movement and, by generating friction, determine hyperthermia. The deposition of acoustic energy in the targeted tissue is called sonication [11].

FUS/HIFU can be targeted in volume ranges of mm^3 to cm^3, causing protein denaturation and coagulative necrosis of the treated tissue within seconds when temperatures are between 55 °C and 60 °C [12]. Other mechanical effects also contribute to tissue damage at the focal point, including cavitation and acoustic radiation force. Temperature above 96 °C triggers further mechanisms like tissue boiling and bubble formation, whose effects on surrounding tissues are less predictable, thus 96 °C is the maximum achievable temperature. The size of the coagulative necrosis area depends on the acoustic pressure, exposure time, and tissue composition [14]. The volume of ablation after a single sonication pulse is small (about 6 mm × 25 mm) [15], therefore, several sonications have to be performed in order to achieve ablation of larger tissues, with an interval between the treatments that protect surrounding structures from heat accumulation and thermal damage [14, 16].

11.3 Imaging Guidance

From the 1970s and up to the 1990s, the only imaging modality used for the visualization of target tissues was ultrasounds (ultrasound-guided focused ultrasound surgery, USgFUS) [7]. The imaging guidance in magnetic resonance–guided focused ultrasound surgery (MRgFUS), in addition to the morphological visualization of the organs, provides real-time monitoring of tissue temperature in the form of a "thermal map." The temperature feedback allows to adjust the energy and power of the sonications in order to obtain complete ablation of the lesions avoiding over-sonication and limiting damage to the surrounding structures [17]. Several temperature-sensitive MR parameters can be used for thermal monitoring: the most used one is the phase-mapping method based on the proton resonance frequency (PRF)-shift, which is sensitive even to small variations in temperature. The PRF-shift methods are based on the difference in the nature of hydrogen bonds between water molecules and consequently the difference in the resonance frequency of water protons at different temperatures [18].

11.4 Indications and Contraindications

Since the aim of the MRgFUS procedure is to improve UFs-related symptoms rather than to determine local tumor control, only symptomatic patients are considered eligible for treatment.

In these patients, clinical diagnosis needs to be confirmed by MRI, also in order to rule out the presence of other diseases that could represent a contraindication to treatment. In the same circumstance, given that UFs are often a multifocal pathology, the "dominant" UF needs to be identified: it can be defined as the most likely fibroid to be responsible for symptoms, according to imaging features including size, signal intensity, and vascularization (Fig. 11.1).

So, eligible patients are symptomatic women with an identified dominant UF compatible with the clinical presentation and women with UFs that have MRI features suitable for the treatment.

Absolute exclusion criteria are the following: presence of absolute contraindication to paramagnetic contrast agents, pregnancy, and presence of any other pelvic disease.

Other exclusion criteria are related to some morphological characteristics of UFs. These characteristics can be identified during a preliminary MRI examination performed with the patient

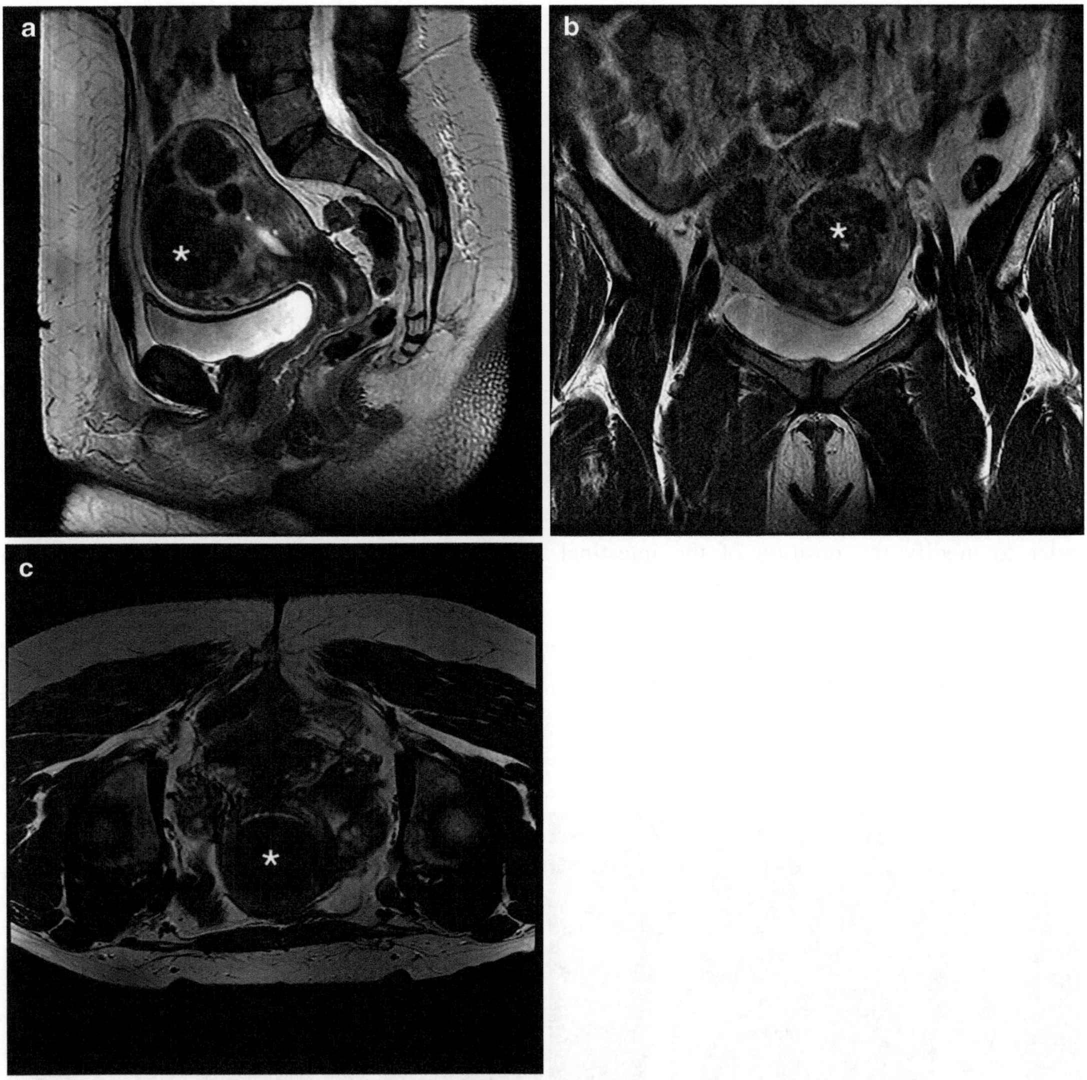

Fig. 11.1 Sagittal (**a**), coronal (**b**), and axial (**c**) T2W pre-treatment MR in a patient with pain due to UFs. The dominant fibroid (*asterisk*) is defined as the most likely fibroid to be responsible for symptoms, according to imaging features including size, signal intensity, and vascularization. From: Napoli, A., Alfieri, G., Andrani, F., Scipione, R., Manganaro, L., Pecorini, F., & Catalano, C. (2021, February). Uterine Myomas: Focused Ultrasound Surgery. In *Seminars in Ultrasound, CT and MRI* (Vol. 42, No. 1, pp. 25–36). WB Saunders

in the prone position [19], which will be the one assumed during treatment.

UFs with a diameter greater than 10–12 cm are generally not treated, in order to avoid excessively long procedures with the possibility of causing discomfort as well as complications such as deep vein thrombosis [20]. However, preliminary treatment with GnRH agonists may allow for fibroid shrinkage, which can result in shortened treatment times [21, 22].

Several other MR characteristics of the lesions have to be considered in order to assess eligibility: hyperintensity of the lesion in the T2-weighted MRI (Funaki type 3) is considered an exclusion criterion due to demonstrated low efficacy of MRgFUS in this category of UFs [23]; pedunculated UFs are not treated since the ablation of the stalk may cause disconnection of the lesion from the uterine wall, requiring surgical treatment to remove free debris into the pelvic cavity; not-enhancing UFs are excluded, since the effect of the treatment is precisely to determine coagulation necrosis, which in non-vascularized UFs has probably already occurred; the presence of a calcified envelope may determine complete reflection of the ultrasound energy, with scarce clinical results and unpredictable side effects.

The interposition of the bowel between the transducer and the targeted lesion may represent an obstacle to the ultrasound beam path, since the sonication of bowel loops can cause bowel injury and, at worst, perforation. Filling the rectal ampulla and/or bladder with ultrasound gel, in order to modify the position of the intestinal loops, or employing an angled ultrasound beam are techniques used in order to avoid the interposition of structures that could be damaged: However, when these mitigation techniques are not applicable or ineffective, bowel interposition is considered a contraindication to MRgFUS.

It is also necessary to evaluate the distance between the midpoint of the lesion and the skin surface: a distance greater than or equal to 12 cm is a contraindication, due to the limited penetration depth of the ultrasound beam. The proximity of the lesions to the sacrum is another contraindication, since heat accumulation in the bone can be transferred to the perineural fat and adjacent nerves, determining nerve injury: the safety distance between the target area and the sacrum should be at least 4 cm. Even in these cases, mitigation techniques such as rectum filling can be used (Fig. 11.2).

The presence of skin scars is another relative contraindication, since cutaneous scars can absorb ultrasounds, thus causing skin burns. Changing the beam angulation can sometimes prevent this event [24].

Relative and absolute contraindications are summarized in Tables 11.1 and 11.2.

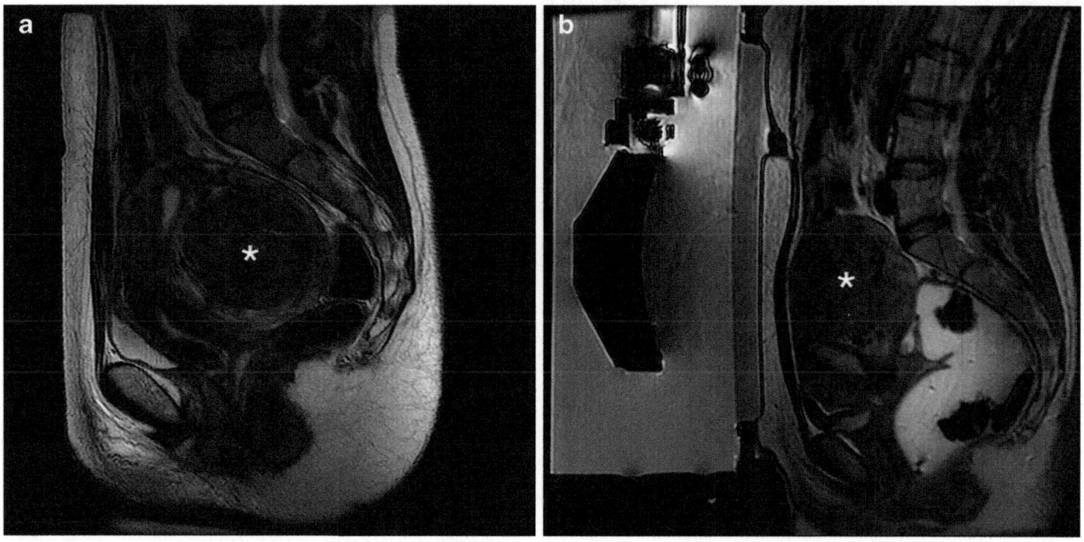

Fig. 11.2 Sagittal (**a**) T2W pre-treatment MR performed in the prone position in a patient with a 6 cm UF (*asterisk*). The fibroid is less than 4 cm distant from the sacrum. Filling the rectal ampulla with the ultrasound gel displaces the uterus anteriorly, thus increasing the distance between the lesion and sacrum, as shown in the T2W sagittal image (**b**). From: Napoli, A., Alfieri, G., Andrani, F., Scipione, R., Manganaro, L., Pecorini, F., & Catalano, C. (2021, February). Uterine Myomas: Focused Ultrasound Surgery. In *Seminars in Ultrasound, CT and MRI* (Vol. 42, No. 1, pp. 25–36). WB Saunders

Table 11.1 General contraindications in MRgFUS for UFs

Absolute contraindications	Relative contraindications
MRI contraindications	Cutaneous scars
Pregnancy	
Other pelvic diseases	

Table 11.2 MRI exclusion criteria in MRgFUS for UFs

Absolute contraindications	Relative contraindications
Fibroid diameter >10 cm	Bowel interposition
Funaki 3 fibroids	Distance from the sacrum <4 cm
Pedunculated or calcified fibroids	Distance skin—Midpoint of fibroid >12 cm
Not-enhancing fibroids	

11.5 Procedure

A typical MRgFUS treatment comprises three steps with an MRI prescan for delineation of the UFs and subsequent treatment planning, the FUS treatment as such, and a contrast-enhanced MRI post-treatment scan to evaluate the treated volume.

MRgFUS can be performed in an outpatient setting. Before treatment, the patient undergoes a trichotomy of the skin from the umbilical to the pubis; an intravenous access and a Foley urinary catheter are placed.

The procedure is performed with the patient in a prone position on a dedicated MR table, with the abdomen lying in a water bath of deionized degassed water, in contact with an acoustic coupling gel pad located above the ultrasound transducer.

In this phase, patients are informed about the possibility of experiencing discomfort in the pelvic area during the procedure: in case of severe acute pain, neurological symptoms, and skin-burning sensation, they can report it verbally or via an emergency button, immediately interrupting sonication.

A moderate sedation is administered to help relax, prevent movement, and minimize discomfort during the procedure.

Right before starting a procedure, baseline T2-weighted MR images in axial, coronal, and sagittal planes are obtained for treatment planning. The region of treatment (ROT) is defined and drawn by the radiologist in all three planes; critical structures, such as bone tissue, nerves, and intestinal loops, are marked in order to avoid their sonication. The operator also establishes anatomical landmarks to identify and possibly compensate for the patient's physiological or accidental movements during the procedure. At this stage, the bladder and/or the rectus can be filled, if necessary.

Once treatment planning is defined, a few low-energy sonications are performed for final targeting calibration.

At this point, the actual clinical treatment can start; the procedure is performed with multiple therapeutic sonications until a sufficient fibroid volume is covered [25]. Each sonication lasts 20–40 s with a cooling period between subsequent sonications lasting up to 90 s [15]. Real-time MR thermometry will reveal any potentially dangerous heating or unwanted exposure (Fig. 11.3).

At the end of the procedure, T1-weighted images are acquired before and after the intravenous administration of the paramagnetic contrast medium to assess the extent of the ablated area. A specific parameter that is helpful in evaluating the percentage of therapeutic necrosis is the non-perfused volume (NPV): it represents the ratio between the non-perfused tissue volume after treatment and the pretreatment volume of the lesion (Fig. 11.4).

A post-procedure clinical evaluation makes it possible to detect the presence of complications.

Most patients can return to work a few days after the treatment.

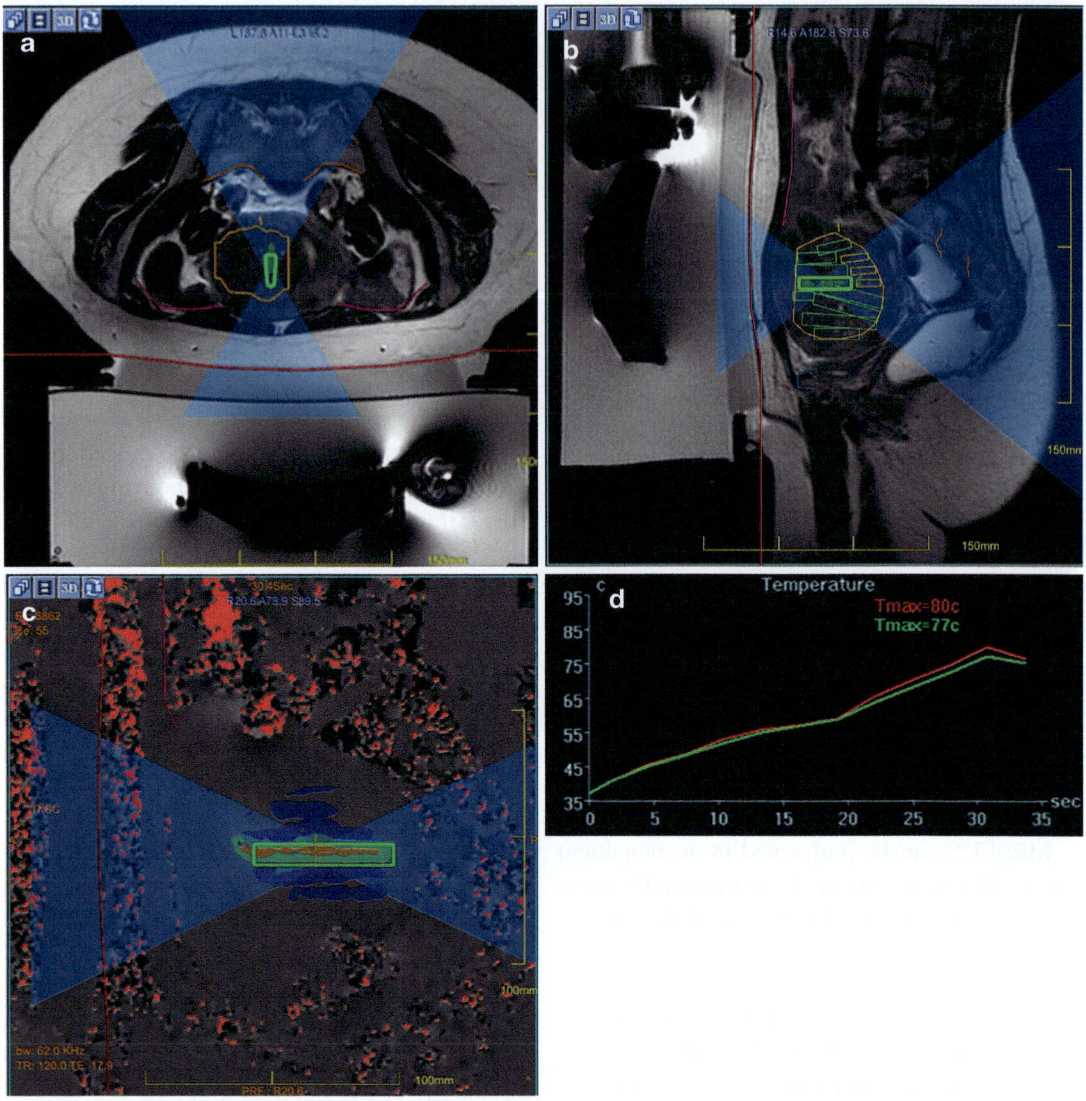

Fig. 11.3 Axial (**a**) and sagittal (**b**) MRI images acquired during the planning phase of the MRgFUS procedure. The non-pass region marker along the surface of the sacrum and around bowel loops is drawn; the region of treatment is bordered. Once all these regions are manually marked, the software automatically splits the region of treatment into several discrete sonication areas (boxes): the operator can change automatic parameters at any time during the procedure. (**c**) Real-time thermometric map obtained at the end of a single sonication during the procedure using proton resonance frequency sequences; the central area represents the site where the critical threshold for coagulative necrosis has been reached. (**d**) Temperature trend in the treated area during the sonication time. From: Napoli, A., Alfieri, G., Andrani, F., Scipione, R., Manganaro, L., Pecorini, F., & Catalano, C. (2021, February). Uterine Myomas: Focused Ultrasound Surgery. In *Seminars in Ultrasound, CT and MRI* (Vol. 42, No. 1, pp. 25–36). WB Saunders

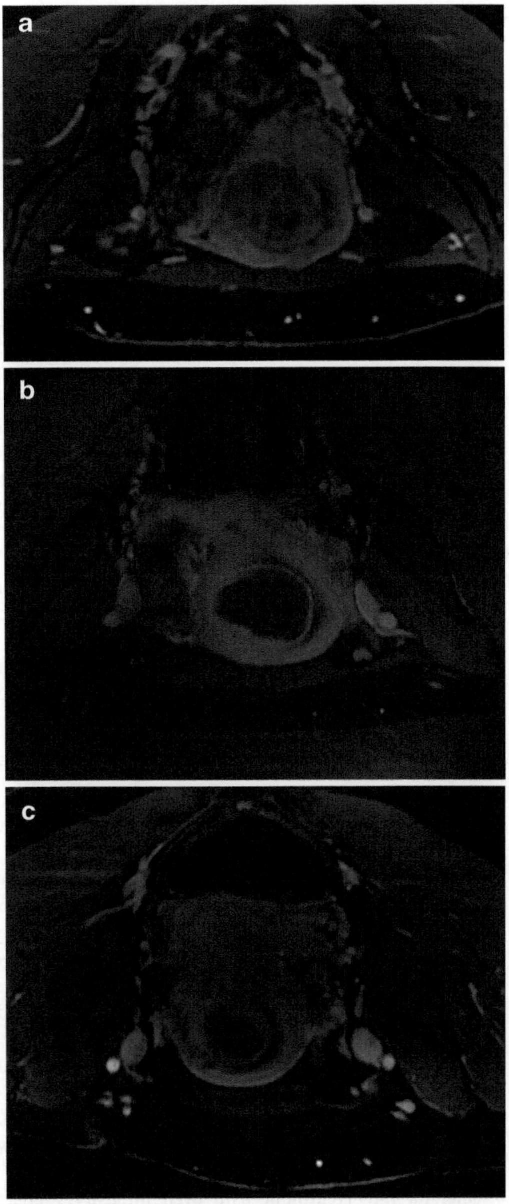

Fig. 11.4 Pre- and post-treatment contrast-enhanced axial MR images of a patient who underwent MRgFUS treatment for UF. (**a**) Preprocedural scan demonstrates the presence of an enhancing lesion with a diameter of 4 cm. (**b**) Postprocedural image shows the necrotic area within the lesion (NPV was about 80% of the initial volume). (**c**) Three months after the treatment the volume of the whole lesion decreased, with a maximum diameter of 3 cm; the nonperfused area is still present within the fibroid. From: Napoli, A., Alfieri, G., Andrani, F., Scipione, R., Manganaro, L., Pecorini, F., & Catalano, C. (2021, February). Uterine Myomas: Focused Ultrasound Surgery. In *Seminars in Ultrasound, CT and MRI* (Vol. 42, No. 1, pp. 25–36). WB Saunders

11.6 Literature Data

Numerous scientific evidence have confirmed the efficacy of MRgFUS in the management of UFs, during the first 12 months following treatment. Two recent reviews demonstrated that HIFU ablation is more effective than surgical interventions regarding the improvement of QoL, requiring shorter hospital stay and recovery time [25, 26].

The re-intervention rate after MRgFUS treatment, defined as the need for any additional intervention including secondary HIFU, myomectomy, hysterectomy, or hormone treatment, is about 13–14% at 24 months [27], with some studies reporting no significant difference between MRgFUS and conventional surgery in reintervention rate [25].

HIFU-related adverse reactions are few and mild, most resolving spontaneously. The reported adverse event rate is 8.7%, most of which is due to minor side effects [27]. The most common complication of FUS is dermal toxicity along the acoustic path, which is manifested by skin blister or induration [28]. Such injuries can be avoided by ensuring that there is no interposition of air between the transducer and the patient's skin during the procedure. Other reported adverse events are vaginal discharge lasting 3–14 days, uterus bleeding, transient lower abdominal pain, odynuria or hematuria, cystitis, urinary retention, transient leg or buttock pain, constitutional symptoms, fever, and blurred vision. Major adverse events occur in 0.2% of patients: deep vein thrombosis, high-degree skin burn, intestinal perforation, and sciatic nerve injury have been reported [27–29]. These data support the overall safety of MRgFUS treatment when compared to UAE and myomectomy, in which the adverse event rate rises to 19% and 25%, respectively, with 2.9% of major complications after UAE [30, 31]. Moreover, the improvement of FUS technologies and operator learning curves have determined a further reduction of adverse events compared to early reports, as suggested in more recent works [27].

MRgFUS is a relatively safe noninvasive method which seems not to deteriorate fertility compared to pre-treatment status. Surgical myomectomy, that was considered the standard of care for treating symptomatic UFs in women who wish to preserve their fertility, exposes patients to a high risk of obstetric complications [32] and is associated with classical surgical complications such as pelvic adhesions that may decrease the reproductive potentials [33]; experts agree that UAE is associated with lower pregnancy rates, higher miscarriage rates, and more adverse pregnancy outcomes in comparison with myomectomies [34].

Available data prove that there is no impairment of the ovarian function [35] and of the possibility to conceive after the FUS therapy for UFs [36–41]: pregnancy is possible after the treatment, with no increased rate of spontaneous abortions or pregnancy complications [32]. In 2015, FDA approved MRgFUS with a next-generation ExAblate system for the treatment of symptomatic UFs and changed the labeling to allow consideration for women who desire to maintain fertility. However, in accordance with the recent Radiological-Gynecological Expert Meeting, due to the lack of large-scale prospective clinical trials, a recommendation on the use of MRgFUS in pregnancy cannot be made and, in women wishing to become pregnant, an interval of at least 6 months from treatment is recommended [42].

11.7 Conclusions

MRgFUS represents an efficacious treatment in relieving symptoms related to UFs with a low rate of complications. Moreover, the improvement of technology and the experience of physicians over time have led to a progressive reduction in the adverse event rate. MRgFUS is repeatable and does not seem to impair the possibility to conceive and the obstetrical outcome in case of pregnancy. The main disadvantage is that only a few patients are eligible.

The treatment of UFs requires an individualized, patient-tailored approach and is dependent on the patient's age, symptoms, UF location and size, the expectations of the patient concerning reproductive plans, the desire for the preservation of the uterus, physician experience, and patient preference.

References

1. Stewart EA, Cookson CL, Gandolfo RA, Schulze-Rath R. Epidemiology of uterine fibroids: a systematic review. BJOG Int J Obstet Gynaecol. 2017;124(10):1501–12.
2. Stewart EA. Uterine fibroids. Lancet. 2001;357(9252):293–8.
3. Clarke-Pearson DL, Geller EJ. Complications of hysterectomy. Obstet Gynecol. 2013;121(3):654–73.
4. Donnez J, Dolmans M. Uterine fibroid management: from the present to the future. Hum Reprod Update. 2016;22(6):665–86. https://doi.org/10.1093/humupd/dmw023.
5. Hsiao YH, Kuo SJ, Tsai HD, Chou MC, Yeh GP. Clinical application of high-intensity focused ultrasound in cancer therapy. J Cancer. 2016;7(3):225.
6. Focused ultrasound foundation: the Technology, State of the Technology. https://www.fusfoundation.org/the-technology/state-of-the-technology. Accessed 25 Sept 2021.
7. Ebbini ES, Ter Haar G. Ultrasound-guided therapeutic focused ultrasound: current status and future directions. Int J Hyperth. 2015;31(2):77–89.
8. Focused ultrasound foundation: diseases and conditions, miscellaneous. https://fusfoundation.org/diseases-and-conditions/overview. Accessed 25 Sept 2021.
9. Napoli A, Scipione R, Hans-Peter E, Marrocchio C, Dababou S. Uterus-sparing treatment options for the Management of Fibroids. Obstet Gynecol Cases Rev. 2018;5:131.
10. Napoli A, Bazzocchi A, Scipione R, Anzidei M, Saba L, Ghanouni P, Catalano C. Noninvasive therapy for osteoid osteoma: a prospective developmental study with MR imaging–guided high-intensity focused ultrasound. Radiology. 2017;285(1):186–96.
11. Ter Haar G. Therapeutic ultrasound. Eur J Ultrasound. 1999;9(1):3–9.
12. Mihcin S, Melzer A. Principles of focused ultrasound. Minim Invasive Ther Allied Technol. 2018;27(1):41–50. https://doi.org/10.1080/13645706.2017.1414063.
13. Mason TJ. Therapeutic ultrasound an overview. Ultrason Sonochem. 2011;18(4):847–52.
14. Shehata IA. Treatment with high intensity focused ultrasound: secrets revealed. Eur J Radiol. 2012;81(3):534–41.
15. Roberts A. Magnetic resonance-guided focused ultrasound for uterine fibroids. Semin Intervent Radiol. 2008;25(4):394–405. https://doi.org/10.1055/s-0028-1102999.
16. Al-Bataineh O, Jenne J, Huber P. Clinical and future applications of high intensity focused ultrasound in cancer. Cancer Treat Rev. 2012;38(5):346–53.
17. Wang Y, Wang ZB, Xu YH. Efficacy, efficiency, and safety of magnetic resonance-guided high-intensity focused ultrasound for ablation of uterine fibroids: comparison with ultrasound-guided method. Korean J Radiol. 2018;19(4):724–32.

18. Rieke V, Butts Pauly K. MR thermometry. J Magn Reason Imaging. 2008;27(2):376–90.
19. Duc NM, Keserci B. Review of influential clinical factors in reducing the risk of unsuccessful MRI-guided HIFU treatment outcome of uterine fibroids. Diagn Interv Radiol. 2018;24(5):283.
20. Nguyen MD, Huynh QH, Keserci B. Adverse events of focused ultrasound surgery for uterine fibroids and adenomyosis. Rep Med Imaging. 2018;11:15.
21. Smart OC, Hindley JT, Regan L, Gedroyc WG. Gonadotrophin-releasing hormone and magnetic-resonance–guided ultrasound surgery for uterine leiomyomata. Obstet Gynecol. 2006;108(1):49–54.
22. Lethaby A, Vollenhoven B, Sowter M. Efficacy of pre-operative gonadotropin hormone releasing analogues for women with uterine fibroids undergoing hysterectomy or myomectomy: a systematic review. Obstet Gynecol Surv. 2003;58(5):323–4.
23. Kim YS, Lee JW, Choi CH, Kim BG, Bae DS, Rhim H, Lim HK. Uterine fibroids: correlation of T2 signal intensity with semiquantitative perfusion MR parameters in patients screened for MR-guided high-intensity focused ultrasound ablation. Radiology. 2015;278(3):925–35.
24. Geraci L, Napoli A, Catalano C, Midiri M, Gagliardo C. Magnetic resonance imaging-guided focused ultrasound surgery for the treatment of symptomatic uterine fibroids. Case Rep Radiol, vol. 2017; 2017. p. 2520989.
25. Tsai MC, Chang LT, Tam KW. Comparison of high-intensity focused ultrasound and conventional surgery for patients with uterine myomas: a systematic review and meta-analysis. J Minim Invasive Gynecol. 2021;28(10):1712–24.
26. Gao H, Li T, Fu D, Wei J. Uterine artery embolization, surgery and high intensity focused ultrasound in the treatment of uterine fibroids: a network meta-analysis. Quant Imaging Med Surg. 2021;11(9):4125–36. https://doi.org/10.21037/qims-20-1331.
27. Verpalen IM, Anneveldt KJ, Nijholt IM, Schutte JM, Dijkstra JR, Franx A, Boomsma MF. Magnetic resonance-high intensity focused ultrasound (MR-HIFU) therapy of symptomatic uterine fibroids with unrestrictive treatment protocols: a systematic review and meta-analysis. Eur J Radiol. 2019;120:108700.
28. Chen J, Chen W, Zhang L, et al. Safety of ultrasound-guided ultra- sound ablation for uterine fibroids and adenomyosis: a review of 9988 cases. Ultrason Sonochem. 2015;27:671–6.
29. National Institute for Health and Care Excellence. Magnetic resonance image-guided transcutaneous focused ultrasound for uterine fibroids. 2017. https://www.nice.org.uk/guidance/ipg413. Accessed 28 Sept 2021.
30. Toor SS, Jaberi A, Macdonald DB, McInnes MD, Schweitzer ME, Rasuli P. Complication rates and effectiveness of uterine artery embolization in the treatment of symptomatic leiomyomas: a systematic review and meta-analysis. Am J Roentgenol. 2012;199(5):1153–63.
31. Moss JG, Cooper KG, Khaund A, Murray LS, Murray GD, Wu O, Lumsden MA. Randomised comparison of uterine artery embolization (UAE) with surgical treatment in patients with symptomatic uterine fibroids (REST trial): 5-year results. BJOG Int J Obstet Gynaecol. 2011;118(8):936–44.
32. Milazzo GN, Catalano A, Badia V, et al. Myoma and myomectomy: poor evidence concern in pregnancy. J Obstet Gynaecol Res. 2017;43:1789–804.
33. Kumakiri J, Kikuchi I, Kitade M, et al. Association between uterine repair at laparoscopic myomectomy and postoperative adhesions. Acta Obstet Gynecol Scand. 2012;91:331–7.
34. Carranza-Mamane B, Havelock J, Hemmings R, Cheung A, Sierra S, Case A, Vause T. The management of uterine fibroids in women with otherwise unexplained infertility. J Obstet Gynaecol Can. 2015;37(3):277–85.
35. Cheung VY, Lam TP, Jenkins CR, Cheung GK, Chan SS, Choi WK. Ovarian reserve after ultrasound-guided high-intensity focused ultrasound for uterine fibroids: preliminary experience. J Obstet Gynaecol Can. 2016;38(4):357–61.
36. Stanford Health Care. Risks of the MRgFUS procedure. 2019. https://stanfordhealthcare.org/medical-treatments/m/mr-guided-focused-ultrasound/complications.html. Accessed 28 Sept 2021.
37. Yin N, Hu L, Xiao ZB, et al. Factors influencing thermal injury to skin and abdominal wall structures in HIFU ablation of uterine fibroids. Int J Hyperth. 2018;34:1298–303.
38. Machtinger R, Inbar Y, Cohen-Eylon S, et al. MR-guided focus ultrasound (MRgFUS) for symptomatic uterine fibroids: predictors of treatment success. Hum Reprod. 2012;27:3425–31.
39. Schlesinger D, Benedict S, Diederich C, et al. MR-guided focused ultrasound surgery, present and future. Med Phys. 2013;40:080901.
40. Rabinovici J, David M, Fukunishi H, et al. Pregnancy outcome after magnetic resonance-guided focused ultrasound surgery (MRgFUS) for conservative treatment of uterine fibroids. Fertil Steril. 2010;93:199–209.
41. Łoziński T, Filipowska J, Gurynowicz G, Zgliczyńska M, Kluz T, Jędra R, Ciebiera M. The effect of high-intensity focused ultrasound guided by magnetic resonance therapy on obstetrical outcomes in patients with uterine fibroids–experiences from the main polish center and a review of current data. Int J Hyperth. 2019;36(1):582–90.
42. Qu K, Mao S, Li J, Wang J, Ouyang G, Wang Z, Wang Z, Xiong Y, Zhang L. The impact of ultrasound-guided high-intensity focused ultrasound for uterine fibroids on ovarian reserve. Int J Hyperth. 2020;37(1):399–403. https://doi.org/10.1080/02656736.2020.1754473.

12 Embolization of Uterine Arteriovenous Malformations

Cristina Mosconi, Renato D'Onofrio, Alberta Cappelli, Violante Mulas, Antonio De Cinque, Francesco Modestino, Antonio Basile, Massimo Venturini, and Rita Golfieri

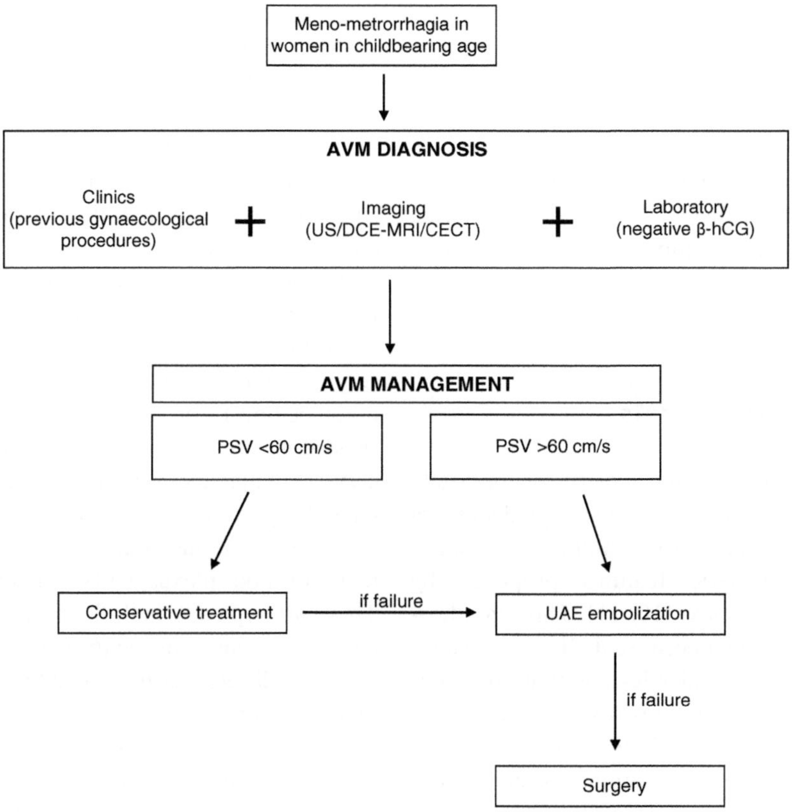

C. Mosconi (✉) · R. D'Onofrio · A. Cappelli
V. Mulas · A. De Cinque · F. Modestino · R. Golfieri
Department of Radiology, IRCCS Azienda Ospedaliero-Universitaria di Bologna, Bologna, Italy
e-mail: cristina.mosconi@aosp.bo.it; renato.donofrio@studio.unibo.it; alberta.cappelli@aosp.bo.it; francesco.modestino@aosp.bo.it; rita.golfieri@unibo.it

A. Basile
Unit of Radiology 1, Policlinico Rodolico, Catania, Italy

M. Venturini
Department of Diagnostic and Interventional Radiology, Circolo Hospital, Insubria University, Varese, Italy
e-mail: massimo.venturini@uninsubria.it

R. Niola et al. (eds.), *Diagnostic and Interventional Radiology in Gynecological and Obstetric Diseases*, https://doi.org/10.1007/978-3-031-11910-1_12

12.1 Introduction

Arteriovenous malformations (AVMs) are vascular anomalies where direct communication is established between arteries and veins, without a capillary circulation [1]. Uterine AVMs represent rare peripheral localization but can result in potentially fatal vaginal bleeding [2, 3], accounting for 1–2% of intraperitoneal hemorrhages [4, 5]. These are typical of women of reproductive age, often multiparous; however, some cases have been reported in both adolescent and postmenopausal women. Pregnancy and associated hormonal status appear to play an important role in the pathogenesis [3, 6]. The major symptom is vaginal bleeding, which is often intermittent and torrential, typical of high vascular flow, and can represent a life-threatening condition. Pelvic pain, anemia, and hypotension, secondary to blood loss, may be present with a possible need for a blood transfusion. Nevertheless, uterine AVMs can remain asymptomatic and diagnosed incidentally [7–9].

12.2 Pathophysiology of Uterine AVMs

In 1982, the International Society for the Study of Vascular Anomalies (ISSVA) adopted a binary classification system for vascular anomalies based on pathologic features proposed by Mulliken and Glowacki [10, 11]. This classification is very important because it allows a systematic approach to vascular lesions that correlates predictably with clinical history, disease course, and treatment options, making it clinically useful [12]. The ISSVA classification system divides vascular anomalies into two (binary) primary biological categories: (1) vasoproliferative or vascular neoplasms and (2) vascular malformations. While the former has an increase in endothelial cell turnover (i.e., they proliferate and undergo mitosis) because they are neoplasms, the latter does not have an increase in endothelial cell turnover. Vascular malformations, on the other hand, are structural anomalies of the capillary, venous, lymphatic, and arterial systems that grow in proportion to the child [10–12].

Furthermore, vascular malformations can be further classified according to their vascularity characteristics: AVM with a direct fistulous connection of the arteries and venous structures in the absence of a high-flow nidus or AVM characterized by a high-pressure gradient across the arterial and venous system that allows a high vascular flow through the nidus, the interposed network of communicating vessels arteries to veins.

Uterine AVMs are rare, but they can determine severe recurring and intermittent menorrhagia. Uterine AVMs are also further classified based on origin and divided into congenital and acquired AVMs. Congenital AVMs arise from a defect in capillary differentiation during fetal angiogenesis, resulting in multiple thin arteriovenous connections organized in a nest, with frequent involvement of extrauterine structures [2, 13]. These are typically low-flow AVMs without an early venous drainage.

In contradistinction, acquired AVMs are vascular abnormalities secondary to reparative processes following previous pregnancies, pelvic trauma, surgery (dilatation and curettage, cesarean section, myomectomy), or gynecological malignancies (gestational trophoblastic disease, endometrial and cervical malignancy). Therefore, these are characterized by a large and single communication between the uterine artery branches and the myometrial venous plexus, without an interposed nest. These are typically high-flow AVMs and present an early venous drainage [6, 8, 14].

These differences mean that the term "vascular malformation" is exclusively characteristic of congenital forms because of fetal development origin, whereas terms such as "arteriovenous fistula," "traumatic uterine arteriovenous malformation," and "arteriovenous shunt" are used in the literature, despite their differences, to describe such acquired pathology which may be difficult to differentiate [15]. However, all these terms were all collectively included in the concept of acquired uterine AVM though the exact underlying pathophysiology has not yet been understood. It is likely that during surgery, packing and locking for hemostats control can cause blood to shunt from the capillary plexus to the less resistant venous system possibly resulting in fistula formation after uterine procedures [16]. Moreover, uterine dilation and curettage (D&C), cesarean section, and myomectomy or pathologic processes (such as infection or trophoblastic disease) are associated with acquired AVM. Furthermore, hormones appear to play an important role in the physiology of uterine AVMs, because worsening of symptoms has been observed during pregnancy; in particular, Beta Human Chorionic Gonadotropin (β-hCG) seems to be crucial because provoking a proliferation of otherwise latent AVMs through an unclear mechanism [17]. Similarly, in women undergoing fertility treatments, elevated estrogen levels can cause endothelial proliferation and differentiation with higher risk AVMs [17].

The occurrence of uterine AVM is rare but should always be considered in the case of a young patient with uterine hemorrhage, especially nowadays with the increasing number of uterine interventions. The differential diagnosis is broad [18] and only the synthesis of anamnestic, clinical-laboratory, and imaging data allows the diagnosis of uterine AVM [8]. In the past, this diagnosis was obtained on the operative piece after hysterectomy [6].

12.3 Clinical Presentation

Multiparous childbearing age women are typical patients with uterine AVMs; according to a systematic review by Peitsidis et al. [19] the mean age of women diagnosed with a uterine AVM was 30 years. Women without children and previous gynecological procedures rarely have acquired uterine AVM [19].

Menorrhagia and metrorrhagia are the most common symptoms of uterine AVM. Bleeding could be intermittent and torrential [9]. The different pressure gradient between the arterial and venous systems causes the high vascular flow through the AVM and consequently the bleeding. Menorrhagia and metrorrhagia are often associated with anemia and hypotension, due to acute blood loss, requiring in approximately 50% of patients blood transfusion [19]; other described symptoms are vague pelvic discomfort, urinary symptoms, including polyuria and incontinence, and dyspareunia [9]. However, some patients may remain asymptomatic for a long time and develop the first symptoms only after trauma or secondary to hormonal changes related to pregnancy or the menstrual cycle.

12.4 Diagnosis

The occurrence of uterine AVM is rare but should always be considered in the case of a young patient with uterine hemorrhage, especially nowadays with the increasing number of uterine interventions. The differential diagnosis is broad [18] and only the synthesis of anamnestic, clinical-laboratory, and imaging data allows the diagnosis of uterine AVM [8]. In the past, this diagnosis was obtained on the operative piece after hysterectomy [6].

12.4.1 Laboratory Findings

The main laboratory finding is the presence of a negative β-hCG test, which allows the differential diagnosis, often difficult with the imaging alone, between uterine AVM and other gynecological disorders where the β-hCG test is positive and shows a progressive decline in case of retained products of conception or abnormal placentation and gestational trophoblastic disease [20]. The main aspect of the difficult differential diagnosis is the different treatment: dilation and curettage (D&C) is one of the treatments of retained product of conceptions, but it can lead to a worsening of the AVM, complicating the AVM angioarchitecture, and creating new fistulous connections. Therefore, negative β-hCG tests associated with imaging are crucial in the diagnosis of uterine AVM.

The other parameter to consider is the possible reduction of hemoglobin, especially in significant menometrorrhagia.

12.4.2 Transvaginal Ultrasound

Transvaginal Ultrasound (US) is the first-line method in case of abnormal vaginal bleeding; however, Doppler imaging is necessary for the diagnosis because the grayscale ultrasound alone is not enough for a definitive diagnosis. The typical appearance of uterine AVM is the presence of hypoechogenic tubular structures within the myometrium, characterized by pronounced vascularization and turbulence [13, 21]. For the detection of these US findings, the use of color Doppler is necessary, without which the risk of misdiagnosis is high; the identification of uterine high-velocity blood flow with low impedance by Doppler ultrasound is highly suggestive for a uterine AVM [22]. Color Doppler US also provides significant diagnostic and prognostic information through flow parameters: in case of uterine AVM with PSV (Peak Systolic Velocity) <40 cm/s and without significant bleeding, periodic follow-up is expected; with PSV 40–60 cm/s, treatment is medical provided that the bleeding is not severe and stops; with PSV >60–70 cm/s, uterine artery embolization (UAE) or surgery is indicated [13, 22, 23].

However, hypervascularity and turbulent flow are typical aspects also of subinvolution of the placental bed and adenomyosis in patients with menorrhagia, and there are no specific criteria for the differential diagnosis between the two pathologies. Moreover, a differential diagnosis should be made also with hypervascularized tumors (sarcoma) and pseudoaneurysms.

12.4.3 DCE-MRI and CECT

Dynamic Contrast-Enhanced Magnetic Resonance Imaging (DCE-MRI) is the second-level examination after US and allows an accurate abdominopelvic anatomical definition [24]. Typical imaging includes serpiginous structures with characteristic signal void and early enhancement after contrast injection (Fig. 12.1a–f). Moreover, better than US,

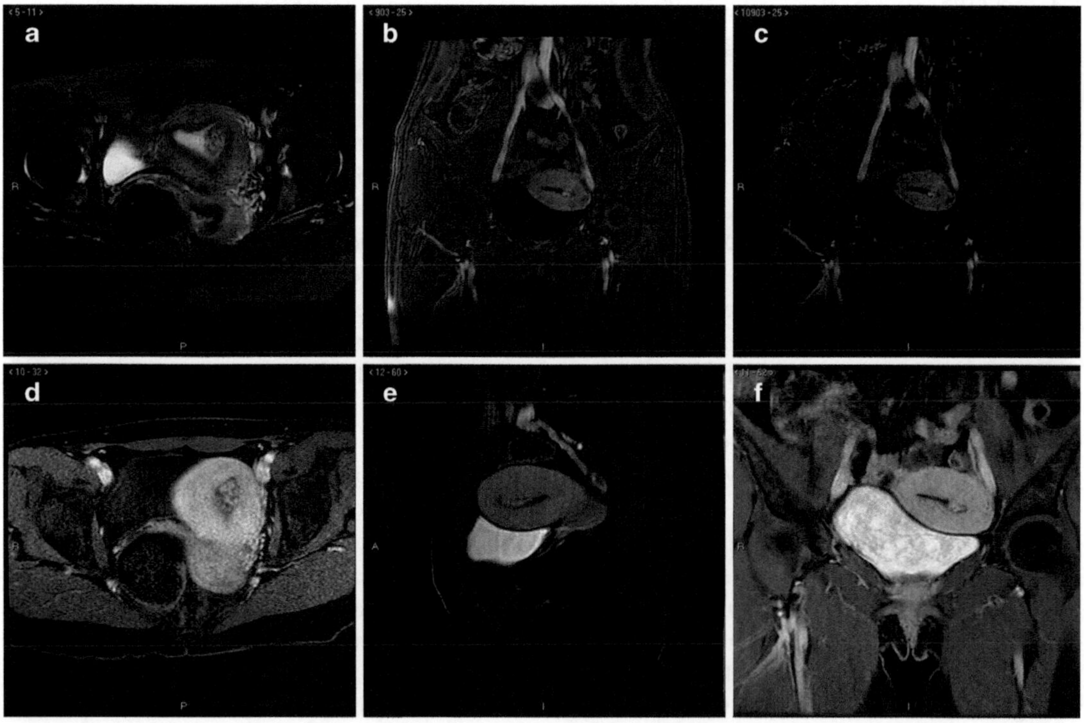

Fig. 12.1 (**a–f**) A uterine acquired AVM after IVG curettage in a 38-year-old patient; she had a history of two previous cesareans. Two months after curettage, she had anemia with menorrhagia and metrorrhagia. The preprocedural MR images (pre- and post-contrast medium on three planes) show the AVM protruding intraluminally at the level of the body in the left paramedian site

MRI allows higher tissue contrast, possible quantification of extrauterine involvement, suggestive of congenital AVM, and endometrial involvement, more likely related to retained product of conception (RPC).

Contrast-Enhanced Computer Tomography (CECT) can assess the degree of involvement of the surrounding visceral structures, but it is not always a method of choice because of the radiant exposure for young patients of reproductive age and does not add significant information compared to MRI. A typical CECT finding is a hypervascularized soft density mass [6, 8, 25].

12.4.4 Angiography

Angiography is nowadays the gold standard for diagnosis [19]. It is performed directly before UAE and allows to study the extent of the lesion, the presence or absence of a central nidus, the arterial supply, the venous drainage, and the connection with the pelvic vascularization [26]. The arteries vessels are often tortuous, and the outflow veins are dilated with early contrast filling [15].

12.5 Conservative Treatment

Conservative treatment is applied in cases of minor blood loss, with small uterine AVMs and PSV < 60 cm/s; it should be kept in mind that asymptomatic lesions may regress spontaneously [8]. Some medications can be used in the case of AVMs: methotrexate, misoprostol, methylergometrine maleate, and GnRH agonists [22]. Recently the effectiveness of an oral norethisterone (a progesterone derivative) has been proven [23] in bleeding resolution in around 90% of cases of postabortal patients, and therefore its use could also be indicated in uterine AVM.

12.6 Endovascular Treatment (UAE)

In the past, the treatment of uterine AVMs was surgical with hysterectomy; in the late 1980s, Wilms et al. [27] described the first case of uterine AVM embolization. Since then, UAE has proved to be safe and effective and represents the treatment of choice, in particular when lesions are large and very vascular with PSV > 60–70 cm/s. Moreover, UAE has the advantage of being a minimally invasive approach and, above all, of allowing patients to maintain the uterus and childbearing capacity [14, 28].

The technical and clinical success rate is high, between 71% and 93% [8]; sometimes, to achieve complete success, multiple embolizations are required and for this reason, Yoon et al. [6] reported in their review a primary success rate with symptom control of 61% and a secondary success rate of 91% after repeated treatment [6]. Based on the literature search, there are no definitive treatment guidelines for patients who fail initial embolization. Further, there have been no studies completed comparing the effectiveness of repeat embolization versus medical therapy versus hysterectomy for persistent bleeding after initial embolization. In total, transcatheter embolization (TCE) and a combination of medical therapy resulted in the eventual resolution of symptoms in 46 (85%) out of 54 patients without more invasive surgical procedures.

To obtain high clinical success, the goal is to embolize the point of fistula or the nidus and a proximal embolization should be avoided for the high risk of recurrence. To perform a complete embolization, the treatment must be well planned, both by carefully analyzing contrast-enhanced MR or CT distinguish the AVM arterial feeders and venous drainages, both by performing a panoramic aorto-iliac arteriogram during the initial diagnostic arteriography to confirm bilateral or non-bilateral and multiple supply arteries compared to CT or MRI [8]. UAE, therefore, is planned according to the vascular anatomy of both arterial supply and venous drainage, which largely depends on the type of uterine AVM. Acquired AVMs are usually supplied by one or both uterine arteries and venous drainage is usually in the hypogastric veins; both anterior hypogastric trunks and uterine arteries must be investigated selectively. The anatomical complexity is higher for congenital uterine AVMs because the lesions have more complex angioarchitecture, with possible multiple pelvic and extra-pelvic arterial supply (ovarian, lumbar, mesenteric, and epigastric) and multiple venous drainages [8]. In these cases, beyond what is described for the MAVs acquired, an abdominal aortography is necessary because the arterial afferents can be multiple as well as the venous drainages. Congenital AVMs, especially those large, often require multiple treatments, whereas for acquired AVMs a single treatment is usually sufficient [6], with a mean time interval between the traumatic event and the embolization treatment of 19.5 months (range: 6 weeks–6 years) [14].

The approach can be unilateral, by choosing the dominant side of the artery supplying, or bilateral, which depends on the clinical context and the preference of the interventional radiologist. It has been hypothesized that the higher rate of retreatment in the case of a bilateral approach is associated with the greater extent or depth of the lesion [6]. The standard procedure is performed with a right common femoral approach using the Seldinger technique with a 5 French valve introducer. An aortogram is first performed to obtain an overview of the pelvic vascularization, after that the hypogastric arteries and then the uterine arteries are selectively catheterized using catheters and microcatheters. The dominant uterine artery is identified and embolized first, usually followed by the contralateral and the extrauterine branches, if present. The procedure is considered completed if the AVM nidus is completely obliterated with no persistent early venous drainage [14, 15] (Fig. 12.2a–d). Obviously, the preliminary step to UAE is to obtain the patient's informed consent, check coagulation parameters and renal function, and rule out any allergy (if present, premedication is necessary).

A variety of embolic agents and a combination of embolic agents are reported in the literature and the choices of the embolic agents were usually based on the preference of the interventional radiologists. Various types of embolization techniques and embolizing agents including glues, gelatin sponge, coils, microspheres, and PVA (Polyvinyl Alcohol Particles) are reported in the literature; based on this literature search there has been no study comparing the efficacy of each embolic agent, or combinations [6].

However, metallic agents may produce a too proximal occlusion with the risk of ineffective treatment due to the inability to completely embolize the nidus while particulated agents present a possible risk of venous migration and pulmonary embolism [8]; gelatin sponge is correlated to high risk of recanalization as it is a reabsorbable element and it plays a role in temporary bleeding control or presurgical purpose; therefore, it is not preferable to use the embolizers described above. Liquid agents like glues seem to provide a better permanent embolization than other embolic agents; recently, the dymethilsulfoxide family agents are generally preferred [14, 29–31]. It is a liquid agent that derives from neurointerventions and, compared to glues, presents some relevant advantages. The manipulation and injection are much more controllable than glue, as it does not depend on the vascular flow but on the thrust imposed by the operator and does not present the risk of entrapment of the microcatheter. It also allows good embolization of the nidus without the risk of outflow into the venous system.

A retrograde transvenous approach was also described, due to multiple arterial afferents and the torturous aspect of the arteries themselves [32]. It is necessary to use a balloon catheter positioned at the level of the venous system which, once inflated, avoids the outflow into the pulmonary circulation; then the embolizing agent is injected with the aim of embolizing the nidus.

However, to date, despite the various options and combinations, with the limitations of the dif-

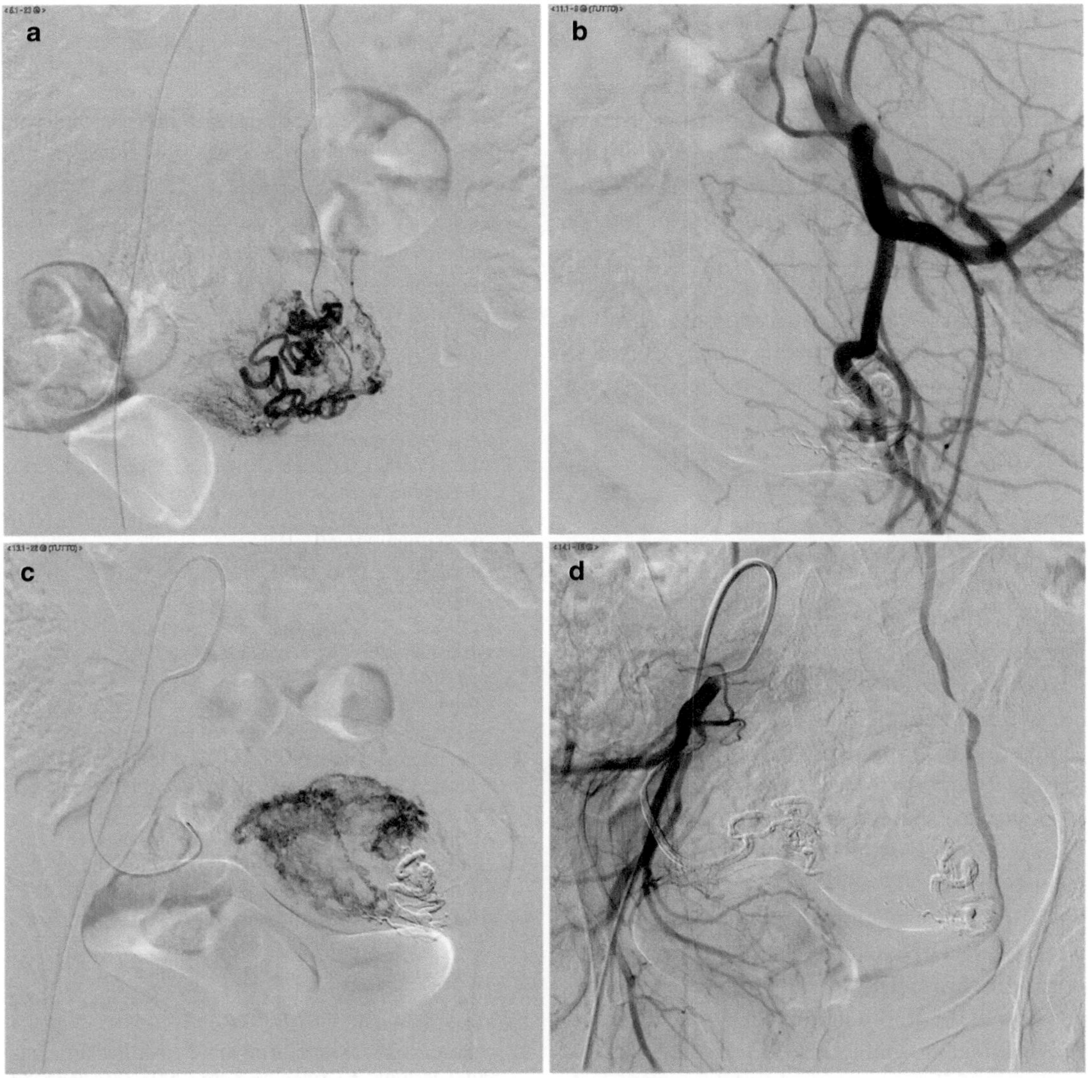

Fig. 12.2 (**a–d**) With unilateral right femoral 5Fr access, both uterine arteries were embolized with Onyx. The patient had clinical benefit and was discharged after 2 days

ferent approaches and the small number of cases reported, no significant differences in retreatment rate have emerged between the various techniques. Thereby, there is no equivocal consensus in either the choice of the technique or embolizing agent; this means that the choice is often based on the preference of the interventional radiologist [6, 15].

After UAE, patients may present with mild general symptoms related to post-procedure syndrome (pelvic pain, fever, fatigue, and nausea) which can be resolved with medical therapy in the first 48–72 h. No significant mid- to long-term complication rates have been reported in the literature [6, 19].

Clinical and radiological follow-up is recommended, at least up to 3 months after treatment [8].

The possibility of carrying a pregnancy to term after treatment has now been widely demonstrated, with an average interval between UAE and delivery of 15.6 months (range: 11–28 months) [33]. An increased risk of placental abnormalities has been observed in pregnancies after endovascular treatment, especially placenta accreta [34, 35].

12.7 Surgical Treatment

The surgical approach was the elective therapy in the pre-embolization era. Nowadays it is reserved for cases where endovascular treatment fails, for example, in case of recanalization of treated vessels or channeling of collateral vessels; in such cases, hysterectomy is recommended [36].

In literature, there have been reported some surgical fertility preserving approaches in the form of case reports, consisting mainly of laparoscopic ligation of the uterine arteries, sometimes associated with electrosurgical resection of the AVM bed [37–39].

12.8 Conclusion

Uterine AVMs are a rare but potentially life-threatening cause of vaginal bleeding, which necessitates proper diagnostic evaluation. There are two forms of uterine AVMs, congenital and acquired, which differ in etiopathogenesis, anatomical complexity, extra-pelvic extension, rate of recurrence, and retreatment.

The instrumental diagnosis is based on documentation with US with Doppler and DCE MRI or CECT of an abnormal uterine vascular network characterized by high-flow tortuous vessels. Endovascular treatment is nowadays considered the gold standard, due to the high success rate and the young age of the patients. If this treatment fails, surgery with hysterectomy is recommended.

References

1. Grivell RM, Reid KM, Mellor A. Uterine arteriovenous malformations: a review of the current literature. Obstet Gynecol Surv. 2005;60(11):761–7. https://doi.org/10.1097/01.ogx.0000183684.67656.ba.
2. Aziz N, Lenzi TA, Jeffrey RB Jr, Lyell DJ. Postpartum uterine arteriovenous fistula. Obstet Gynecol. 2004;103(5 Pt 2):1076–8. https://doi.org/10.1097/01.AOG.0000123241.44401.01.
3. Kelly SM, Belli AM, Campbell S. Arteriovenous malformation of the uterus associated with secondary postpartum hemorrhage. Ultrasound Obstet Gynecol. 2003;21(6):602–5. https://doi.org/10.1002/uog.148.
4. Newlands ES, Bagshawe KD, Begent RH, Rustin GJ, Holden L, Dent J. Developments in chemotherapy for medium- and high-risk patients with gestational trophoblastic tumours (1979–1984). Br J Obstet Gynaecol. 1986;93(1):63–9. https://doi.org/10.1111/j.1471-0528.1986.tb07815.x.
5. McIvor J, Cameron EW. Pregnancy after uterine artery embolization to control haemorrhage from gestational trophoblastic tumour. Br J Radiol. 1996;69(823):624–9. https://doi.org/10.1259/0007-1285-69-823-624.
6. Yoon DJ, Jones M, Taani JA, Buhimschi C, Dowell JD. A systematic review of acquired uterine arteriovenous malformations: pathophysiology, diagnosis, and transcatheter treatment. AJP Rep. 2016;6(1):e6–e14. https://doi.org/10.1055/s-0035-1563721.
7. Ahn HY, Park IY, Lee G, Kim SJ, Shin JC. Uterine arteriovenous malformation. Arch Gynecol Obstet. 2005;271(2):172–5. https://doi.org/10.1007/s00404-003-0588-4.
8. Giurazza F, Corvino F, Silvestre M, Cavaglià E, Amodio F, Cangiano G, De Magistris G, Niola R. Uterine arteriovenous malformations. Semin Ultrasound CT MR. 2021;42(1):37–45. https://doi.org/10.1053/j.sult.2020.08.002.
9. Molvi SN, Dash K, Rastogi H, Khanna SB. Transcatheter embolization of uterine arteriovenous malformation: report of 2 cases and review of literature. J Minim Invasive Gynecol. 2011;18(6):812–9. https://doi.org/10.1016/j.jmig.2011.07.007.
10. Mulliken JB, Glowacki J. Hemangiomas and vascular malformations in infants and children: a classification based on endothelial characteristics. Plast Reconstr Surg. 1982;69(3):412–22. https://doi.org/10.1097/00006534-198203000-00002.
11. Mulliken JB, Glowacki J. Classification of pediatric vascular lesions. Plast Reconstr Surg. 1982;70(1):120–1.
12. Van Aalst JA, Bhuller A, Sadove AM. Pediatric vascular lesions. J Craniofac Surg. 2003;14(4):566–83. https://doi.org/10.1097/00001665-200307000-00032.
13. Timmerman D, Wauters J, Van Calenbergh S, Van Schoubroeck D, Maleux G, Van Den Bosch T, Spitz B. Color Doppler imaging is a valuable tool for the diagnosis and management of uterine vascular malformations. Ultrasound Obstet Gynecol. 2003;21(6):570–7. https://doi.org/10.1002/uog.159.
14. Barral PA, Saeed-Kilani M, Tradi F, Dabadie A, Izaaryene J, Soussan J, Bartoli JM, Vidal V. Transcatheter arterial embolization with ethylene vinyl alcohol copolymer (onyx) for the treatment of hemorrhage due to uterine arteriovenous malformations. Diagn Interv Imaging. 2017;98(5):415–21. https://doi.org/10.1016/j.diii.2016.09.003.
15. Ghai S, Rajan DK, Asch MR, Muradali D, Simons ME, TerBrugge KG. Efficacy of embolization in traumatic uterine vascular malformations. J Vasc

Interv Radiol. 2003;14(11):1401–8. https://doi.org/10.1097/01.rvi.0000096761.74047.7d.
16. Verma SK, Bergin D, Gonsalves CF, Mitchell DG. MRI detection of a female pelvic arteriovenous fistula after hysterectomy: treatment with superselective coil embolisation. Br J Radiol. 2008;81(969):e221–4. https://doi.org/10.1259/bjr/53820918.
17. Rebarber A, Fox NS, Eckstein DA, Lookstein RA, Saltzman DH. Successful bilateral uterine artery embolization during an ongoing pregnancy. Obstet Gynecol. 2009;113(2 Pt 2):554–6. https://doi.org/10.1097/AOG.0b013e318193bfdf.
18. Albers JR, Hull SK, Wesley RM. Abnormal uterine bleeding. Am Fam Physician. 2004;69(8):1915–26.
19. Peitsidis P, Manolakos E, Tsekoura V, Kreienberg R, Schwentner L. Uterine arteriovenous malformations induced after diagnostic curettage: a systematic review. Arch Gynecol Obstet. 2011;284(5):1137–51. https://doi.org/10.1007/s00404-011-2067-7.
20. Huang MW, Muradali D, Thurston WA, Burns PN, Wilson SR. Uterine arteriovenous malformations: gray-scale and Doppler US features with MR imaging correlation. Radiology. 1998;206(1):115–23. https://doi.org/10.1148/radiology.206.1.9423660.
21. Rangarajan RD, Moloney JC, Anderson HJ. Diagnosis and nonsurgical management of uterine arteriovenous malformation. Cardiovasc Intervent Radiol. 2007;30(6):1267–70. https://doi.org/10.1007/s00270-007-9100-z.
22. Timor-Tritsch IE, Haynes MC, Monteagudo A, Khatib N, Kovács S. Ultrasound diagnosis and management of acquired uterine enhanced myometrial vascularity/arteriovenous malformations. Am J Obstet Gynecol. 2016;214(6):731.e1–731.e10. https://doi.org/10.1016/j.ajog.2015.12.024.
23. Taneja A, Chopra I, Kaur H, Naik SS, Aggarwal R, Sachdeva E, Kaur P. Successful management of abnormal uterine bleeding from uterine arteriovenous malformations with progesterone in postabortal patients. J Obstet Gynaecol Res. 2019;45(6):1114–7. https://doi.org/10.1111/jog.13939.
24. Nasu K, Fujisawa K, Yoshimatsu J, Miyakawa I. Uterine arteriovenous malformation: ultrasonographic, magnetic resonance and radiological findings. Gynecol Obstet Investig. 2002;53(3):191–4. https://doi.org/10.1159/000058373.
25. Sellmyer MA, Desser TS, Maturen KE, Jeffrey RB Jr, Kamaya A. Physiologic, histologic, and imaging features of retained products of conception. Radiographics. 2013;33(3):781–96. https://doi.org/10.1148/rg.333125177.
26. Cura M, Martinez N, Cura A, Dalsaso TJ, Elmerhi F. Arteriovenous malformations of the uterus. Acta Radiol. 2009;50(7):823–9. https://doi.org/10.1080/02841850903008792.
27. Wilms GE, Favril A, Baert AL, Poppe W, Van Assche FA. Transcatheter embolization of uterine arteriovenous malformations. Cardiovasc Intervent Radiol. 1986;9(2):61–4. https://doi.org/10.1007/BF02577901.
28. Manolitsas T, Hurley V, Gilford E. Uterine arteriovenous malformation—a rare cause of uterine haemorrhage. Aust N Z J Obstet Gynaecol. 1994;34(2):197–9. https://doi.org/10.1111/j.1479-828x.1994.tb02691.x.
29. Giurazza F, Corvino F, Paladini A, Borzelli A, Scognamiglio D, Frauenfelder G, Albano G, Sirimarco F, Niola R. Uterine arteriovenous fistula with concomitant pelvic varicocele: endovascular embolization with Onyx-18®. Case Rep Vasc Med. 2017;2017:3548271. https://doi.org/10.1155/2017/3548271.
30. Giurazza F, Corvino F, Cangiano G, Cavaglià E, Amodio F, Silvestre M, De Magistris G, Niola R. Transarterial embolization of peripheral high-flow arteriovenous malformation with ethylene vinyl alcohol copolymer (onyx®): single-center 10-year experience. Radiol Med. 2019;124(2):154–62. https://doi.org/10.1007/s11547-018-0948-6.
31. Saeed Kilani M, Lepennec V, Petit P, Magalon G, Casanova D, Bartoli JM, Vidal V. Embolization of peripheral high-flow arteriovenous malformations with onyx. Diagn Interv Imaging. 2017;98(3):217–26. https://doi.org/10.1016/j.diii.2016.06.017.
32. Kishino M, Miyasaka N, Takeguchi Y, Ohashi I. Retrograde transvenous obliteration for uterine arteriovenous malformation. Obstet Gynecol. 2014;123(2 Pt 2 Suppl 2):427–30. https://doi.org/10.1097/AOG.0000000000000083.
33. Maleux G, Timmerman D, Heye S, Wilms G. Acquired uterine vascular malformations: radiological and clinical outcome after transcatheter embolotherapy. Eur Radiol. 2006;16(2):299–306. https://doi.org/10.1007/s00330-005-2799-5.
34. Kanter G, Packard L, Sit AS. Placenta accreta in a patient with a history of uterine artery embolization for postpartum hemorrhage. J Perinatol. 2013;33(6):482–3. https://doi.org/10.1038/jp.2012.99.
35. Soeda S, Kyozuka H, Suzuki S, Yasuda S, Nomura Y, Fujimori K. Uterine artery embolization for uterine arteriovenous malformation is associated with placental abnormalities in the subsequent pregnancy: two cases report. Fukushima J Med Sci. 2014;60(1):86–90. https://doi.org/10.5387/fms.2013-13.
36. Patton EW, Moy I, Milad MP, Vogezang R. Fertility-preserving management of a uterine arteriovenous malformation: a case report of uterine artery embolization (UAE) followed by laparoscopic resection. J Minim Invasive Gynecol. 2015;22(1):137–41. https://doi.org/10.1016/j.jmig.2014.07.016.
37. Levy-Zaubermann Y, Capmas P, Legendre G, Fernandez H. Laparoscopic management of uterine arteriovenous malformation via occlusion of internal iliac arteries. J Minim Invasive Gynecol. 2012;19(6):785–8. https://doi.org/10.1016/j.jmig.2012.07.009.
38. Dauer LT, Thornton RH, Miller DL, Damilakis J, Dixon RG, Marx MV, Schueler BA, Vañó E,

Venkatesan A, Bartal G, Tsetis D, Cardella JF, Society of Interventional Radiology Safety and Health Committee; Cardiovascular and Interventional Radiology Society of Europe Standards of Practice Committee. Radiation management for interventions using fluoroscopic or computed tomographic guidance during pregnancy: a joint guideline of the Society of Interventional Radiology and the Cardiovascular and Interventional Radiological Society of Europe with Endorsement by the Canadian Interventional Radiology Association. J Vasc Interv Radiol. 2012;23(1):19–32. https://doi.org/10.1016/j.jvir.2011.09.007.
39. Kim TH, Kim NK, Kim SK, Lee JR, Jee BC, Kim YB, Kim SH. Uterine arteriovenous malformation treated by hysteroscopic excision. Gynecol Minim Invasive Ther. 2019;8(3):132–4. https://doi.org/10.4103/GMIT.GMIT_114_18.

Malignancies: Collections Drainage, Biopsies, and Endovascular Bail-Out Treatments

13

Domenico Patanè, Giovanni Coniglio, Stefania Bonomo, Giovanni Failla, Francesco Camerano, Flavio Arcerito, Serafino Santonocito, and Pierantonio Malfa

13.1 Introduction

The management of advanced gynecological malignancies is now in the domain of a multidisciplinary management where Interventional Radiology (IR) occupies a prominent role [1, 2].

After a diagnosis of malignancies IR involvement begins with their minimally invasive treatment often in combination with other modalities. IR has also assumed an important place in the management of malignancy complications, which may result from the malignancy itself or from the treatment's consequences.

The most common origin of gynecological malignancy requiring the IR team intervention is ovarian, endometrial, and cervical.

Ovarian cancer has low prevalence but high mortality because it is often diagnosed in the late stages, and there is currently no effective screening method to analyze. At 5 years after diagnosis, 60% of patients will have recurrence after the initial remission [3, 4] and clinical manifestations of complications of the disease.

Initial surgery for ovarian cancer is prognostic as well as therapeutic. Ovarian cancer is surgically staged based on the Federation of Gynecology and Obstetrics (FIGO) staging criteria. Prognosis is strongly correlated with the initial disease stage, as 10-year overall survival ranges from 73% for the stage I disease to less than 5% for the stage IV [5].

First-line therapy often includes surgery and chemotherapy, a combination of cisplatin or carboplatin and paclitaxel. There are currently no standards of care for second-line regimens [6].

Endometrial cancer is the most common malignancy of the female genital tract; it is often diagnosed and treated in the early stages and has a five-year survival rate of 81.5% [7].

Endometrial cancer is classically characterized as either type I (related to excess estrogen) or type II (not associated with hyperestrogenism, worse prognosis, more aggressive histologies such as high-grade endometrioid, papillary serous, or clear cell).

Surgery is the typical first-line therapy, and a surgical sampling of designated areas defines staging according to the 2009 FIGO staging criteria. Adjuvant radiation and chemotherapy may be recommended on the basis of tumor size, histologic subtype, and extent of disease spread.

Gynecologists typically do endometrial biopsy except in rare and particular situations; more frequently, IR is involved in treating advanced-stage complications, primarily due to the tumor spread via direct extension into surrounding pelvic tissue.

Cervical cancer is still the most prevalent gynecological cancer worldwide; however, it is far less prevalent in industrialized countries.

D. Patanè · G. Coniglio (✉) · S. Bonomo · G. Failla
F. Camerano · F. Arcerito · S. Santonocito · P. Malfa
Radiology Department, Azienda Ospedaliera Cannizzaro, Catania, Italy

R. Niola et al. (eds.), *Diagnostic and Interventional Radiology in Gynecological and Obstetric Diseases*, https://doi.org/10.1007/978-3-031-11910-1_13

Most cervical cancer originates from high-risk human papillomavirus (HPV), which is a sexually transmitted infection; HPV 16 and 18 are detected in 95% of cases [8, 9].

Other risk factors include demographic risks (ethnicity, socioeconomic status, age); behavioral risks (early coitarche, multiple sexual partners, smoking); and medical risk factors (immunosuppression, inadequate Papanicolaou screening, increased parity).

The majority of cervical cancers are squamous, originating at the squamocolumnar junction of the cervix, with the second most common being adenocarcinoma arising from the endocervical columnar cells. Cervical cancer is staged clinically.

Primary therapy depends on the stage at diagnosis; early-stage disease is often treated with radical hysterectomy and pelvic lymphadenectomy, while advanced disease is treated with the combination of cisplatin chemotherapy and radiation [10].

As already mentioned for endometrial cancer, and also for the cervix one, the role of IR is confined to the treatment of complications of advanced stages due to the spread of the tumor, which occurs more frequently by the lymphatic route and within the paracervical and parametrial tissue and nearby organs (vagina, ureter, bladder, rectum).

Malignancy can induce dysfunction of many organs and body systems [11]. Progression to multi-organ failure may occur spontaneously either through disease progression, by extension of the malignancy, or more acutely through infection, bleeding, and thromboembolic complications [12]. Though debilitating, a significant portion of these complications are reversible, many of them by minimally invasive IR procedures. Such treatment can relieve symptoms, alleviate pain, and improve the operability of patients, thus having a significant positive impact on the quality of life [11].

IR utilizes minimally invasive advanced image-guided percutaneous techniques in gynecologic treatment, including biopsies, fluid aspiration, drainage catheter placement, and pelvic arterial embolization.

Gynecological biopsies are often requested for the diagnosis of malignancy or, in the case of known malignancy, for further characterization; they may also be helpful in the differential diagnosis of peritoneal carcinomatosis and in case of suspected gynecologic cancer recurrences. Patients with refractory malignant ascites, pleural effusion, postoperative fluid collections (abscess, seroma, or lymphocele), or with urinary and biliary tracts infiltrations may benefit from percutaneous aspiration of fluid collections with or without placement of drainage catheters [13, 14]; those with uncontrolled postoperative or oncological advanced mass bleeding can be effectively managed with transarterial pelvic embolization, both in the acute and chronic setting.

13.2 Collections Drainage

Fluid collection is a common condition among patients affected by gynecological malignancies that may occur either as a surgical complication or as cancer progression. Surgical complications involve debulking procedures leading to a contained or free refractory ascites, seroma, urinoma, biloma, hematomas, lymphocele, abscess, and empyema.

Cancer progression is the most frequent condition since malignancy may develop local progression or disseminate in other organs: A fluid collection can be generated whenever tumor cells infiltrate fluid-producing structures, such as the urinary tract, bile, and lymphatic ducts and peritoneum [11, 15]. The vessel's invasion causes pseudo-encapsulated hematomas that may initially be sterile but may evolve into an abscess [16], especially in immunocompromised patients who often undergo intense cycles of chemotherapy that are less responsive to antibiotic treatment.

Discomfort mass-related or inflammation-related is usually the main symptom.

13.2.1 IR Treatment

IR plays a crucial role in the management of fluid collection. Mini-invasive techniques, such as imaging-guided percutaneous drainage, quickly result in symptom relief. It is an excellent achievement for the patient. The treatment only requires local anesthesia, avoiding both the risks of surgical-related morbidity and general anesthesia and offering an ideal benefit-cost ratio that fits at its best the patient needs.

Image-guided placement of percutaneous drainage catheters is very suitable in oncological patients proving to be curative between 80% and 90% of cases. Most pelvic fluid collections can easily be sampled or drained under ultrasound guidance performed even in bedside conditions, either temporarily or long-term.

The management of drainage catheters in outpatients is easy and well-tolerated, thanks to simple suction bulb attachments and flushing mechanisms [11, 16, 17].

13.2.2 Technique

Mini-invasive treatment consists of the aspiration and drainage of the fluid collection, which can be performed with different approaches, such as the transabdominal (anterior) or the trans-gluteal (posterior), depending on the collection characteristics [15]. In general, a drainage catheter of proper size is placed into the collection under imaging techniques and left in situ so that the fluid can flow out toward some specific draining bags; the procedure usually lasts until the collection walls are entirely cleansed, and at that point, the fluid production should be over.

The catheter size should not exceed 6 Fr when the aspiration is solely performed, and it can drain the collection if the fluid will be not viscous, such as seromas, pleural effusions, lymphoceles. A more significant catheter ranging in size from 8 Fr to 12 Fr is suitable whether the fluid collection is dense or the collection is phlogistic or an abscess in order to ease the fluid flowing out [18, 19].

Sometimes the local sclerotherapy of the capsule's inner surface is required to complete the procedure: alcoholic and antibiotic solutions are more suitable than the absolute alcohol, which is painful for the patient.

In any case, the fluid should be sampled for the bacteriological test by performing an antibiogram and a cytological examination to detect any tumoral cells.

Transabdominal percutaneous drainage may be performed with US or CT for guidance [11].

The US is generally preferred whenever it allows adequate visualization of the entire cavity. It requires less time, enables real-time guidance, and allows more flexible access to a collection from multiple angles. Patients without a safe aspiration pathway (deep collection, organs at risk in the pathway, poor quality visibility of the collection with ultrasound) should undergo a CT-guided procedure even though it takes longer. It may be necessary for transabdominal drainage if the targeted collection is not visible in the US or is obscured by overlying structures, such as the bowel.

Drainage may be performed by using a direct trocar technique, in which a catheter loaded onto a sharp stylet is advanced directly into the collection during imaging visualization. Alternatively, the Seldinger technique may be used with limited fluoroscopic guidance for manipulation of the wire.

The procedure can be divided into steps: a 21 G needle is inserted into the collection sonographically guided, the 0.21 guidewire is then placed under fluoroscopy followed by a non-invasive introducer system; then, through a 0.38 guidewire, catheter drainage is placed into the collection.

Some pelvic collections may not be amenable to transabdominal drainage; the bladder, vessels, bowel, or bone may obscure the target. In such cases, when transgluteal access is possible, CT-guided transgluteal drainage is a safer and more effective alternative [17]. In general, a catheter path is chosen as close to the sacrococcygeal margin and inferior to the piriformis muscle to avoid injuries to the sciatic nerve and gluteal vessels and minimize the risk of pain and bleeding. A tandem trocar or Seldinger technique may be used [18, 19].

The size and type of the drainage catheter should be chosen appropriately according to the nature of the fluid to be drained.

13.2.3 Ascites

Malignant ascites arises from various malignancies such as ovarian or endometrial cancer and is associated with significant morbidity and deterioration in the quality of life (Fig. 13.1a). Approximately 60% of patients with malignant ascites are symptomatic and present with abdominal swelling, pain, nausea/vomiting, anorexia, and fatigue [17, 20, 21]. Although systemic chemotherapy and debulking surgery can be performed for underlying cancer, most malignant ascites requires palliative treatment. Local palliative treatment options include paracentesis, non-tunneled drainage catheters, long-term tunneled drainage catheters, and peritoneal-venous shunts.

Repeated outpatient paracentesis is the most commonly performed and effective procedure since it is safe and provides rapid relief of symptoms. This is important in patients with bowel adhesions, omental and peritoneal disease, or loculated collections [22, 23].

When multiple repeated paracenteses are required from rapid fluid creation, some patients benefit from placement of a non-tunneled drainage catheter (Fig. 13.1b). Non-tunneled pigtail catheters can provide temporary and more durable symptom relief compared with simple paracentesis. There is a higher rate of complications associated with long-term pigtail catheter drainage; therefore, it is often recommended to place a non-tunneled catheter for a short life expectancy. Abdominal fluid shouldn't be drained too fast: After 1000 cc of drained fluid, the drainage should be closed for a while (approximately 1 h) to avoid electrolytic and proteic complications. Then the drainage could be reopened and drain another 1000 cc. There are no absolute contraindications to non-tunneled pigtail catheters. Relative contraindications are coagulopathy and thrombocytopenia, which should be corrected before the procedure to avoid bleeding complications.

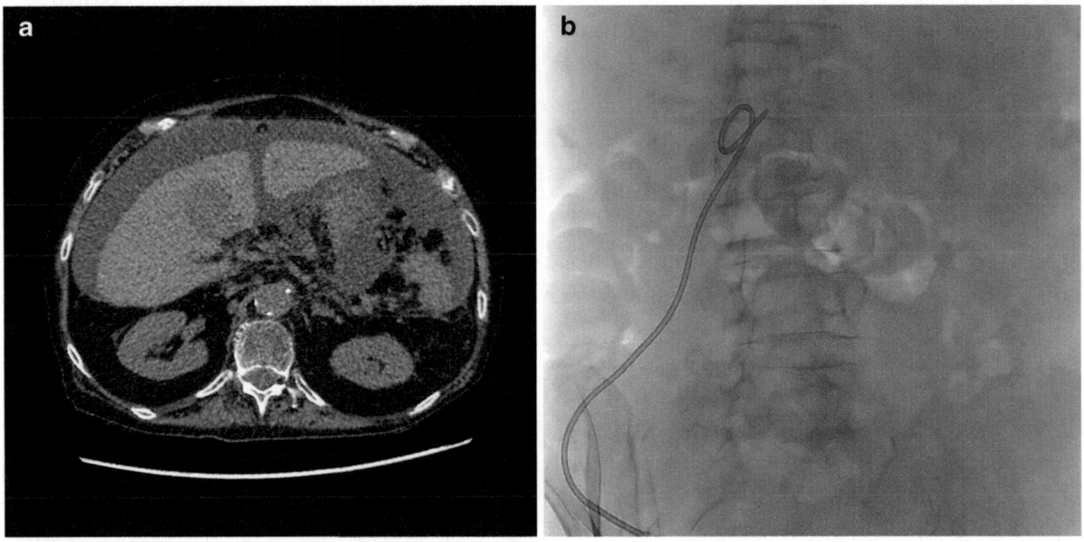

Fig. 13.1 CT scan showing malignant ascites from primary ovarian neoplasm with peritoneal carcinosis (**a**). Peritoneal catheter drainage placement (**b**)

13.2.4 Lymphocele

Lymphocele is defined as an abnormal collection of lymph fluid without an epithelial lining occurring after surgical procedures such as lymphadenectomy for gynecologic malignancy (Fig. 13.2a). A lymphocele in the pelvis poses a unique situation if it causes pressure and pain symptoms [24]. Aspiration alone may not collapse the lymphocytes (Fig. 13.2b). Longer-term drainage catheter insertion and injection of sclerosant agents, such as dehydrated alcohol and sodium tetradecyl sulfate, have been attempted to reduce lymphatic leakage (Fig. 13.2c, d) [24, 25].

13.2.5 Abscess

The incidence of pelvic abscesses is still approximately 4% in patients with gynecology malignancy undergoing major pelvic surgery (Fig. 13.3a). These patients require drainage of the infected fluid (Fig. 13.3b). Minimally invasive percutaneous drainage under image guidance is considered the primary management method for the most infected abdominal or pelvic fluid collections (Fig. 13.3c). These complications lengthen hospitalization and additional interventions with overall increased health care expenses [19]. Percutaneous drainage enables decompression of the abscess cavity, allowing its

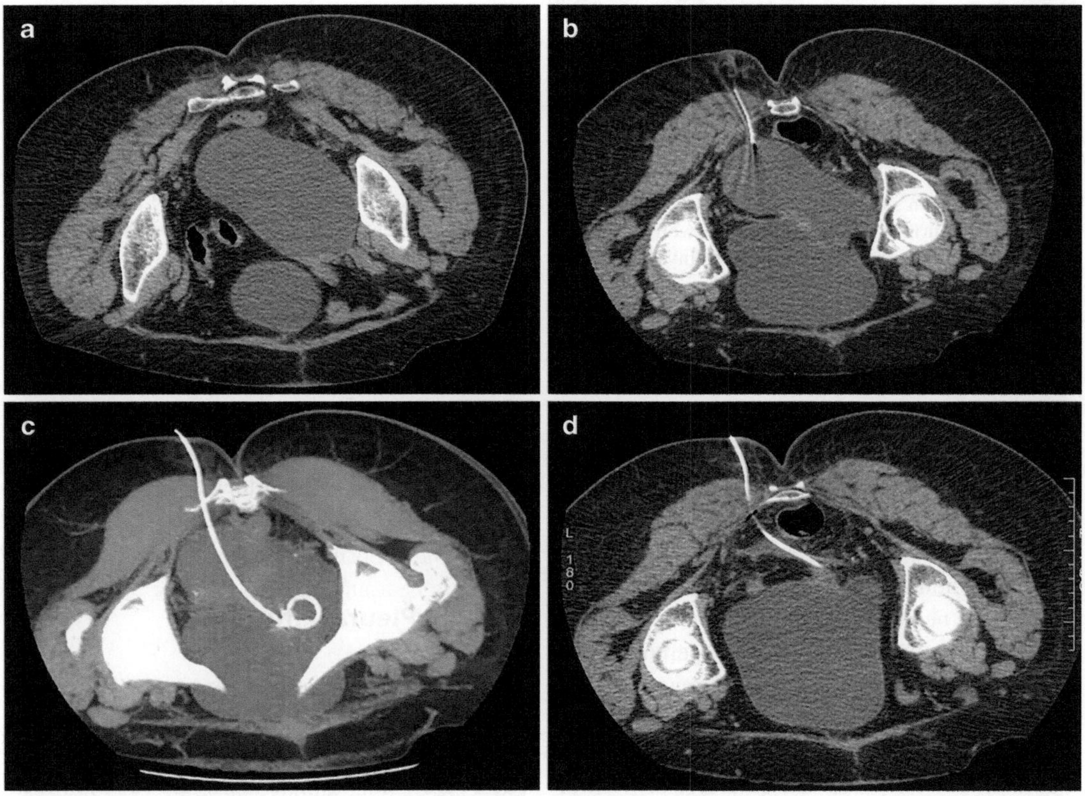

Fig. 13.2 CT images show a pelvic lymphocele in a 72-year-old woman treated with surgical hysteroannessectomy for ovarian cancer (**a**). Percutaneous CT-guided positioning of an introducer sheath set (**b**) with the placement of 8 Fr drainage (**c**) and CT scan after fluid aspiration (**d**)

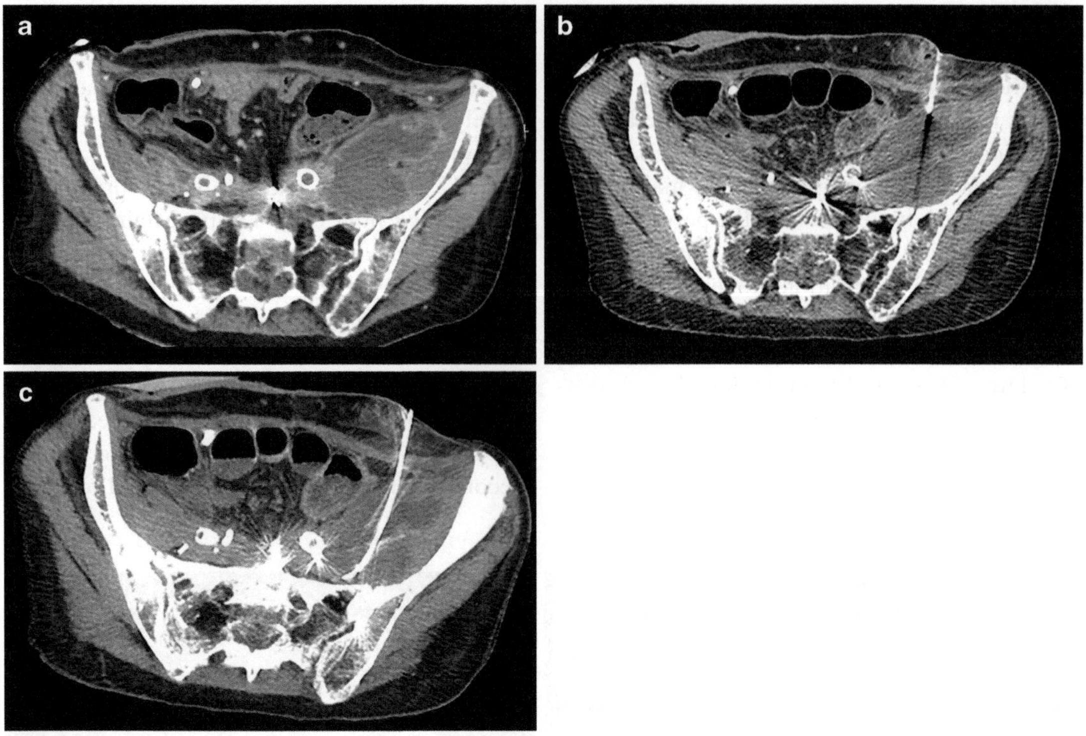

Fig. 13.3 CT scan shows an abscess in the left iliopsoas secondary to a urinoma in a 46-year-old woman with a previous history of hysterectomy, cystectomy, and radiotherapy with cutaneous ureteroileostomy for endometrial cancer (**a**). Percutaneous CT puncture (**b**) then placement of 8 Fr drainage (**c**)

walls to adhere and promoting healing. In conjunction with drainage, antibiotic therapy is essential and is tailored to treat microorganisms that have been cultured from specimens collected at the time of drainage. Superinfected hematomas may evolve in collections. In addition, bladder or ureteral injury as a complication of surgery may result in urinomas; in some cases, urinary diversion may be necessary in conjunction with drainage of the urinoma and or percutaneous nephrostomy. Imaging-guided drainage is the preferred treatment choice in most instances, such as postoperative collections found in the abdomen, pelvis, psoas musculature, or ventral abdominal wall.

Contraindications to the procedure may include coagulopathy, lack of safe percutaneous route for access, and phlegmon. Since most of these conditions can be corrected to an acceptable range, the lack of a safe access route is considered the only absolute contraindication. The incidence of significant complications associated with the procedure is less than 10% and includes bleeding, bowel perforation, sepsis, bacteremia, and superinfection of sterile fluid collection [19, 26].

13.2.6 Pleural Effusion

Malignant pleural effusions, often related to pleural and lymphatic involvement, presenting with dyspnea, cough, chest pain, and feelings of chest pressure or heaviness are a significant source of morbidity in these oncology patients. Although it is most commonly associated with ovarian cancer, any gynecologic malignancy can result in malignant pleural effusion. Image-guided needle aspiration of pleural fluid collections may easily be performed by IR, and successful drainage can be achieved with catheter placement under ultrasound, fluoroscopic, or CT guidance [11, 18, 27]. As a malignant pleural effusion is a preterminal event, the usual aim of treatment is palliation, relief of symptoms, and prevention of recollection with minimal discomfort to improve the quality of life. The fluid may be evaluated for the presence of malignant cells using cytology, aiding the initial diagnosis of malignancy or staging of known disease. In any case, therapeutic thoracocentesis provides temporary symptomatic relief until the effusion reaccumulates, often in the setting of malignant effusions, necessitating a repeated procedure [28–30]. The thoracentesis is the first step in managing pleural effusions: the process can be performed at the bedside with US imaging guidance. Ultrasound use may avoid potential complications if the effusion is small and facilitates drainage in patients with loculated effusions. The difficulties associated with thoracentesis include post-procedure pneumothorax, pneumothorax ex vacuo, hemothorax, re-expansion pulmonary edema, and organ laceration. When performing large-volume thoracentesis, it is recommended to stop removing fluid if the patient develops chest discomfort, pain, or cough to reduce the risk of complications. No more than 1500 mL of fluid is removed to avoid re-expansion pulmonary edema [31–34]. For patients with shorter life expectancy, a non-tunneled drainage catheter may be placed to manage symptomatic malignant pleural effusion. The drainage catheter is connected to a sterile plastic pleural drainage system. The catheter is flushed periodically with sterile saline to maintain the patency.

13.2.7 Urinary Tract

A wide range of gynecologic malignancies frequently causes ureteral obstruction due to extrinsic tumor compression, retroperitoneal adenopathy, or direct tumor invasion (Fig. 13.4a). Ureteral obstruction may be unilateral or bilateral (Fig. 13.4b, c). Management requires urinary decompression using percutaneous nephrostomy [11, 18]. This is the most common renal intervention performed by IR. The provision of direct access to the urinary tract allows the drainage of tract contents and provides access for further intervention via the route established. Indications for nephrostomy in the emergent setting include urinary tract sepsis, pyonephrosis, deteriorating renal function, or electrolyte disturbances such as hyperkalemia and metabolic acidosis. Percutaneous nephrostomy may be performed using an oblique prone position under US guidance [35–38]. If difficulty is encountered in US visualization or wire manipulation, it is possible to use fluoroscopy support. A 21- or 22-gauge needle is advanced into a selected calyx with US guidance (Fig. 13.4e). Removal of the needle stylet may allow urine to be aspirated; subsequently, an 0.018-inch wire is moved into the collecting system. The needle is then removed, and a 5- or 6-Fr dilator-sheath assembly is advanced into the collecting system. The dilator is removed, and the 0.018-inch wire is exchanged for a 0.035-inch (3-mm) J-tip wire. The sheath is then exchanged for an 8-Fr nephrostomy tube (Fig. 13.4e). Percutaneous nephrostomy in pregnant patients has been performed during intravenous sedation with opiates and with local anesthesia alone [27, 35–37].

Possible complications of the procedure include septic shock in the setting of urosepsis, as well as hematuria; major hemorrhage is rare [39]. Other complications include tube dislodgement and tube obstruction [39–43].

In some cases, an antegrade approach may overcome the obstruction by using a guide and a hydrophilic catheter to place a double J stent in order to re-establish the physiological urinary tract.

Sometimes it is necessary to perform a percutaneous dilatation of the structure anterogradely through the PCN tract. Under fluoroscopic guidance, a balloon catheter is manipulated across the stenotic region, and the lesion is progressively dilated by inflating balloons of appropriate diameter and length. After dilatation, an internal ureteral stent or internal-external nephron-ureteral catheter is placed to prevent restenosis [44].

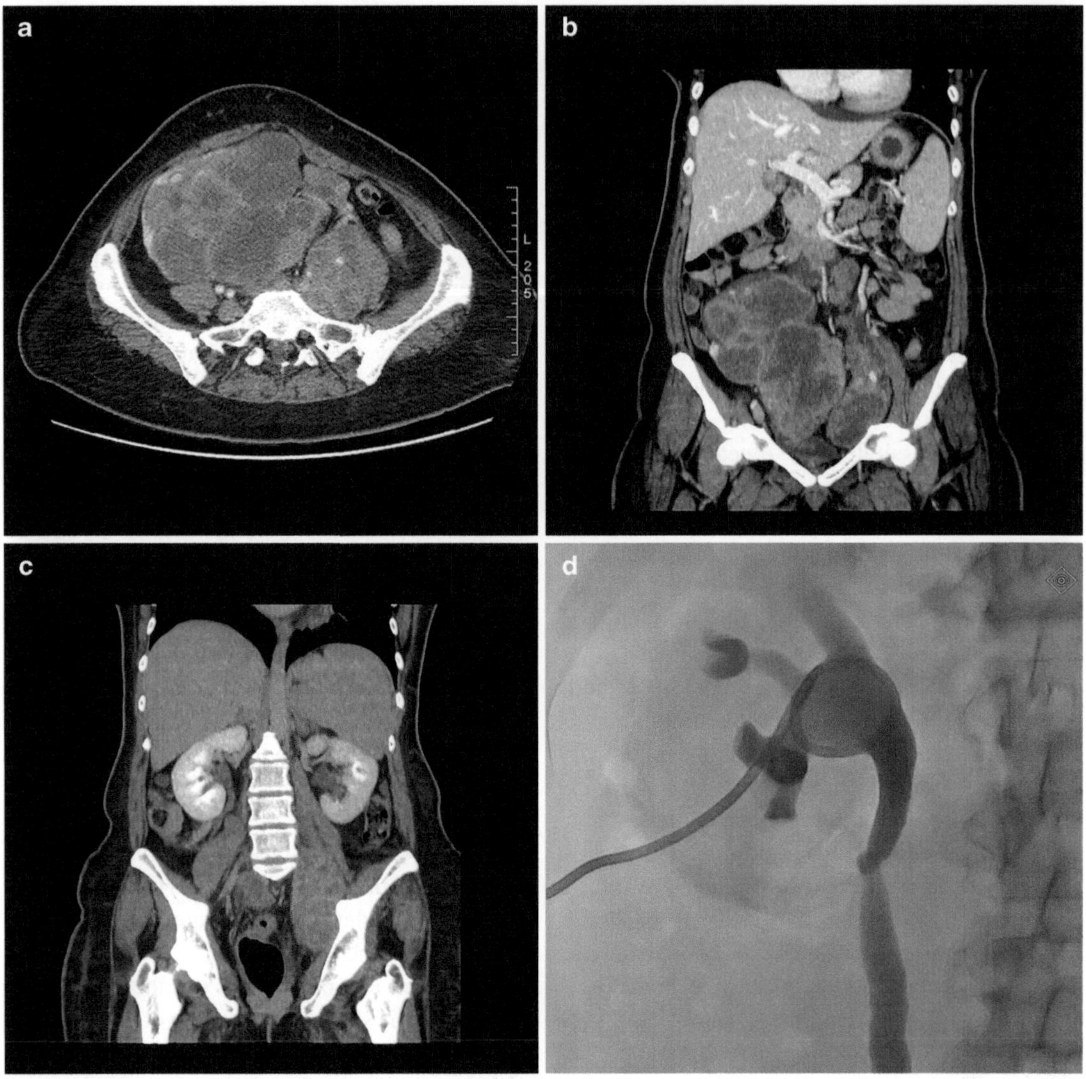

Fig. 13.4 Axial CT scan with a contrast medium that shows an adnexal mass within the pelvis which causes compression on the posterior retroperitoneal structures (**a**). Coronal reconstruction of CT scan demonstrates the extension of the retroperitoneal lesion (**b**) and the presence of bilateral hydronephrosis (**c**). The patient has undergone nephrostomy drainage placement: an ultrasound-guided puncture with 21 G Chiba needle of the lower calyceal group of the left kidney and percutaneous approach and consequent placement of 8 Fr nephrostomy drainage with a curled distal end of the catheter in the pyelocaliceal cavity (**d**)

Nephrostomy has to be performed in cases of iatrogenic or infiltrative injuries causing urine extravasation [35] or ureterovaginal fistulas to keep the lesion dry and promote the healing; then a double J stent has to be placed to allow the scarring. The initial step is to provide an alternative route for urinary drainage through bilateral percutaneous nephrostomies. It usually allows the healing of the fistula.

13.2.8 Biliary Tract

Metastatic disease at the hepatic hilar nodes or in the peripancreatic nodes may cause obstructive jaundice from extrinsic pressure on the proximal portions of the biliary tree and may require percutaneous intervention (Percutaneous Biliary Drainage, PBD) if less invasive endoscopic means fails to achieve adequate biliary decompression

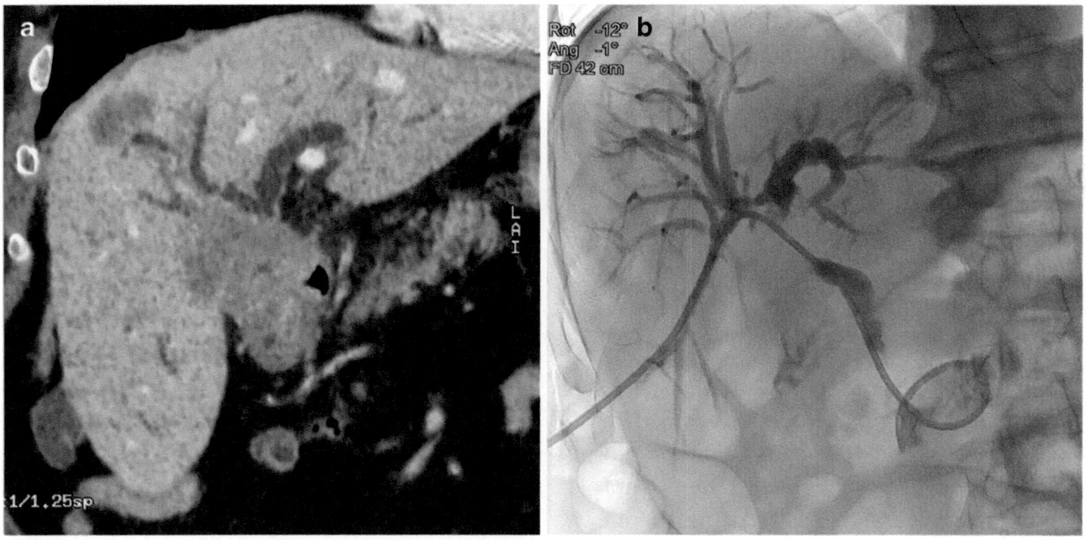

Fig. 13.5 Coronal CT reconstruction of hepatic hilum metastasis causing biliary tree dilatation and jaundice (**a**). Placement of internal-external percutaneous biliary drainage (**b**)

(Fig. 13.5a, b). PBD can be associated with major complications, including sepsis, hemorrhage, and localized infective and inflammatory processes (abscess, peritonitis, cholecystitis, and pancreatitis) [45]. The incidence of complications is higher in oncology than in the general population, perhaps related to advanced malignancy and the potential presence of coexisting immunosuppression [45, 46]. The incidence of cholangitis in oncology patients undergoing PBD approaches 50%. Such infection is more common in those with internal and external drainage than in those with external drainage alone [47]. The longer the duration of PBD, the more likely the patient is to develop cholangitis [48]. The incidence of infected bile in patients with malignant biliary obstruction is 25–36% [49].

13.3 Biopsies

Gynecological biopsies are often requested for the diagnosis of malignancy or, in the case of known malignancy, for further characterization; the most common origin for gynecological malignancy biopsy requests to the interventional radiologist are ovarian, endometrial, and cervical [10].

Although the primary diagnosis of most ovarian cystic lesions should be performed with surgical procedures, several subgroups of patients with cystic ovarian or other adnexal lesions are ideal candidates for less invasive percutaneous or transvaginal procedures [50].

The biopsy may also be helpful in the differential diagnosis of peritoneal carcinomatosis that may be caused by ovary, breast, colon, appendix, pancreas, and stomach cancers, among others; the treatment of these tumors varies, and surgery is contraindicated in some patients. Gynecologists typically do an endometrial biopsy, but in some situations it is challenging to access the endometrial cavity; in these cases, the transvaginal ultrasound approach can be considered [51].

More in general, any pelvic mass in women requires a definitive cytological or histological diagnosis and an accurate staging of the disease to determine the right treatment options; this is especially important when patients need treatments that can have a significant risk of morbidity [13].

While non-invasive imaging techniques have improved assessment and staging for cancer, histologic confirmation remains the gold standard for the definitive diagnosis of many tumors [11].

Before the procedure, evaluation of all pertinent imaging is necessary to determine whether a safe biopsy window is available; in these cases, biopsies to establish histological diagnosis are increasingly performed using minimally invasive techniques by interventional radiologists [52], enabling rapidity of diagnosis and the formulation of cancer treatment plans [13].

13.3.1 Indications

The first aim of the biopsy of a mass suspected of gynecological origin is to clarify whether it's malignant or not and what its origin is. Not all pelvic masses are malignant tumors, not all tumors are primary (metastases from stomach, colorectal, breast), and some inflammatory-infectious pathologies (TBC and mycobacteria) resemble tumor masses [10].

Among incidental findings, it is common to find ovarian mass, and although the majority of incidentally detected ovarian masses are benign [13, 51], many of these masses cannot be definitively characterized with serum tumor markers and imaging, so the patients are referred for surgical resection. Hence, a less invasive method for pursuing a tissue diagnosis in an incidental ovarian mass would be helpful [53].

The surgical and chemotherapy treatments of gynecological malignancies remained the first choice over the past few decades; however, more recently, the ability to perform molecular profiling has led to advancements in treatment through pathway-targeted agents [10, 54].

Modern histology techniques, including immunohistochemistry, enable a site-specific diagnosis in more than 93% of biopsies taken [55].

A definitive histological diagnosis is crucial when patients undergo treatments that can have a significant risk of morbidity [13] and when patients are poor surgical candidates with pre-existing comorbidities [50].

Sometimes a biopsy of suspected gynecologic cancer recurrences can be requested to confirm the diagnosis (due to a rising tumor marker, cancer antigen 125 (CA-125), or to an area of concern on CT scan or PET/CT with the unclear origin of the tumor.

Similarly, if there is a clinical recurrence but no rise in tumor markers, a biopsy may provide more relevant information for the discrepancy. If there is a significant length of time from the initial treatment or the anatomic location of recurrence is atypical for the pelvic malignancy, a biopsy may help reveal a new primary malignancy [10] or metastases to the ovaries or peritoneum or non-genital tumors [56].

In the context of ovarian cancer research, the molecular profiling of tumor is becoming increasingly important; the goals of this practice are to improve diagnosis through the use of biomarkers (measuring complementary DNA and the messenger RNA expression of a large number of genes) and to aid in treatment by both predicting chemotherapy response as well as identifying chemotherapy resistance [10, 54, 57].

In some cases, women with ovarian or peritoneal carcinoma can be managed with primary chemotherapy followed by interval debulking surgery, which shows the same survival rates but much lower morbidity [58–60].

In order to give the appropriate primary chemotherapy, it becomes necessary to obtain a biopsy to confirm the tumor type [61].

Another target of tissue biopsy is to characterize subtypes of ovarian malignancies further to develop a hierarchy of ovarian cancers similar to that developed for breast cancers [62].

Moreover, metastatic gastrointestinal tumors such as colon, gastric, and pancreatic adenocarcinomas and, on occasion, breast cancer mimic ovarian cancer on presentation [63]. Therefore, tissue sampling has become necessary to plan therapy even when imaging indicates a malignant ovarian mass [53].

Endometrial biopsy is typically done by gynecologists (with the Pipelle suction technique or at hysteroscopy), but in some situations it is challenging to access the endometrial cavity; in these cases, an alternative is to undertake transvaginal ultrasonography-guided access to the endometrial cavity [51].

Moreover, similar to ovarian cancers, molecular profiling of endometrial cancer has been used for diagnosis, treatment, and further classification. The knowledge of the genetic profiles and the study of their related pathways have led to tumor-specific therapies for endometrial cancer.

The role of IR in cervical biopsies is minimal. Some rare indications reported in the literature are cervical tumors not accessible vaginally and tumors in hysterotomy scar [56].

The value of molecular profiling is poor in this district as well, since it is the only aspect studied in patients with HPV infection, which may progress to cervical cancer [10].

13.3.2 Sampling, Guide, and Technique

13.3.2.1 Sampling

Image-guided needle biopsy represents a minimally invasive method to obtain aspirate and core samples for pathologic analysis and [53] molecular analysis, which may allow targeted therapy [10].

Although both fine-needle aspiration and core biopsy are widely used for confirming the presence of malignancy, core biopsy has been proven to be more sensitive [13] as it provides a sample with preserved tissue architecture, allowing comprehensive histological evaluation including immunohistochemistry (which could play a crucial role in the differential diagnosis, especially of colon and ovarian cancer) [10, 56, 64] and molecular profiling providing important information about therapy and prognosis (a biopsy sample can be used to identify resistance to the standard platinum-based therapy and to tailor the regimen to the tumor genotype) [53].

Studies have shown that needle core biopsy techniques outperform fine-needle aspiration cytology in diagnostic rates without changing the risk of complications [55]; therefore, it is preferable to obtain a core needle biopsy for histology rather than ascites for cytology [10].

Cytologic analysis of the ascites represents an even less invasive option but yields poor predictive value for an organ-specific cancer diagnosis compared with core needle biopsy [65].

The sensitivity of fine needle aspiration is likely limited by insufficient cells in the aspirates, especially for low-grade or borderline tumors. In contrast, core needle samples yield more tissue and would also allow for the diagnosis of benign masses [57, 66].

Seeding remains the major risk for percutaneous biopsies. Therefore, each procedure must always be preceded by a careful assessment of the individual case, the risks, and the benefits.

13.3.2.2 Image-guidance

The choice of image guidance modality is multifactorial (location, safe access, comorbidity, operator experience), and there are many available options, including ultrasound, CT, MRI, and a digitally directed angiographic approach [11, 56, 67].

When lesions are visible by ultrasound, with suitable equipment and appropriate operator experience, this modality can provide equivalent or superior guidance to CT at the time of biopsy [67, 68]. The US procedure is quicker and more reliable. In fact, it offers high flexibility in the choice of biopsy approach (transabdominal, transvaginal, transrectal) [56] and the benefit of real-time imaging, allowing accurate monitoring of the needle trajectory through tissues en route to the target lesion, with the dual advantage of avoiding patient and staff exposure to ionizing radiation during the biopsy [68]. Precise guidance of the needle tip during the whole procedure also reduces the risk of bleeding complications.

In combination with color Doppler imaging, it also facilitates the choice of a vital part of the tumor for biopsy [56].

CT guidance offers enhanced anatomical detailing and delineation with more precise needle localization when compared to ultrasound [68]; CT-guided percutaneous biopsy has been established as an efficient and safe procedure in the evaluation of retroperitoneal and abdominal masses [69–75], but it has certain limitations in the case of deep pelvic masses due to limited transabdominal accessibility or limited imaging in the osseous pelvic space. In such cases, the US is better suited for reaching deep pelvic masses through the transvaginal and endorectal approaches [67].

MRI is used only rarely, despite its imaging benefits, as it requires special non-magnetic equipment and experience [76].

The staging CT or MR imaging scan is invaluable in planning any biopsy [51] and in establishing the approach, which can be: anterior, posterior, transgluteal (CT), transvaginal, and endorectal (US) [67].

When evaluation of the diagnostic imaging study shows that direct anterior, posterior, and lateral approaches to the lesions are obstructed by small or large bowel loops, the bladder, bony structures, external or internal iliac vessels, or a combination of these, the CT-guided coaxial needle biopsy by an anterolateral approach through the iliopsoas muscle, with the use of a curved needle, seems to be safe and effective for obtaining samples from deep pelvic lesions. This approach is particularly useful for external iliac, internal iliac, and obturator nodes, but it poses a theoretical risk of injury to the femoral nerve, the deep circumflex iliac vessels, and the ureter [77].

Zikan et al. tested several variables as potential factors influencing adequacy of ultrasound true-cut biopsy: age, body mass index (BMI), CA 125 level, indication group, operator, histology, biopsy site, biopsy approach, and ascites [56].

In particular, higher adequacy has been proven for:

- Transvaginal biopsies (vs. transabdominal), probably due to the proximity of the biopsy lesion to guide the biopsy probe more precisely into the vital parts of the tumor
- CA 125 levels and the presence of ascites; maybe for the large tumor load in these cases
- Carcinomatosis, as a biopsy site that is often easily accessible transvaginally in the pouch of Douglas and transabdominally by a peritoneal approach through the anterior abdominal wall
- The serous histotype of ovarian cancer, which is often present as solid nodules of carcinomatosis and a large tumor load in advanced inoperable cases
- Inoperable/suboptimally operable tumor

On the other hand, non-ovarian tumors are a strong negative predictor.

13.3.2.3 Technique

All patients are tested for the coagulation parameters and platelet counts to ensure that they do not have any hemorrhagic diathesis.

Some procedures are carried out under conscious sedation (intravenous administration of midazolam and fentanyl) with pulse oximetry and hemodynamic monitoring.

Local anesthesia by infiltration of the abdominal wall with lidocaine is used for transabdominal biopsy; there is no need for anesthesia for vaginal biopsy.

For transvaginal procedures, antibiotic therapy is administered intravenously immediately before the procedure and after the procedure; [50] likewise, antibiotic prophylaxis before biopsies must be used with an endorectal approach due to the risk of infection.

Antibiotic prophylaxis before biopsies is likewise by the endorectal approach. The antibiotic is necessary for the risk of infection.

For a core-cut biopsy, an automatic biopsy system with needle 18–16 G and the appropriate length may be used.

For fine-needle aspiration biopsy (FNAB), a thin needle of 19–22 G ($\leq$0.9 mm) is used to obtain tissue or cells by aspiration.

In the transvaginal approach is used a special needle guide similar to that used for oocyte retrieval, attached to the vaginal ultrasound probe [56].

Usually, a minimum of two passes was performed on each lesion.

For masses containing cystic components, solid portions are targeted (e.g., cyst wall or mural nodule). The tip of the biopsy needle is carefully visualized during the whole procedure to achieve optimal sampling and patient safety. At the end of the biopsy procedure, bleeding from the biopsy site needs to be checked.

When biopsy of a predominantly cystic mass is performed, care should be taken to aspirate the fluid component completely prior to the acquisition of the tissue samples; complete aspiration will decrease the likelihood of superinfection of residual cyst contents and should increase the yield of solid material with the core biopsy of the cyst wall [50].

13.3.2.4 Complications

Seeding of a tumor along the biopsy track or into the peritoneum is a potential risk. Hence, percutaneous biopsy should not be done in pelvic malignancy unless there is already evidence of spread from the primary tumor [51] or after a gynecologic oncologist has weighed the potential risk of seeding in the context of the patient's overall prognosis, morbidities, and treatment plan [53].

Other possible complications are infectious in nature (especially in patients who underwent biopsy by the endorectal approach with sonographic guidance) [67], bleeding, bowel injury, and inadequate needle positioning [50, 56].

Image-guided (with US or CT) needle biopsy represents a minimally invasive method to obtain aspirate and core samples for pathologic analysis; it is a safe and technically successful procedure with high sensitivity and specificity for the detection of malignancy. It yields accurate histologic diagnosis for benign and malignant masses [53].

Biopsy represents a reliable and less invasive alternative to surgery for obtaining an accurate tissue diagnosis in presumed benign and malignant lesions [51] and in the management of advanced, recurrent, or atypical abdominopelvic tumors where unnecessary laparotomy or laparoscopy can be avoided [56].

The minimally invasive nature of outpatient biopsy techniques allows rapidity of diagnosis and the formulation of cancer treatment plans [13].

Havrilesky et al. demonstrated that aside from the observed potential clinical benefit to the patient, there might also be an overall reduced cost of therapy [78].

However, because the management of these patients is quite complex, this approach should be undertaken when one is working with a gynecologic oncologist. The care of patients with negative or benign biopsy results requires close follow-up and detailed knowledge of gynecologic disease processes [50].

13.4 Endovascular Bail-Out Treatment

There are many, often concomitant, conditions leading to bleeding in patients with malignancy. First, malignancies themselves are a risk factor of coagulopathy such as neovascularization due to growth factors, metastatic bone marrow invasion, thrombotic microangiopathy, disseminated intravascular coagulation, or macrophage activation syndrome. Furthermore, iatrogenic causes are often involved: chemotherapy causing aplasia, prevention of thromboembolic disease, postoperative pseudoaneurysms, and a fragile vascular bed following radiotherapy. Lastly, cancer mass may cause direct vascular injuries. In the case of hyper vascularization, tumor rupture may lead to catastrophic bleeding.

The malignant tissue can erode adjacent vessels (Fig. 13.6a) through mechanical invasion and local inflammatory reaction (Fig. 13.6b–d); in addition, the tumor mass may obstruct venous circulation, causing an increase in proximal hydrostatic pressure and resulting in varices and shunts, which may finally rupture.

Internal iliac artery bleeding due to pelvic neoplasm treated with transarterial catheter embolization was first described 40 years ago [79, 80].

During the years, endovascular embolization applications in the pelvic region have expanded with the inclusion of treatment of benign diseases such as myomas, the prevention and control in perioperative bleeding during gynecological and obstetrics surgery, and the control of massive hemorrhage from pelvic tumors and trauma [18, 81–85]. Gynecological tumors can present with massive vaginal bleeding (Fig. 13.7a); in other cases, life-threatening hemorrhages can occur as a consequence of other treatments like surgery and radiotherapy. Delay in the treatment of hemorrhage can also delay the treatment of the malignancy itself. Thus, early and effective control of bleeding is mandatory (Fig. 13.7b).

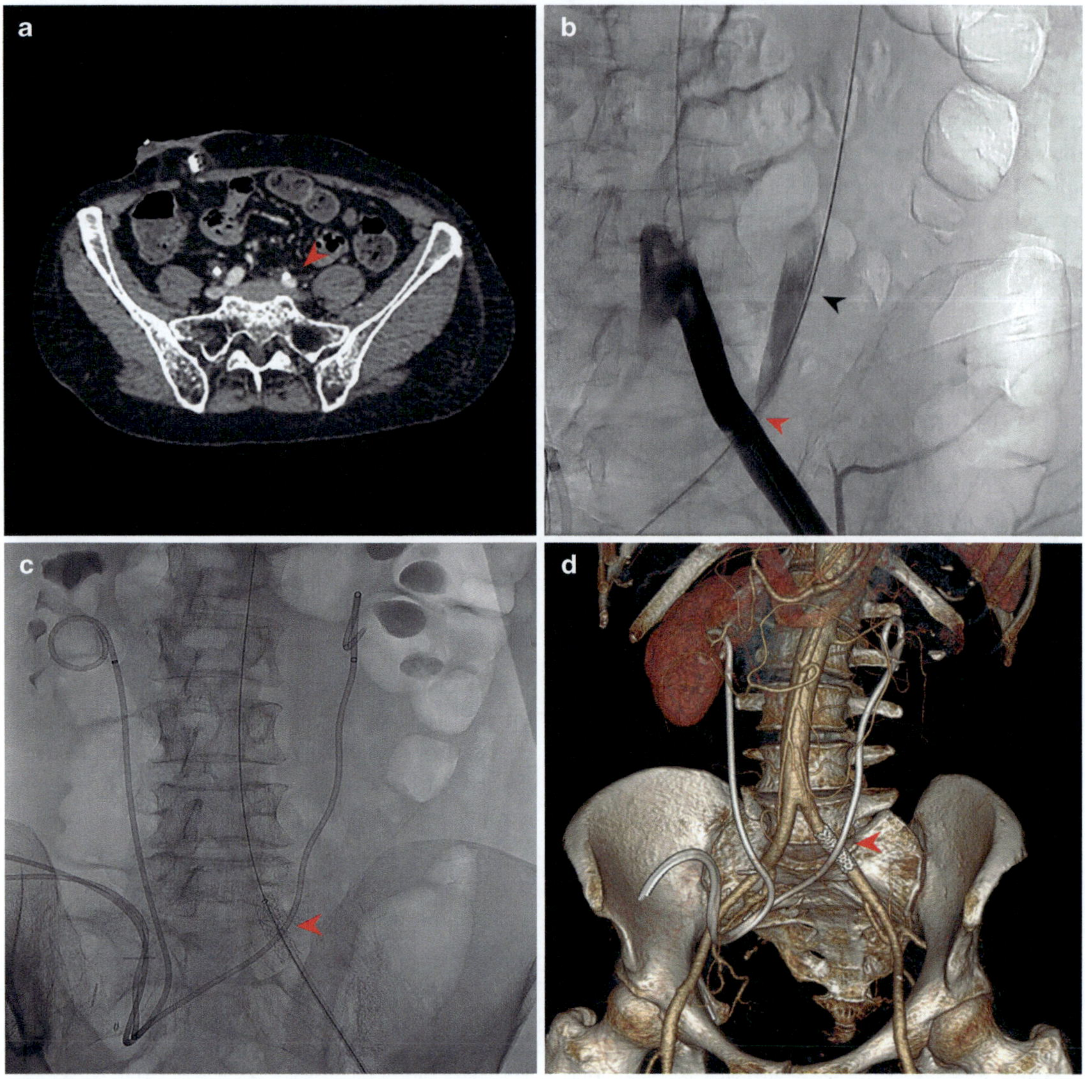

Fig. 13.6 A 46-year-old woman with a previous history of hysterectomy, cystectomy, and radiotherapy with uretero-ileo-cutaneostomy for endometrial cancer. The patient is also a carrier of ureteral stents, the left of which lies on the left common iliac artery: contact point between the ureteral catheter and the anterior wall of the left common iliac artery (**a**, *red arrowhead*). The patient presents to the emergency room for conspicuous bleeding from the stoma associated with pain and a drop in blood pressure. Left common iliac arteriography is performed urgently after removal of the ipsilateral ureteral catheter with a safety guide maintained: selective arteriography demonstrates the simultaneous opacification of the ipsilateral ureter (**b**, *black arrowhead*) from the crossing point (**b**, *red arrowhead*). The iliac-covered stent is placed in the arterio-ureteral fistula point (**c**, *red arrowhead*). Volume rendering reconstructions of the control CT demonstrate closure of the arterial ureteral fistula after placement of endoprostheses (**d**, *red arrowhead*)

Transcatheter embolization of the internal iliac arteries was described in endometrial or cervical cancers as well as in advanced uterine cancers (Fig. 13.7c, d) [86–88]. All experiences reported rapid control of bleeding, a reduced incidence of re-bleeding, and improvement in the patient's general conditions. Intractable hemorrhages rate has been reported to be less

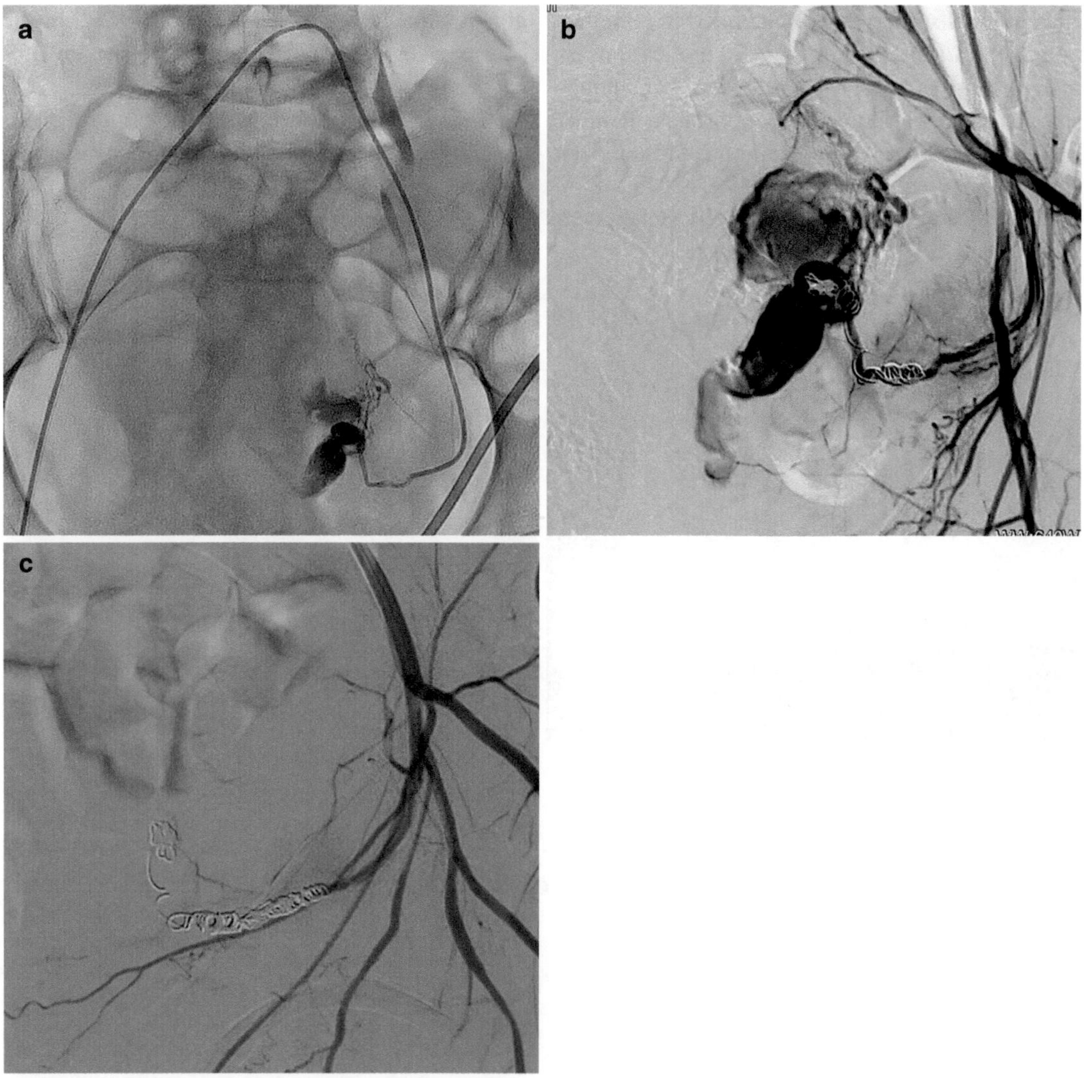

Fig. 13.7 A 46-year-old patient with cervical cancer and blood loss: DSA images of the hypogastric artery and then cervical trunk show massive vaginal bleeding (**a**); progressive embolization with coils of that vessel (**b**). Final angiogram after the procedure that confirms complete exclusion of the bleeding (**c**)

than 1% in an extensive series of gynecological oncologic patients [88]. The accurate assessment of the amount of vaginal blood loss is complex and the transfusion amounts prior to arterial embolization serve only as an indicator of blood loss.

Identification of the arterial supply of a solid tumor by preoperative contrast-enhanced CT facilitates devascularization of neoplastic tissue by transcatheter embolization.

Mechanical occlusion can be achieved by polyvinyl alcohol (PVA), Amplatzer occlusion devices, coils, and embospheres introduced into the tumor bed and lodged in the feeding vessel following fluoroscopic guided selective arterial catheterization [89–91]. This technique can be used alone as the primary modality of treatment, where interruption of the afferent blood supply to the tumor induces hypoxia and inhibits tumor growth; on the other hand, ablative treatments or conventional surgery may be applied in conjunction [89]. In acute hemorrhagic complications of malignancies (as massive hemoptysis, hematemesis, pleural or peritoneal/retroperitoneal hemorrhages), transarterial embolization is the standard goal treatment (Fig. 13.8a, b) [13, 91]. Diagnostic selective angiography at the beginning of the procedure is mandatory (Fig. 13.8c, d).

Endovascular approaches involving either parent vessel occlusion, embolization of vascular

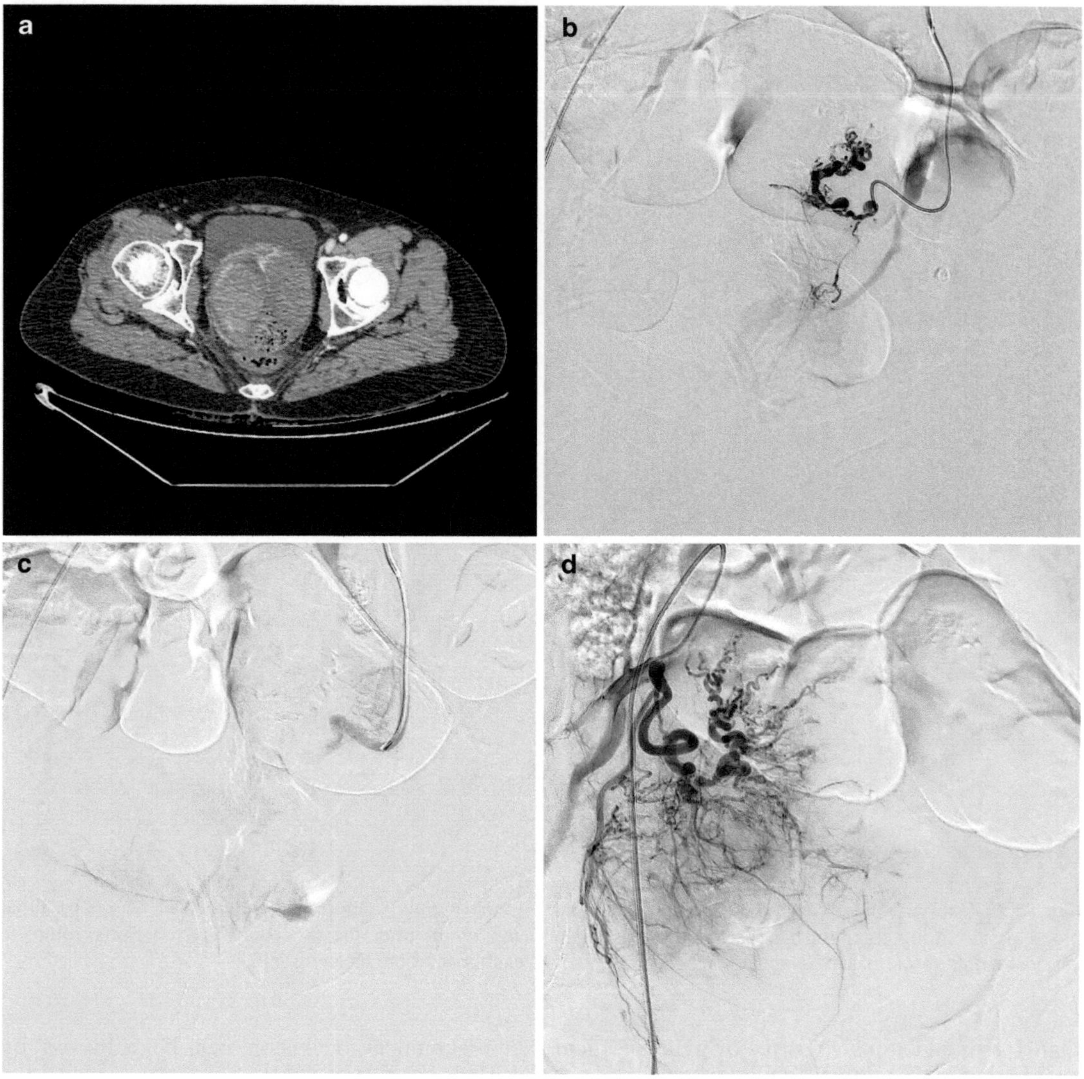

Fig. 13.8 A 50-year-old woman with a history of pelvic pain, metrorrhagia, and a drop in hemoglobin. A contrast-enhanced CT scan demonstrates a heterogeneous mass that surrounds the uterine cervix with multiple bleeding foci (**a**). Superselective angiography of left uterine artery performed with microcatheter: intra-arterial injection confirms the presence of multiple bleeding foci and hypervascularization (**b**). Transcatheter arterial embolization with 300–500 μm microspheres: following angiogram demonstrates no residual vascularity within the lesion on the left side (**c**). Selective right hypogastric arteriogram also shows the contralateral presence of rich hypervascularization with fine, tortuous, and irregular vessels caused by structural subversion that are demonstrated in the early phase (**d**). Selective arteriogram of distal right uterine artery: transcatheter embolization with 300–500 μm microspheres: the first angiogram during embolization demonstrates a massive reduction of vascularity within the lesion (**e**). Post-embolization and selective hypogastric angiography show no residual vascularity homolateral nor opacification of contralateral visceral branches (**f**)

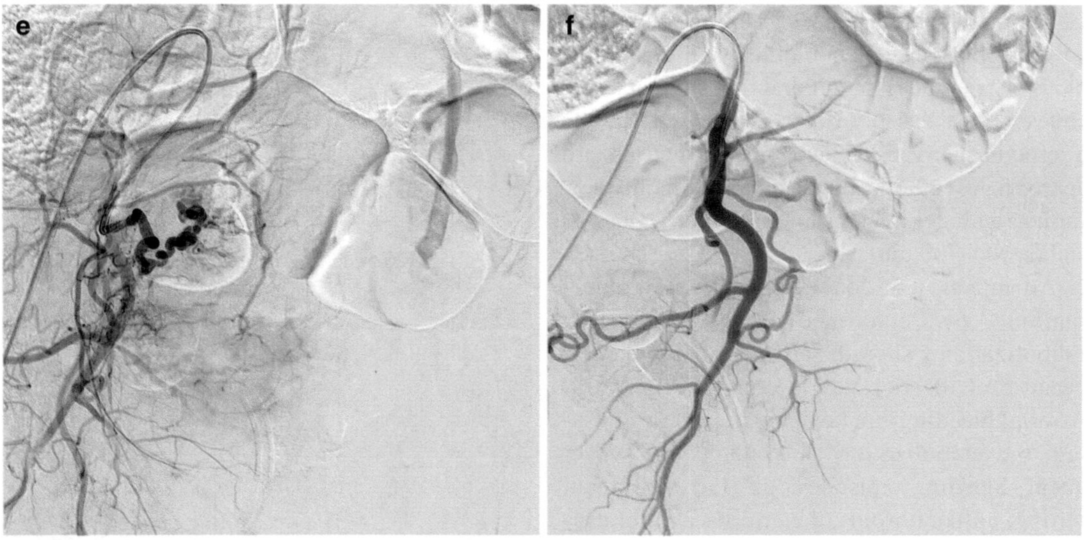

Fig. 13.8 (continued)

injury, or placement of a covered stent have decreased the need for invasive open surgery in high-risk patients, controlling bleeding with high precision, low complication rates, and minimal procedure-related ischemic damage. This technique is a safe and efficacy palliative measure alternative to surgical treatment (Fig. 13.8d–f).

Surgical intervention in these high-risk patients, often expiring, may be challenging owing to hostile anatomy from previous irradiation therapy and/or radical dissections, and it is associated with high rates of major morbidity, especially if performed in an emergent setting. Endovascular treatment could also be an adjunctive part of surgical treatment. The vast collateral blood supply to the pelvis is the reason why proximal ligation of the hypogastric artery may fail to control bleeding in patients with intractable tumoral vaginal bleeding.

Although metrorrhagia is a common presenting feature of cervical cancer, it is infrequent for this to be hemodynamically threatening [12]. Any vaginal packing should be removed during DSA to allow visualization of the bleeding point. Permanent spheres ranging from 300 to 900 microns supplemented by absorbable gel foam and metallic micro coils can be adopted for selective embolization (Fig. 13.8). The smallest spheres are first injected to occlude the capillary vessels; coils should be used to occlude distal vessels with super selectively catheterization technique; indeed, embolization of proximal vessels may promote the development of collaterals with further bleeding. Failure to identify the site of bleeding does not preclude the embolization procedure: In these cases, empiric embolization can be performed as in pelvic trauma, based on the clinical status and CT findings.

All patients should perform a CT scan: after the basal acquisition, contrast enhancement ones were acquired at 30s, 70–80 s, and 180 s after intravenous injection.

CT images allowed to detect active bleeding or vascular damage but also to obtain a vascular map to plan the embolization strategy.

All procedures should be performed with femoral access through a 5 Fr- introducer sheath. Based on CT findings, a diagnostic pelvic arteriogram was performed with 5 Fr diagnostic catheters to detect the origin of the main vessel supplying the malignancy. Both hypogastric districts must be examined.

The procedure should also be performed by selective catheterization of the anterior division of the internal iliac artery and super-selective with the use of a 2.7 Fr microcatheter to navigate of the “usual suspects,” such as uterine and cervicovaginal arteries that could have a thin and tortuous aspect due to tumoral neoangiogenesis. Unless a focal vascular defect is detected, such as a pseudoaneurysm in which micro coils are appropriate, embolization is most commonly performed with gel foam or microspheres (300–500 and/or 600–700 μm).

An injection is conducted until flow interruption is confirmed angiographically. Embolization should always be bilateral because of the rich pelvic collateral network. Arterial bleeding can be episodic and progressing; the embolization can reduce the subsequent bleeding episodes. In the malignant setting, unlike fibroids, the arteries are not usually hypertrophied. Also, prior radiation therapy can cause vascular sclerosis, degrading the arterial supply into a lace-like mesh. From a technical point of view, embolization can be more challenging if the patient has already undergone surgery and/or radiotherapy since anatomic relationships are distorted, and there may be atypical sources of bleeding.

If the vaginal bleeding is related to pelvic cancers, it typically shows slow, intermittent, and persistent bleeding. It is also poorly responsive to surgical interventions or radiotherapy; it can be life-threatening in advanced uterine neoplasms, and it is the immediate cause of death in the 6% of women with cervical cancer.

A less frequent but potentially life-threatening cause of lower gastrointestinal (GI) hemorrhage in the female patient is advanced pelvic neoplasm. Lower GI bleeding arising from the internal iliac artery branches is rare but clinical presentation may be quite dramatic because of the involvement of large pelvic arteries [92]. This may occur when there is an extension of the neoplasm into the adjacent rectum and sigmoid colon (Figs. 13.9 and 13.10). In addition, hemorrhage can be the result of vessel damage from previous radiation therapy. Although transcatheter embolotherapy has a limited role in the management of most causes of lower GI bleeding, embolization techniques can be lifesaving in patients who present massive lower GI bleeding related to advanced pelvic malignancy. Gelfoam, PVA particles, coils, and covered stents have been used to occlude or exclude vessels responsible for the bleeding [93–98].

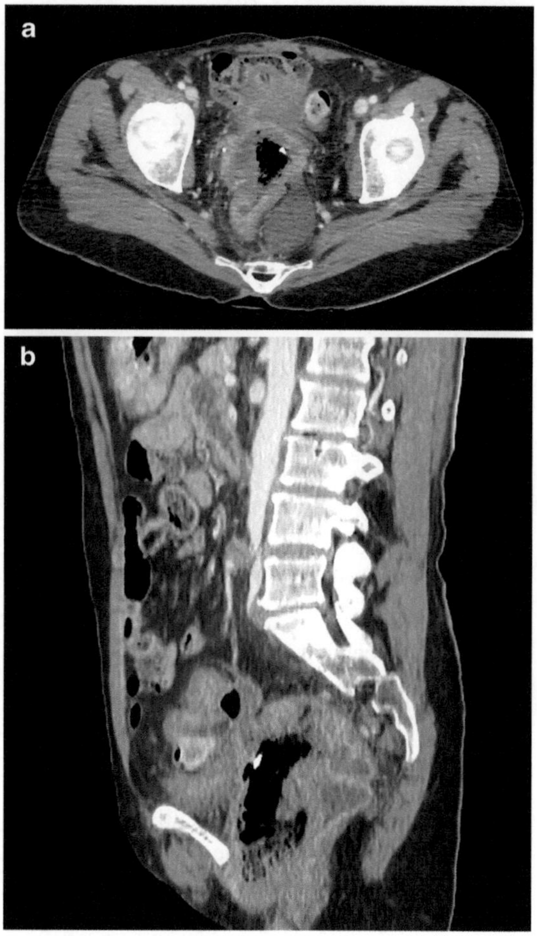

Fig. 13.9 A 51-year-old patient with cervical cancer and rectorragia; CT shows a mass infiltrating the vagina and the sigmoid colon with contrast medium blush from active bleeding originating from the sigmoid arteries (**a**); along sagittal scan (**b**) is appreciated the pathological extent of neoplasia at that level of the sigma and therefore the presence of hematoma in various stages of coagulation

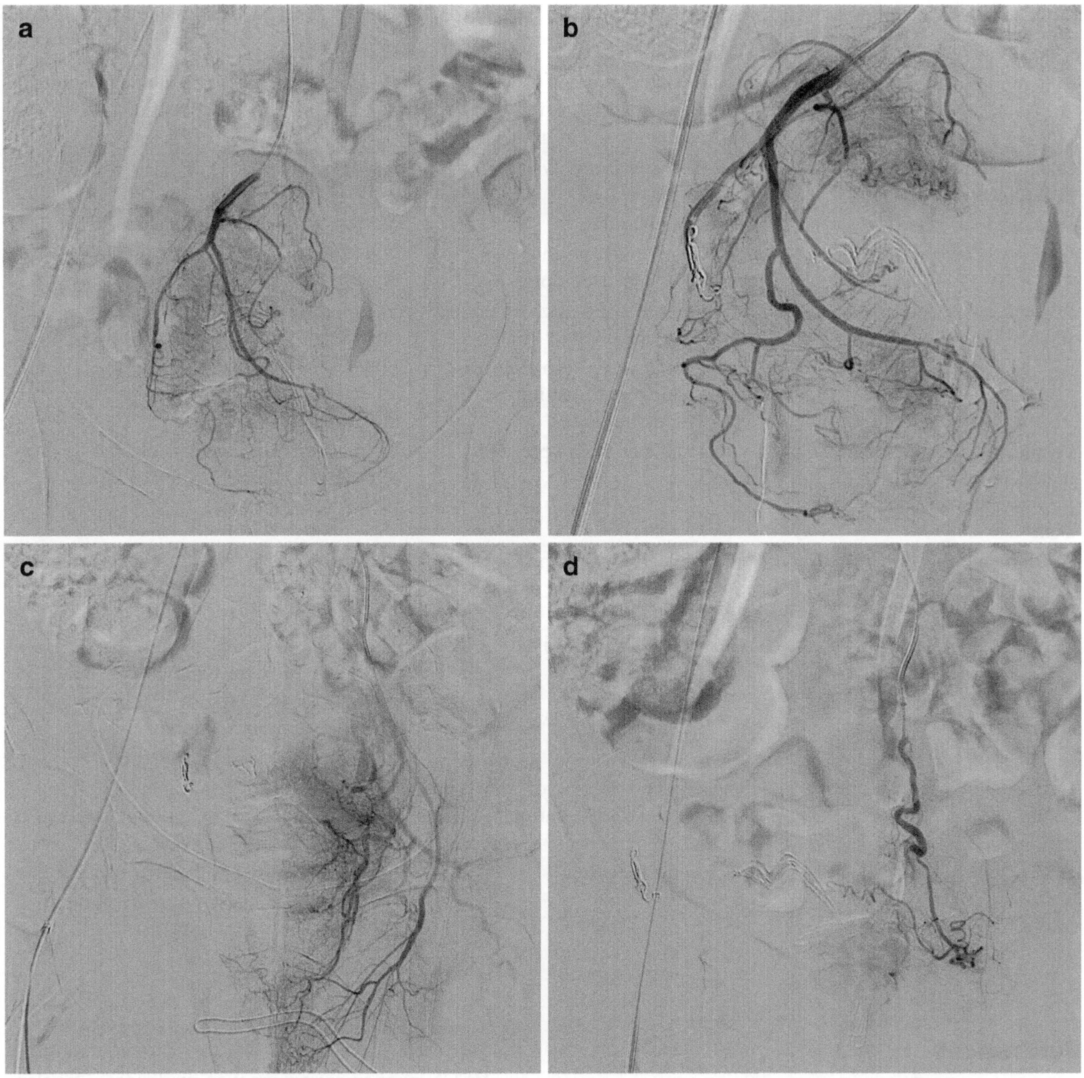

Fig. 13.10 DSA of the inferior mesenteric artery and sigmoid arteries (**a**) confirms the active bleeding and the neoplastic vascularization treated with gel foam injection and coils embolization (**b**); DSA of the left hypogastric trunk and cervical arteries shows a neoplastic vascularization and an interrupted vessel as indirect sign of bleeding (**c**); the latter was treated with gel foam injection (**d**)

13.5 Conclusion

Nowadays, IR offers a wide variety of procedures for the treatment of gynecological malignancies and their complications (Table 13.1). IR utilizing minimally invasive advanced image-guided percutaneous techniques plays an important role in gynecologic malignancies treatment not only in diagnosis with biopsies but in the management of complications like fluid aspiration, drainage catheter placement in pleural or abdominal effusion, and prolonging lifespan with pelvic arterial embolization in bloody malignancies.

The wide availability of materials and multidisciplinary collaboration with gynecologists is essential for the clinical and technical success of these procedures.

Table 13.1 Summary table of IR procedures with indications and risk factors for gynecological malignancies

Procedures	Indications	Risk factors
Imaging-guided paracentesis	– Symptomatic malignant ascites (abdominal swelling, pain, nausea/vomiting, anorexia, fatigue)	Bowel adhesions, omental and peritoneal disease or loculated collections
Imaging-guided percutaneous drainage	Infected abdominal or pelvic fluid collections (abscesses)	Major pelvic surgery
Percutaneous biliary drainage (PBD)	– Obstructive jaundice	Metastatic disease at the hepatic hilar nodes or in the peripancreatic nodes
	– If endoscopy fails to achieve adequate biliary decompression	
Percutaneous nephrostomy (PCN)	– Decompression of malignant ureteral obstruction unilateral or bilateral	Extrinsic tumor compression, retroperitoneal adenopathy or direct tumor invasion
	– Urinary tract sepsis, pyonephrosis, deteriorating renal function or electrolyte disturbances	
Percutaneous dilatation of ureteral stricture and positioning internal ureteral stent	– To treat stenosis and to prevent restenosis	Extrinsic tumor compression, retroperitoneal adenopathy or direct tumor invasion
Arterial embolization	– Massive bleeding from pelvic neoplasms (endometrial or cervical cancers)	– Coagulopathy related to malignancy
	– Preoperative devascularization	– Iatrogenic causes (chemotherapy, radiotherapy, postoperative pseudoaneurysms)
		– Hypervascularized tumor
		– Mechanical vascular invasion
Occlusion of arterio-ureteric fistula	– Hematuria microscopic or macroscopic (often recurrent)	– Previous history of abdominal or pelvic oncologic or vascular surgery, urinary shunt surgery
	– Catastrophic bleeding	– Prolonged use of a bladder catheter
		– PREVIOUS history of radiotherapy

References

1. Chow DS, Itagaki MW. Interventional oncology research in the United States: slowing growth, limited focus, and a low level of funding. Radiology. 2010;257:410–7. https://doi.org/10.1148/radiol.10100070.
2. Mahnken AH, Bruners P, Günther RW. Techniques of interventional tumor therapy. Dtsch Arztebl Int. 2008;105:646–53. https://doi.org/10.3238/arztebl.2008.0646.
3. Cannistra SA. Cancer of the ovary. N Engl J Med. 2004;351(24):2519–29.
4. Siegel R, Naishadham D, Jemal A. Cancer statistics, 2012. CA Cancer J Clin. 2012;62(1):10–29.
5. Benedet JL, Bender H, Jones H III, et al. FIGO Committee on Gynecologic Oncology. FIGO staging classifications and clinical practice guidelines in the management of gynecologic cancers. Int J Gynaecol Obstet. 2000;70(2):209–62.
6. Morgan RJ Jr, Copeland L, Gershenson D, et al. The National Comprehensive Cancer Network. NCCN ovarian cancer practice guidelines. Oncology (Williston Park). 1996;10(11, Suppl):293–310.
7. NNA H, Krapcho M, Garshell J, et al., editors. SEER cancer statistics review, 1975–2010. Bethesda, MD: National Cancer Institute; 2013. Based on November 2012 SEER data submission, posted to the SEER Website: http://seer.cancer.gov/csr/1975_2010/.
8. Walboomers JM, Jacobs MV, Manos MM, et al. Human papillomavirus is a necessary cause of invasive cervical cancer worldwide. J Pathol. 1999;189(1):12–9.
9. Scheurer ME, Tortolero-Luna G, Adler-Storthz K. Human papillomavirus infection: biology, epidemiology, and prevention. Int J Gynecol Cancer. 2005;15(5):727–46.
10. CorrBR, BehbakhtK, SpillmanMA. Gynecologic biopsy for molecular profiling: a review for the interventional radiologist. Semin Intervent Radiol. 2013;30(4):417–24. https://doi.org/10.1055/s-0033-1359738.

11. O'Neill SB, O'Connor OJ, Ryan MF, et al. Interventional radiology and the care of the oncology patient. Radiol Res Pract. 2011;2011:160867. https://doi.org/10.1155/2011/160867.
12. Revel-Mouroz P, Mokrane FZ, Collot S, et al. Hemostatic embolization in oncology. Diagn Interv Imaging. 2015;96:807–21. https://doi.org/10.1016/j.diii.2015.06.008.
13. Yu H, Stavas JM. The role of interventional radiology in the management of benign and malignant gynecologic diseases. Obstet Gynecol Surv. 2013;68:691–701. https://doi.org/10.1097/OGX.0b013e3182a878c6.
14. Singh H. Interventional radiology in the gynecological oncology patient. Best Pract Res Clin Obstet Gynaecol. 2001;15:279–90. https://doi.org/10.1053/beog.2000.0168.
15. Mahnken AH, Bruners P. Günther RW: techniques of interventional tumor therapy. Deutsches Arzteblatt. 2008;105(38):646–53.
16. Yu H, Stavas JM. The role of interventional radiology in the management of benign and malignant gynecologic diseases. Obstet Gynecol Surv Oct. 2013;68(10):691–701. https://doi.org/10.1097/OGX.0b013e3182a878c6.
17. Stokes LS. Percutaneous management of malignant fluid collections. Semin Interv Radiol. 2007;24:398–408.
18. Singh H. Interventional radiology in the gynaecological oncology patient. Best Pract Res Clin Obstet Gynaecol. 2001;15(2):279–90. https://doi.org/10.1053/beog.2000.0168.
19. Fagotti A, Costantini B, Fanfani F, et al. Risk of postoperative pelvic abscess in major gynecologic oncology surgery: one-year single-institution experience. Ann Surg Oncol. 2010;17:2452–8.
20. Ayantunde AA, Parsons SL. Pattern and prognostic factors in patients with malignant ascites: a retrospective study. Ann Oncol. 2007;18:945–9.
21. Lee CW, Bociek G, Faught W. A survey of practice in the management of malignant ascites. J Pain Symptom Manage. 1998;16:96–101.
22. Runyon BA. Care of patients with ascites. N Engl J Med. 1994;330:337–42.
23. Parsons SL, Watson SA, Steele RJ. Malignant ascites. Br J Surg. 1996;83:6–14.
24. Mahrer A, Ramchandani P, Trerotola SO, et al. Sclerotherapy in the management of postoperative lymphocele. J Vasc Interv Radiol. 2010;21:1050–3.
25. Todokoro T, Furniss D, Oda K, et al. Effective treatment of pelvic lymphocele by lymphaticovenular anastomosis. Gynecol Oncol. 2013;128:209–14.
26. Campbell JJ, Gervais DA. Percutaneous drainage of abscesses in the abdomen and pelvis. In: Mauro MA, KPJ M, Thomson KR, et al., editors. Image-guided interventions. Philadelphia: Saunders Elsevier; 2008. p. 1321–32.
27. O'Connor OJ, Buckley JM, Maher MM. Interventional radiology in oncology. Cancer Treat Res. 2008;143:493–511.
28. Uzbek MH, Almeida FA, Sarkis MG, et al. Management of malignant pleural Effusions. Adv Ther. 2010;27(6):334–47.
29. Seaton KG, Patz EF, Goodman PC. Palliative treatment of malignant pleural effusions: value of smallbore catheter thoracostomy and doxycycline sclerotherapy. Am J Roentgenol. 1995;164(3):589–91.
30. Lombardi G, Zustovich F, Nicoletto MO, Donach M, Artioli G, Pastorelli D. Diagnosis and treatment of malignant pleural effusion: a systematic literature review and new approaches. Am J Clin Oncol. 2010;33(4):420–3.
31. Mironov O, Ishill NM, Mironov S, et al. Pleural effusion detected at CT prior to primary cytoreduction for stage III or IV ovarian carcinoma: effect on survival. Radiology. 2011;258:776–84.
32. Pollak JS, Burdge CM, Rosenblatt M, et al. Treatment of malignant pleural effusions with tunneled long-term drainage catheters. J Vasc Interv Radiol. 2001;12:201–8.
33. Pollak JS. Malignant pleural effusions: treatment with tunneled long-term drainage catheters. Curr Opin Pulm Med. 2002;8:302–7.
34. Whitworth JM, Schneider KE, Fauci JM, et al. Outcomes of patients with gynecologic malignancies undergoing video-assisted thoracoscopic surgery (VATS) and pleurodesis for malignant pleural effusion. Gynecol Oncol. 2012;125:646–8.
35. Russo P. Urologic emergencies in the cancer patient. Semin Oncol. 2000;27(3):284–98.
36. Park BK, Kim SH, Moon MH. Nonvascular interventions of the urinary tract. J Korean Med Sci. 2002;17(6):727–36.
37. Kim SH, Park JH, Han MC. Antegrade balloon dilatation and ureteral stenting for the benign ureteral strictures. J Korean Radiol Soc. 1994;30:57–63.
38. McAleer SJ, Loughlin KR. Nephrolithiasis and pregnancy. Curr Opin Urol. 2004;14(2):123–7.
39. Dyer RB, Regan JD, Kavanagh PV, Khatod EG, Chen MY, Zagoria RJ. Percutaneous nephrostomy with extensions of the technique: step by step. Radiographics. 2002;22(3):503–25.
40. Kalogeropoulou C, Kallidonis P, Liatsikos EN. Imaging in percutaneous nephrolithotomy. J Endourol. 2009;23(10):1571–7.
41. Wong LM, Cleeve LK, Milner AD, Pitman AG. Malignant ureteral obstruction: outcomes after intervention. Have things changed? J Urol. 2007;178(1):178–83.
42. Harrington KJ, Pandha HS, Kelly SA, et al. Palliation of obstructive nephropathy due to malignancy. Br J Urol. 1995;76:101–7.
43. Fallon B, Olney L, Culp DA. Nephrostomy in cancer patients: to do or not to do? Br J Urol. 1980;52:237–42.
44. Shekarriz B, Shekarriz H, Upadhyay J, et al. Outcome of palliative urinary diversion in the treatment of advanced malignancies. Cancer. 1999;85:998–1003.
45. Rossi P, Bezzi M, Rossi M, et al. Metallic stents in malignant biliary obstruction: results of a multicenter

European study of 240 patients. J Vasc Interv Radiol. 1994;5(2):279–85.
46. Becker CD, Glättli A, Maibach R, Baer HU. Percutaneous palliation of malignant obstructive jaundice with the Wallstent endoprosthesis: follow-up and reintervention in patients with hilar and non-hilar obstruction. J Vasc Interv Radiol. 1993;4(5):597–604.
47. Carrasco CH, Zornoza J, Bechtel WJ. Malignant biliary obstruction: complications of percutaneous biliary drainage. Radiology. 1984;152(2):343–6.
48. Nomura T, Shirai Y, Hatakeyama K. Bacteribilia and cholangitis after percutaneous transhepatic biliary drainage for malignant biliary obstruction. Dig Dis Sci. 1999;44(3):542–6.
49. Nichols DA, MacCarty R, Gaffey TA. Cholangiographic evaluation of bile duct carcinoma. Am J Roentgenol. 1983;141(6):1291–4.
50. O'Neill MJ, Rafferty EA, Lee SI, et al. Transvaginal interventional procedures: aspiration, biopsy, and catheter drainage. Radiographics. 2001;21(3):657–72. https://doi.org/10.1148/radiographics.21.3.g01ma20657.
51. Weston M, Soyer P, Barral M, et al. Role of interventional procedures in obstetrics and gynecology. Radiol Clin N Am. 2020;58(2):445–62. https://doi.org/10.1016/j.rcl.2019.11.006.
52. Gupta S, Wallace MJ, Cardella JF, et al. Quality improvement guidelines for percutaneous needle biopsy. J Vasc Interv Radiol. 2010;21(7):969–75.
53. Thabet A, Somarouthu B, Oliva E, et al. Image-guided ovarian mass biopsy: efficacy and safety. J Vasc Interv Radiol. 2014;25(12):1922–1927.e1. https://doi.org/10.1016/j.jvir.2014.08.009.
54. Varadhachary GR, Abbruzzese JL, Lenzi R. Diagnostic strategies for unknown primary cancer. Cancer. 2004;100(9):1776–85.
55. Spencer JA, Swift SE, Wilkinson N, et al. Peritoneal carcinomatosis: image-guided peritoneal core biopsy for tumor type and patient care. Radiology. 2001;221(1):173–7.
56. Zikan M, Fischerova D, Pinkavova I, et al. Ultrasound-guided true-cut biopsy of abdominal and pelvic tumors in gynecology. Ultrasound Obstet Gynecol. 2010;36(6):767–72. https://doi.org/10.1002/uog.8803.
57. Griffin N, Grant LA, Freeman SJ, et al. Image-guided biopsy in patients with suspected ovarian carcinoma: a safe and effective technique? Eur Radiol. 2009;19:230–5.
58. Kobal B, Noventa M, Cvjeticanin B, et al. Primary debulking surgery versus primary neoadjuvant chemotherapy for high grade advanced-stage ovarian cancer: comparison of survivals. Radiol Oncol. 2018;52(3):307–19.
59. Van der Burg ME, van Lent M, Buyse M, et al. The effect of debulking surgery after induction chemotherapy on the prognosis in advanced epithelial ovarian cancer: gynecological cancer cooperative Group of the European Organization for research and treatment of cancer. N Engl J Med. 1995;332:629–34.
60. Rose PG, Nerenstone S, Brady MF, et al. Secondary surgical cytoreduction for advanced ovarian carcinoma. N Engl J Med. 2004;351:2489–97.
61. Hewitt M, Anderson K, Hall G, et al. Women with peritoneal carcinomatosis of unknown origin: efficacy of image-guided biopsy to determine site-specific diagnosis. BLOG. 2006;114(1):46–50.
62. Prat A, Perou CM. Deconstructing the molecular portraits of breast cancer. Mol Oncol. 2011;5(1):5–23.
63. Walkey MM, Freidman AC, Sohotra AC, et al. CT manifestations of peritoneal carcinomatosis. AJR Am J Roentgenol. 1988;150:1035–41.
64. Malmstrom H. Fine-needle aspiration cytology versus core biopsies in the evaluation of recurrent gynecologic malignancies. Gynecol Oncol. 1997;65:69–73.
65. Karoo RO, Lloyd TD, Garcea G, et al. How valuable is ascitic cytology in the detection and management of malignancy? Postgrad Med J. 2003;79:292–4.
66. Oge T, Yalcin OT, Ozalp SS, et al. Sonographically guided core biopsy: a minimally invasive procedure for managing adnexal masses. J Ultrasound Med. 2013;32(11):2023–7. https://doi.org/10.7863/ultra.32.11.2023.
67. Yarram SG, Nghiem HV, Higgins E, et al. Evaluation of imaging-guided core biopsy of pelvic masses. AJR Am J Roentgenol. 2007;188(5):1208–11. https://doi.org/10.2214/AJR.05.1393.
68. Arellano RS, Maher M, Gervais DA, et al. The difficult biopsy: let's make it easier. Curr Probl Diagn Radiol. 2003;32(5):218–26.
69. Chojniak R, Isberner RK, Viana LM, et al. Computed tomography-guided needle biopsy: experience from 1,300 procedures. Sao Paulo Med J. 2006;124:10–4.
70. Bdour M, Hourani S, Mefleh W, et al. Comparison between fine-needle aspiration cytology and true-cut biopsy in the diagnosis of breast cancer. J Surg Pak (Int). 2008;13:19–21.
71. Charboneau JW, Reading CC, Welch TJ. CT and sonographically guided needle biopsy: current techniques and new innovations. AJR. 1990;154:1–1.
72. Scanlan KA, Propeck PA, Lee FT Jr. Invasive procedures in the female pelvis: the value of transabdominal, endovaginal, and endorectal US guidance. Radiographics. 2001;21:491–506.
73. Dodd GD III, Esola CC, Memel DS, et al. Sonography: the undiscovered jewel of interventional radiology. Radiographics. 1996;16:1271–88.
74. Memel DS, Dodd GD III, Esola CC. Efficacy of sonography as a guidance technique for biopsy of abdominal, pelvic, and retroperitoneal lymph nodes. AJR. 1996;167:957–62.
75. Bret PM, Guibaud L, Atri M, et al. Transvaginal US-guided aspiration of ovarian cysts and pelvic masses. Radiology. 1992;185:377–80.
76. Gupta S, Nguyen HL, Morello FA Jr, et al. Various approaches for CT- guided percutaneous biopsy of deep pelvic lesions: anatomic and technical considerations. Radiographics. 2004;24:175–89.
77. Gupta S, Madoff DC, Ahrar K, et al. CT-guided needle biopsy of deep pelvic lesions by extraperito-

neal approach through iliopsoas muscle. Cardiovasc Intervent Radiol. 2003;26(6):534–8. https://doi.org/10.1007/s00270-003-0035-8.
78. Havrilesky LJ, Krivak TC, Mucenski JW, et al. Impact of a chemoresponse assay on treatment costs for recurrent ovarian cancer. Am J Obstet Gynecol. 2010;203(2):e1–7.
79. Bree RL, Goldstein HM, Wallace S. Transcatheter embolization of the internal iliac artery in the management of neoplasms of the pelvis. Surg Gynecol Obstet. 1976;143:597–601.
80. Grace DM, Pitt DF, Gold RE. Vascular embolization and occlusion by angiographic techniques as an aid or alternative to operation. Surg Gynecol Obstet. 1976;143:469–82.
81. Hendrickx P, Orth G, Grunert J. Embolisation of pelvic bleeding lesions from benign origin—long-term results. J Belg Radiol. 1995;78:339–41.
82. Hutchins FL Jr, Worthington-Kirsch R. Embolotherapy for myoma-induced menorrhagia. Obstet Gynecol Clin North Am. 2000;27:397. https://doi.org/10.1016/s0889-8545(00)80030-3.
83. Baakdah H, Tulandi T. Uterine fibroid embolization. Clin Obstet Gynecol. 2005;48:361–8. https://doi.org/10.1097/01.grf.0000159542.19598.ea.
84. Li X, Wang Z, Chen J, et al. Uterine artery embolization for the management of secondary postpartum haemorrhage associated with placenta accreta. Clin Radiol. 2012;67:e71–6. https://doi.org/10.1016/j.crad.2012.07.021.
85. Hori A. Complications following transcatheter arterial embolization for haemorrhage associated with pelvic fracture. Nihon Igaku Hoshasen Gakkai Zasshi. 1991;51:365–74.
86. Mihmanli I, Cantasdemir M, Kantarci F, et al. Percutaneous embolization in the management of intractable vaginal bleeding. Arch Gynecol Obstet. 2001;264:211–4. https://doi.org/10.1007/s004040000119.
87. Tinelli A, Prudenzano R, Malvasi A, et al. Emergency endovascular nanopharmacologic treatment in advanced gynecological cancers. Int J Gynecol Cancer. 2010;20:1250–5. https://doi.org/10.1111/IGC.0b013e3181e4a68d.
88. Albu S, Grigoriu C, Vasiliu C, et al. The role of uterine artery embolization in cervical cancer—single case report. Medica (Buchar). 2011;6:137–40.
89. Cabrera R, Nelson DR. Review article: the management of hepatocellular carcinoma. Aliment Pharmacol Ther. 2010;31:461–76. https://doi.org/10.1111/j.1365-2036.2009.04200.x.
90. Amesur NB, Zajko AB, Carr BI. Chemo-embolization for unresectable hepatocellular carcinoma with different sizes of embolization particles. Dig Dis Sci. 2008;53:1400–4. https://doi.org/10.1007/s10620-007-9995-x.
91. Rodríguez Carvajal R, Orgaz A, Leal JI, et al. Renal embolization and nephrectomy in a single surgical act in high-risk renal tumor pathology. Ann Vasc Surg. 2011;25:222–8. https://doi.org/10.1016/j.avsg.2010.03.037.
92. Spinosa DJ, Angle JF, McGraw JK, et al. Transcatheter treatment of life-threatening lower gastrointestinal bleeding due to advanced pelvic malignancy. Cardiovasc Intervent Radiol. 1998;21:503–5. https://doi.org/10.1007/s002709900312.
93. Matsumoto AH, Selby JB Jr, Tegtmeyer CJ. Detachable balloons as peripheral vascular embolic agents. Semin Intervent Radiol. 1992;9:62–71. https://doi.org/10.1055/s-2008-1074671.
94. Marin ML, Veith FJ, Panetta TF, et al. Percutaneous transfemoral insertion of a stented graft to repair a traumatic femoral arteriovenous fistula. J Vasc Surg. 1993;18:299–302.
95. Piazza F, Corvino F, Silvestre M, et al. Role of interventional radiology in obstetric and gynecological diseases. J Radiol Rev. 2020;7:26–38. https://doi.org/10.23736/S2283-8376.20.00253-3.
96. Corvino F, Giurazza F, Cangiano G, et al. Endovascular treatment of peripheral vascular blowout syndrome in end-stage malignancies. Ann Vasc Surg. 2019;58:382.e1–5. https://doi.org/10.1016/j.avsg.2018.10.051.
97. Coppola M, Giurazza F, Corvino F, et al. Severe metrorrhagia in patients with advanced gynecologic cancer: endovascular treatment benefits in acute and chronic setting. Radiol Med. 2021;126(2):277–82. https://doi.org/10.1007/s11547-020-01251-6.
98. Patanè D, Coniglio G, Bonomo S, Camerano F, Arcerito F, Calcara G, Bisceglie P, Malfa P. Gynecological malignancies: bail-out interventional radiology treatments. Semin Ultrasound CT MR. 2021;42(1):95–103. https://doi.org/10.1053/j.sult.2020.09.003.

Part IV

Obstetrical Pathologies

Embolization of Scar Pregnancies and Extrauterine Implants

14

Laura Crocetti, Orsola Perrone, Gianvito Candita, Giulia Lorenzoni, Francesco Giurazza, and Roberto Cioni

14.1 Introduction

Ectopic pregnancy (EP) consists in the implantation of an embryo in a site other than the endometrium of the uterine cavity. It occurs in 1–2% of all reported pregnancies.

The most common extrauterine location is the fallopian tube, which represents 96% of cases. Other usual non-tubal locations are the cervix, ovary, peritoneal cavity, and cesarean scar [1].

Cesarean scar pregnancy (CSP) is a rare occurrence consisting in the implantation of the embryo within the myometrium of a prior cesarean delivery scar, with a reported incidence ratio of CSP to normal pregnancies ranging from 1:1800 to 1:2216 in women with at least one previous cesarean section. Depending on the depth of implantation, we can describe two different types of CSPs: type 1 (or endogenic type), with preferential development of the pregnancy toward the uterine cavity, and type 2 (or exogenic type), progressing toward the bladder [2].

The pathogenesis of this condition is unknown even if it is probably related to abnormal transportation of fertilized ovum within the fallopian tube.

The recognized risk factors include: a history of pelvic inflammatory disease, presence of intrauterine devices, previous tubal surgery (ipsilateral salpingectomy and cornual reanastomosis), cervical conization, Asherman's syndrome (an acquired condition characterized by the formation of scar tissue in the uterine cavity and/or the cervix), in-vitro fertilization, and cesarean section [3]. In the last decades, the Chinese CSP incidence rate has significantly increased because of the augmented cesarean section rate and China's second-child policy [4].

Diagnosis is based on a combination of clinical evaluation (amenorrhea, vaginal bleeding, pelvic pain); measurement of serum β-hCG concentrations (increasing slower than expected); and transvaginal ultrasound (with findings of an embryo in addition to a gestational sac or sizes of adnexal mass) [5]. For equivocal ultrasound results, MRI can be used to determine the location of embryonic implantation and assess the depth of intrusive growth from the gestational sac to the muscular layer [4].

About 15–20% of Eps are burdened by a rupture with internal bleeding, which can lead to severe hemorrhages up to hypovolemic shock and often needs surgical treatment [6]. As the Eps may be fatal, they should be immediately interrupted as soon as possible.

L. Crocetti (✉) · O. Perrone · G. Candita
G. Lorenzoni · R. Cioni
Division of Interventional Radiology, Department of Diagnostic, Interventional Radiology and Nuclear Medicine, Azienda Ospedaliero Universitaria Pisana, University of Pisa, Pisa, Italy
e-mail: laura.crocetti@unipi.it; g.candita@studenti.unipi.it; r.cioni@ao-pisa.toscana.it

F. Giurazza
Vascular and Interventional Radiology Department, Cardarelli Hospital, Naples, Italy

R. Niola et al. (eds.), *Diagnostic and Interventional Radiology in Gynecological and Obstetric Diseases*, https://doi.org/10.1007/978-3-031-11910-1_14

The management of Eps has changed over the years and counts different fertility-preserving options.

Wait-and-see approach is suitable and preferred in asymptomatic patients with low β-hCG values (<10,000 mI U/mL). Since many small and early diagnosed EPs resolve spontaneously, these patients are at risk to be overtreated and should be monitored with sequential β-hCG measurements and sonography [7].

Medical treatment for EP is represented by methotrexate, a folic acid antagonist that is toxic to cells undergoing rapid mitotic division. It causes lysis of fetal cells that can lead to intraperitoneal bleeding with abdominal pain in patients [8]. Since its intramuscular administration is associated with different severe side effects (bone marrow suppression, elevated liver enzymes, rash, alopecia areata, stomatitis, nausea, diarrhea), single-dose regimens with a small loss of effectiveness are preferred. When used, the time to resolution of EP is 3–7 weeks [9]. Methotrexate seems to be effective in the treatment of early EPs, occurring in well-vascularized areas, with β-hCG values <10,000 IU/L and a crown-rump length <10 mm [10].

After methotrexate administration, follow-up is necessary. It is based on serial serum β-hCG measurements on day 4, day 7, and then weekly until β-hCG levels decline to zero. Repeating medical treatment may be required if β-hCG levels do not fall [9].

Among surgical procedures, laparoscopic salpingostomy, with or without fallopian tube removal, is the preferred surgical treatment in tubal EPs. The main purpose is the removal of only the ectopic gestational sac: surgeons try not to remove all the tube in order to preserve fertility. Surgery is mandatory in case of rupture, but it is also performed in some unruptured EPs with β-hCG values >2500 IU/L. Surgical complications (pain, infection, pelvic adhesions) are possible [11].

Surgery may not be suitable for management of non-tubal EPs.

Cornual resection via laparotomy or laparoscopy has been used to treat cornual EPs, causing problems of fertility or hemorrhages because of the rich vascular supply in the interstitial area [3]. A relatively new approach consists in the use of hysteroscopy to endoscopically remove type-2 CSP, offering visually directed treatment, reduced operative bleeding, shorter stay, and better patient compliance [2].

When possible, conservative management such as suction and curettage or interventional procedures is the favored option in women desiring future pregnancies.

In the last years, an important role is played by minimally invasive interventional procedures in the treatment of EPs. Direct administration of chemicals by ultrasound-guided injection into the ectopic implant or endovascular uterine artery chemoembolization (UAE) can be performed to successfully treat EPs and CSPs.

14.2 Direct Chemical Injection

In the treatment of superficial *EPs*, US-guided direct chemical injection of the ectopic gestational sac is a possible alternative to surgery. After antibiotic prophylaxis and cleansing of the vaginal vault with preparatory solution, a needle (e.g., 20-gauge Chiba type) is inserted into the amniotic sac with transvaginal US guidance. Color Doppler imaging helps to avoid vessels along the planned route. Once the needle is carried into the sac, the amniotic fluid is usually aspirated before the chemical is injected in order to mechanically disrupt the sac and to prevent its overdistension and a possible leakage of the chemical [12]. In presence of leakage, the operator may instill Ringer's Lactate solution to dilute the chemotherapeutic agent and minimize any peritoneal effect [8]. The chemical can be injected into the sac or directly into the fetus, depending on the size and the gestational age. The most common chemicals used in this technique include methotrexate (1 mg per kg of body weight), potassium chloride (1–3 mL in a 2 mEq/mL solution), and hyperosmolar glucose (50% solution).

The direct injection of methotrexate into the amniotic sac presents potential advantages as compared to intramuscular therapies. This way it is possible to reach higher local concentrations of the chemical, reducing systemic toxic effects. Direct chemical injection is also suitable in presence of a synchronous uterine implantation, which represents a contraindication to systemic treatment, if the patient desires to carry on the uterine pregnancy.

If there are any contraindications to methotrexate injection (blood dyscrasia, severe pulmonary disease, coexisting hepatic disease, breastfeeding, immunocompromised state), other alternative chemicals may be used to treat EPs. Moreover, in presence of residual fetal cardiac activity, potassium chloride may be preferred to increase the probability of its cessation [12].

The only primary contraindications to direct chemical injection of EPs are hemodynamic instability and hemoperitoneum, which represent an indication of emergency surgery [12].

Extended follow-up after local chemical injection is similar to that after intramuscular injection of methotrexate. For this reason, this procedure is not indicated in those patients who are likely to be lost during the follow-up [3, 12].

The procedure of direct chemical injection is also performed in some *non-tubal EPs* that occur in cornu, cervix, or cesarean section scar. It may be difficult in distal interstitial or isthmic pregnancies. The technique used in these cases is similar to that for injection of a tubal ectopic sac, although interventional radiologists bring adaptations in all the different cases. For example, in the treatment of a cornual pregnancy or CSP, some interventional radiologists perform an endovascular uterine artery embolization immediately before chemical injection, to prevent the comparison of severe post-injection hemorrhages related to the greater vascularization in cornual or scar tissues [12].

14.3 Endovascular Treatment

14.3.1 Introduction

UAE is another minimally invasive procedure used in the treatment of non-tubal EPs [13]. This technique is also used to treat fibroids, myomas, uterine vascular malformations, gynecologic malignancies, or postpartum hemorrhage. It consists in the injection of embolic agents directly into the uterine arteries. The embolization decreases blood flow to the ectopic sac, inducing subsequent trophoblastic degeneration and minimizing bleeding, particularly in cases when the trophoblasts are deeply embedded in the myometrium.

UAE treatment of CSP was first reported in 1999 [14]. Since then, it has been used widely to control hemorrhage and preserve the uterus and it is considered an adjuvant treatment of EP, since it minimizes bleeding, particularly in cases when the trophoblasts are deeply embedded in the myometrium.

14.3.2 Patient Selection Criteria

UAE is mainly performed in CSP patients who fulfill the following criteria:

- Established laboratory and imaging diagnosis of EP
- Age $\geq$ 18 years
- Patients who want to preserve fertility
- Absolute contraindication or unwillingness to undergo methotrexate therapy
- Absolute contraindication (a previous reaction) or unwillingness (Jehovah's witnesses) to blood transfusion
- High arterial flow related to the gestational sac
- Myometrial thickness between the sac and urinary bladder below 2 mm, a gestational sac greater than 5 cm
- Serum b-hCG level more than 10,000 mIU/mL
- Hemodynamic stability
- Absence of contraindication to an angiographic exam (e.g., previous reaction to iodinated contrast media)
- Willingness or ability to be followed up [15, 16]

14.3.3 Pre-treatment Imaging Evaluation

The transvaginal ultrasonography criteria were described by Timor-Tritsch et al. [17] and include:

1. An empty uterine cavity and cervical canal
2. A gestational sac located anteriorly at the level equivalent to the prior lower uterine segment of the cesarean section scar
3. Evidence of functional trophoblastic/placental circulation on Doppler scans
4. A negative sliding organ sign, defined as the inability to displace the gestational sac from its position

A preoperative TVUS is mandatory to confirm the diagnosis of EP and to evaluate the vascularization of the gestational sac.

A preoperative CT/MR evaluation may be performed to accurately assess the location and vascularization of the gestational sac and to exclude the presence of concurrent uterine lesions or hemorrhages, which could contraindicate the procedure. If possible, CT scans should be avoided in young females due to x-ray exposure.

14.3.4 Procedure

After disinfection and local anesthesia (10 mL of lidocaine 2%), the femoral artery is punctured through the Seldinger technique. First, hypogastric arteries and bilateral uterine arteries angiograms are performed to provide interventional radiologists an opportunity to study the vascular anatomy and to rule out the presence of some anastomosis that could complicate the procedure. Once the catheter is appropriately positioned for treatment, the embolization phase starts with the injection of embolic agents separately in both uterine arteries.

The choice of the embolic agent depends on different variables and operator expertise. The most common embolic agent used is absorbable gelatin sponge, a water-insoluble gelatin that allows revascularization within 4 or 6 weeks after the procedure. In the last years, some operators prefer the injection of permanent embolic agents, such as polyvinyl alcohol (PVA) beads, to produce a durable and compact vascular block. It is possible to use both embolic agents in the same procedure: Some authors use PVA particles on the ipsilateral side and gelfoam on the contralateral side [18]. The embolic agents should be always larger than 500 µm to avoid paradoxical embolization of the ovarian artery [19] (Fig. 14.1).

The UAE can be performed alone or in combination with other medical, interventional, or surgical therapies.

Embolization may be used in conjunction with intramuscular methotrexate therapy, or after failed methotrexate therapy, for the successful treatment of cornual and cervical ectopic pregnancies: concurrent systemic methotrexate along with UAE has been proven more effective than UAE alone. Systemic methotrexate should be administered before UAE, since the procedure reduces blood flow to the ectopic sac [20].

UAE is increasingly combined with transcatheter intraarterial methotrexate infusion. Before using embolic agents, 50 mg of methotrexate is injected into each uterine artery as close as possible to a vessel feeding the sac. During the embolization, a supplementary 10-mg dose of methotrexate is injected to ensure a high local concentration of the cytotoxic drug in the implantation area [21].

5-Fluorouracil (5-FU) is another cytotoxic drug, which induces blastocysts apoptosis by interference with nucleotide synthesis. During UAE, a 500-mg dose of 5-FU can be intra-arterially administered with methotrexate, to increase the rate of successful resolution of EPs [22].

In the treatment of treat EPs, ultrasound-guided suction and curettage is a simple and convenient method that removes all the gestational residual tissues, although it presents frequent complications, including massive hemorrhage, uterine rupture, and bladder injuries.

Since UAE blocks the uterine blood flow, it also reduces bleeding during a subsequent curettage of the uterine cavity and reduces the need for traumatic open abdominal surgery. For this rea-

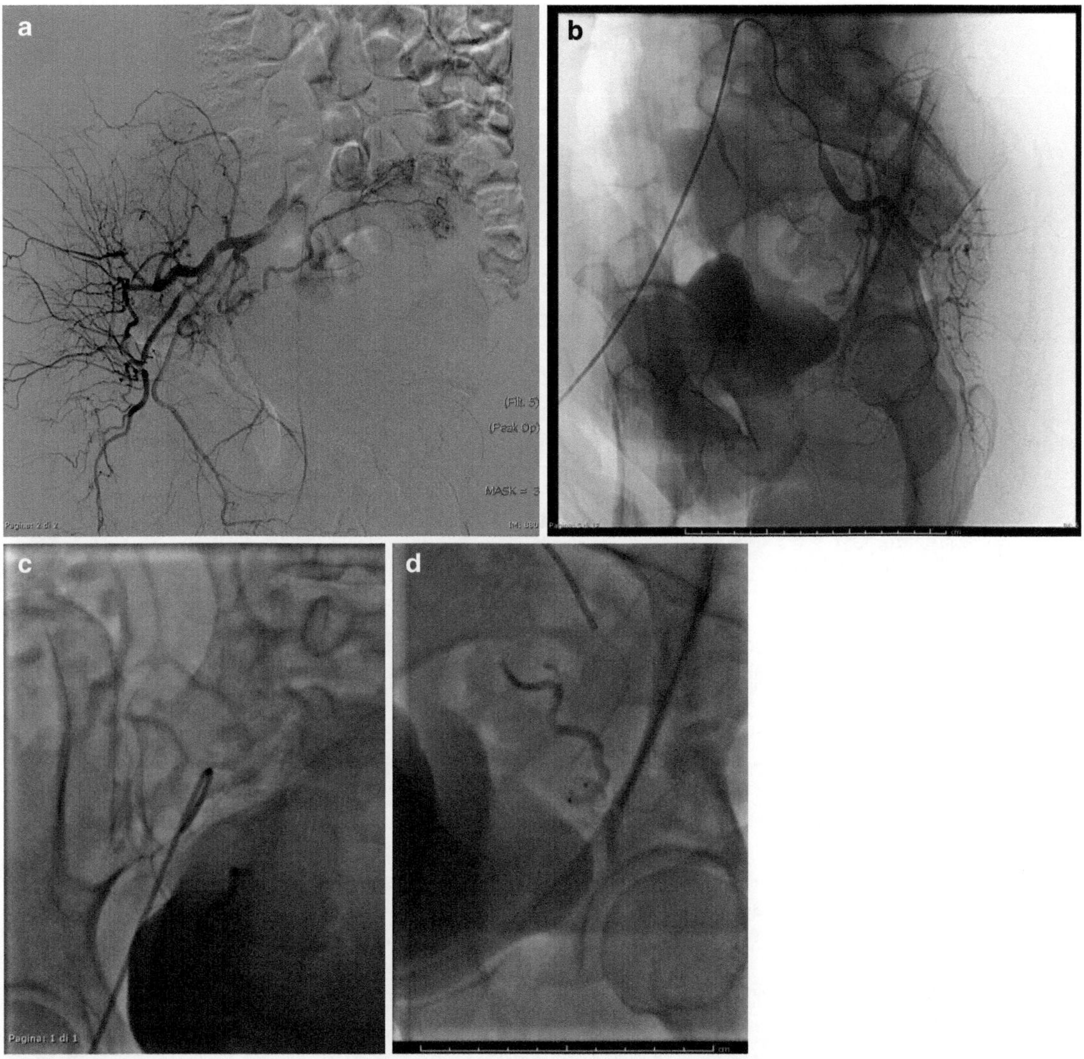

Fig. 14.1 Right femoral access with 5Fr sheath. Angiography of right and left hypogastric artery (**a, b**). Introduction of 2.2Fr microcatheter and embolization of right and left uterine artery with adsorbable gelatin sponge (**c, d**)

son, suction and curettage after UAE has become increasingly accepted by clinics as a conservative treatment method for CSP [23].

After UAE, patients are closely observed for blood β-HCG level decline and gestational sac blood supply changes. UAE may be repeated in selective refractory cases. The dilation and curettage with suction or vacuum aspiration is performed 3–7 days after UAE [19] (Fig. 14.2).

Emergency UAE may be performed for the treatment of severe bleeding after medical or surgical treatment. EP is burdened by a high risk of internal bleeding due to the growth of the sac in a site other than the uterine cavity. This condition is traditionally treated with surgical bilateral hypogastric or uterine ligation, which inevitably leads to infertility. For this reason, it is possible to perform UAE in the management of internal bleeding related to EPs in selected cases of women who want to preserve fertility [24].

The most common complication in UAE is postembolization syndrome. It occurs in 50% of treated patients and is characterized by pain, fever, leukocytosis, and nausea, starting immedi-

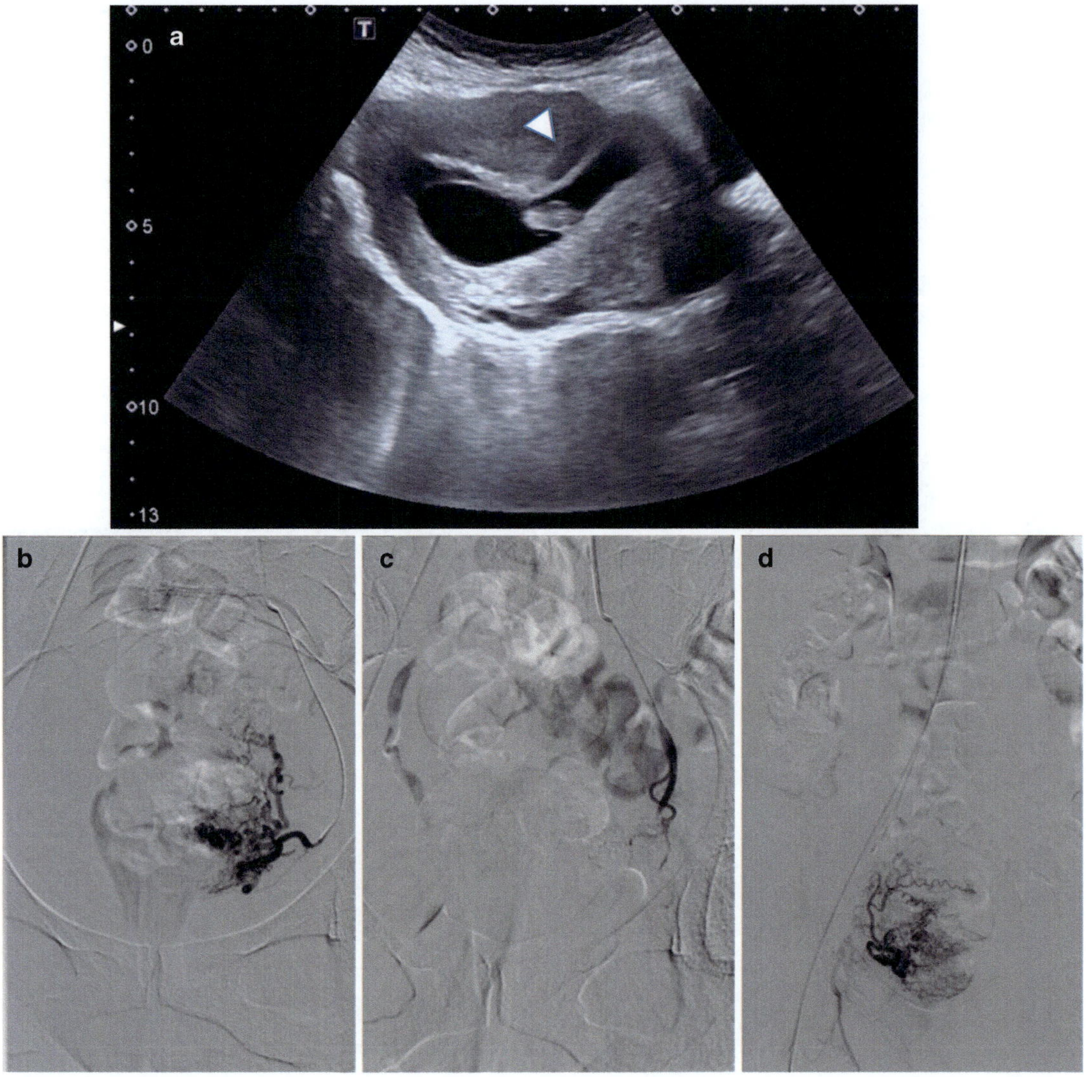

Fig. 14.2 A 27-year-old female with previous cesarean sections and b-HCG values of 13,134 mUI/mL. A transabdominal ultrasound examination detects the presence of CSP (*white arrowhead*) (**a**). After right femoral access with 5Fr sheath, catheterization of left hypogastric artery with Cobra and superselective microcatheterization of tortuous left uterine artery with Progreat 2.7 (**b**). Left UAE with 500–700-micron beads until stop flow (**c**). Subsequently, catheterization of tortuous right uterine artery with Roberts Uterine Catheter (RUC; a long 5Fr tight-curve catheter useful in the catheterization of uterine artery with acute cephalad origin) (**d**). Right UAE with 500–700-micron beads until stop flow. Curettage of uterine cavity three days after bilateral UAE, without hemorrhage. B-HCG values of 3480 mUI/mL five days after UAE

ately after the procedure and lasting for several days. It is treated with analgesic and anti-inflammatory medications [25]. Other rare complications in UAE are uterine infarction or ischemia, necrosis, rupture, sepsis, ovarian abscess, tubal abscess, endometritis, ischemia of adjacent tissues, and ovarian failure. Different studies demonstrate that UAE may be performed in women who wish to preserve fertility, but fertility cannot be guaranteed [3, 18].

Patients who underwent UAE should be followed up with CT or MRI to exclude the appearance of complications and to evaluate the response of endometrium and myometrium.

14.4 HIFU

High-intensity focused ultrasound (HIFU) may become a helpful option for the treatment of EPs. HIFU focuses beams of ultrasound energy accurately on targets deep in the body, producing thermal destruction without damaging surrounding normal tissue [26].

The procedure is usually performed under conscious sedation. A HIFU transducer produces the therapeutic effect. Real-time ultrasound or MRI is used to target the area of the gestational sac and monitor the response.

Hysteroscopy-guided suction and curettage is performed 1–2 h after HIFU [26].

Additional studies are necessary to assess the effectiveness of HIFU in the treatment of EPs.

14.5 Prevention of EP

Interventional Radiology is required also in infertile patients with unilateral or bilateral hydrosalpinx, undergoing in vitro fertilization, before embryo transfer.

Hydrosalpinx afflicts 10–30% of infertile patients undergoing in vitro fertilization. It is related to tubal occlusions, leading to reduced implantation and pregnancy rates with an increased EP and miscarriage rate.

Laparoscopic salpingectomy is the current gold standard for the treatment of this condition, even if this surgery is associated with ovarian failure due to interferences with ovarian blood flow.

In presence of high surgical risk or history of previous multiple abdominal surgeries, advanced stage endometriosis, or major intra-abdominal adhesions, imaging-guided transcervical tubal occlusion with embolization microcoils is preferred.

After a preliminary hysterosalpingography to study tubal anatomy, the interventional radiologist accesses the proximal fallopian tube with a 3-F catheter through a 7-F salpingogram cannula and proceeds to the injection of embolization microcoils, taking about 15–20 min to confirm the exact positioning via fluoroscopy. Microcoils are made of platinum, an ideal obstruction material, and present spaced synthetic fibers. The coils curl within the interstitial portion of the tube to impede migration and prevent a tubal pregnancy, while the synthetic fibers act as a foreign body, leading to adhesion for tubal occlusion.

Recent studies suggest that it is important to avoid the placement of the microcoils in the uterus to decrease the comparison of fluid overload or reduce endometrial receptivity [27].

Summary Table
Ectopic pregnancy (EP) consists in the implantation of the embryo in a site other than the endometrium. Diagnosis is based on a combination of clinical evaluation, measurement of serum β-hCG concentrations, and transvaginal ultrasound.
The most used treatment consists of methotrexate administration and surgery. Suction and curettage or interventional procedures are the favored options in women desiring to preserve fertility.
Direct administration of chemicals by ultrasound-guided injection into the ectopic implant can be considered in superficial EPs.
Bilateral uterine artery embolization (eventually with a trans-catheter administration of methotrexate) is a safe and effective interventional procedure for the treatment of EPs and CSPs.
A tubal injection of embolization microcoils could be evaluated in patients with recurrent EPs.

References

1. Panelli DM, Philips CH, Brady PC. Incidence, diagnosis and management of tubal and nontubal ectopic pregnancies: a review. Fertil Res Pract. 2015;1:15.
2. Sorrentino F, De Feo V, Stabile G, et al. Cesarean scar pregnancy treated by artery embolization combined with diode laser: a novel approach for a rare disease. Medicina. 2021;57:411.
3. Yang SB, Lee SJ, Joe HS, et al. Selective uterine artery embolization for Management of Interstitial Ectopic Pregnancy. Korean J Radiol. 2007;8:176–9.
4. Junhong G, Jiangtao Y, Zhang Q, et al. Clinical efficacy and safety of uterine artery embolization (UAE) versus laparoscopic cesarean scar pregnancy debridement surgery (LCSPDS) in treatment of cesarean scar pregnancy. Med Sci Monit. 2018;24:4659–66.
5. Sivalingam VN, Duncan WC, Kirk E, et al. Diagnosis and management of ectopic pregnancy. J Fam Plann Reprod Health Care. 2011;37(4):231–40.
6. Lee R, Dupuis C, Kim YH, et al. Diagnosing ectopic pregnancy in the emergency setting. Ultrasonography. 2018;37(1):78–87.

7. Levine D. Ectopic pregnancy. Radiology. 2007;245(2):385–97.
8. Nama V, Manyonda I. Tubal ectopic pregnancy: diagnosis and management. Arch Gynecol Obstet. 2009;279:443–53.
9. Lozeau AM, Potter B. Diagnosis and management of ectopic pregnancy. Am Fam Physician. 2005;72(9):1707–14.
10. Zhou Q, Young D, Vingan H. Uterine artery embolization for cervical ectopic pregnancy. Radiol Case Rep. 2015;10:72–5.
11. Taran FA, Kagan KO, Brucker S, et al. The diagnosis and treatment of ectopic pregnancy. Dtsch Arztebl Int. 2015;112(41):693–704.
12. Thabet A, Kalva SP, Liu B, et al. Interventional radiology in pregnancy complications: indications, technique, and methods for minimizing radiation exposure. Radiographics. 2012;32:255–74.
13. Li Z, Xu W, Hu B, et al. Uterine artery embolization in association with methotrexate infusion for the treatment of tubal ectopic pregnancy. J Interv Med. 2018;1(3):182–7.
14. Spies JB, Spector A, Roth AR, et al. Complications after uterine artery embolization for leiomyomas. Obstet Gynecol. 2002;100:873–80.
15. Kanat-Pektas M, Bodur S, Dundar O, et al. Systematic review: what is the best first-line approach for cesarean section ectopic pregnancy? Taiwan J Obstet Gynecol. 2016;55:263–9.
16. Ou J, Peng P, Li C, et al. Assessment of the necessity of uterine artery embolization during suction and curettage for caesarean scar pregnancy: a prospective cohort study. BMC Pregnancy Childbirth. 2020;20(1):378.
17. Timor-Tritsch IE, Monteagudo A, Santos R, et al. The diagnosis, treatment, and follow-up of cesarean scar pregnancy. Am J Obstet Gynecol. 2012;207(1):44.e1–44.e13.
18. Katz MD, Sugay SB, Walker DK, et al. Beyond hemostasis: spectrum of gynecologic and obstetric indications for transcatheter embolization. Radiographics. 2012;32:1713–31.
19. Fornazari VA, Szejnfeld D, Goldman SM, et al. Interventional radiology and endovascular surgery in the treatment of ectopic pregnancies. Einstein. 2015;13(1):167–9.
20. Zakaria MA, Abdallah ME, Kmak DC, et al. Conservative management of cervical ectopic pregnancy: utility of uterine artery embolization. Fertil Steril. 2011;95:872–6.
21. Xiaolin Z, Chengxin Y, Guangxi T, et al. Transcatheter intraarterial methotrexate infusion combined with selective uterine artery embolization as a treatment option for cervical pregnancy. J Vasc Interv Radiol. 2010;21:836–41.
22. Gao J, Li X, Gong W, et al. Uterine artery embolization combined with local infusion of methotrexate and 5-fluorouracil in treating ectopic pregnancy: a CONSORT-compliant article. Medicine (Baltimore). 2018;97(5):e9722.
23. Jie O, Peng P, Chunying L, et al. Assessment of the necessity of uterine artery embolization during suction and curettage for caesarean scar pregnancy: a prospective cohort study. BMC Pregnancy Childbirth. 2020;20:378.
24. Seema S, Abha S, Seema D, et al. Uterine artery embolization: exploring new dimensions in obstetric emergencies. Oman Med J. 2014;29(3):217–9.
25. Kitamura Y, Ascher SM, Cooper C, et al. Imaging manifestations of complications associated with uterine artery embolization. Radiographics. 2005;25:S119–32.
26. He GB, Luo W, Zhou XD, et al. A preliminary clinical study on high-intensity focused ultrasound therapy for tubal pregnancy. Scott Med J. 2011;56(4):214–9.
27. Yang X, Zhu L, Jin F, et al. Proximal fallopian tubal embolization by interventional radiology before embryo transfer in infertile patients with Hydrosalpinx: a prospective study of an off-label treatment. J Minim Invasive Gynecol. 2020;27:107–15.

Interventional Radiology in Postpartum Hemorrhage: Rescue Strategies

15

Mario Vallone, Francesco Giurazza, Fabio Corvino, and Raffaella Niola

15.1 Definitions and Epidemiology

There are many different definitions of postpartum hemorrhage (PPH) between countries but there is a consensus between the most scientific societies' guidelines and World Health Organization (WHO) recommendations to define PPH by blood loss greater than 500 mL or more after vaginal delivery and 1000 mL or more after caesarean delivery [1].

Related to blood loss, PPH can be also minor (500–1000 mL) or major (more than 1000 mL). Major can be further subdivided into moderate (1001–2000 mL) and severe (more than 2000 mL).

Moreover, PPH can be divided into primary (early) and secondary (late) clinical entities. Primary PPH appears during the first 24 h after delivery; secondary PPH is defined as abnormal or excessive bleeding from the birth canal between 24 h and 12 weeks postdelivery.

The PPH incidence is about 5% of deliveries when there is no accurate measurement of blood loss and about 10% when blood loss is quantified [2]. Moreover, severe PPH occurs in about 1% to 2% of deliveries and it is one of the main causes of severe maternal mortality and morbidity; severe PPH is responsible today for the deaths of 150,000 women a year, or else 25% of annual maternal deaths worldwide [3, 4].

15.2 Etiology of PPH

A pregnant woman presents an increase in circulating blood of about 50%: This allows to compensate the physiological hemorrhage occurring during delivery.

In normal conditions, during vaginal delivery, hemostasis derives from effective myometrium contraction compressing the spiral arteries [5]. This process can be alternated by multiple pathological conditions, which can be summarized in the clinical practice by the "4 Ts" [6, 7] (Table 15.1):

- *TONE*: loss of uterine tone, or else uterine atony, is the main responsible event for PPH and accounts for 70% of the cases
- *TISSUE*: retention of placental tissues and/or abnormally invasive placenta, accounting for 10–30% of the cases
- *TRAUMA*: during the delivery phases, traumatic lesions of the uterus wall, cervix, and birth canal account for 15–20% of PPH
- *THROMBIN*: coagulopathies, misdiagnosed or acquired, are the less common cause of PPH and account for less than 1% of the cases

M. Vallone (✉)
Interventional Radiology Department, Ospedale Civico Di Cristina e Benfratelli, Palermo, Italy

F. Giurazza · F. Corvino · R. Niola
Vascular and Interventional Radiology Department, Cardarelli Hospital, Naples, Italy

R. Niola et al. (eds.), *Diagnostic and Interventional Radiology in Gynecological and Obstetric Diseases*, https://doi.org/10.1007/978-3-031-11910-1_15

Table 15.1 The rule of the "4 Ts" causing PPH

"T"	Etiology	Frequency (%)
Tone	Loss of uterine tone	70
Tissue	Retention of placental tissues	10–30
Trauma	Trauma injury during delivery	15–20
Thrombin	Coaguolopathies	<1

Prenatal assessable risk factors for PPH are nowadays well known: increasing age of women at the time of conception, obesity, previous cesarean deliveries, and assisted reproductive techniques [8]; all of these are more frequent in Western countries.

However, it should also be considered that PPH can occur unexpectedly in women without the abovementioned factors.

15.3 Management of PPH

Therapeutic measures should be applied for blood loss greater than 500 and 1000 mL after vaginal and caesarean deliveries, respectively [9, 10].

Multidisciplinary hemorrhage protocols for the management of PPH have been recently advocated by the most important professional societies; these protocols include medical/resuscitative treatments with blood products and intravenous fluids, uterotonic medications, as well as surgical options with external uterine massage, intrauterine balloon and/or curettage.

All measures aim to obtain hemodynamic control of the patient and to identify and treat the cause of hemorrhage.

The evolution of endovascular procedures has established a role for arterial embolization in the setting of uncontrolled PPH. Uterine artery embolization has the advantage of being a minimally invasive treatment that preserves the uterus without eliminating the possibility of future surgical intervention if necessary.

The multiple progressive steps of PPH management are described below in the following subparagraphs:

15.3.1 Prevention

Immediately after delivery, before the occurrence of a possible PPH, preventive administration of uterotonic has proven to reduce PPH by 50%. Other prophylactic maneuvers, such as uterine massage and early cord clamping, do not affect the incidence of PPH[10].

It is of paramount importance to estimate properly the amount of blood loss, using blood collection bags routinely.

15.3.2 First-Line Measures

When a PPH is recognized, an immediate alert of the multidisciplinary team must be activated: obstetrician, anesthesiologist, and surgeon.

Initial steps are: manual uterine exploration, assessment of genital tract, bladder indwelling catheter, temperature maintenance, pulse-blood pressure-respiratory monitoring, oxygen supply, uterine massage, infusion of crystalloids, and use of uterotonic (oxytocin).

If a laceration is individuated during the assessment of the genital tract, suture must be attempted.

15.3.3 Second-Line Measures

If PPH persists despite first-line measures, additional steps are necessary: sulprostone in case oxytocin is ineffective; fluid resuscitation to maintain hemoglobin >8 g/dL, fibrinogen >2 g/L, and platelet count >50,000/μL [9]; tranexamic acid should be taken into account within the first 3 h because it reduces mortality thanks to its antifibrinolytic action [11–13].

Finally, before moving to interventional strategies, intrauterine balloon tamponade should be considered because it has proven to be clinically effective in up to 86% of the cases [14].

15.3.4 Third-Line Measures

When conservative therapies fail, surgical and endovascular strategies are applied.

Surgery includes arterial ligation, uterine sutures, and hysterectomy.

Among the surgical strategies, arterial ligation presents a high rate of failure because of the rich vascular collateral network of the female pelvis, especially developed in pregnancy status: apart from the uterine artery, the blood supply to the placenta derives from several regions such as lumbar, hypogastric, superior epigastric, gonadal, rectal, gluteal, and femoral arteries [15]; uterine sparing surgery with sutures, as B-lynch or Cho sutures, aims to replicate vascular compression [16]; peripartum hysterectomy should be performed as last option, when all other measures failed to manage life-threatening bleeding [17].

On the other hand, endovascular embolization is becoming widely accepted because it allows to preserve the uterus and it can be repeated and performed without general anesthesia; however, at moment, only the guidelines of the French College of Gynaecologists and Obstetricians (CNGOF) clearly recommend embolization as first-choice therapy after failure of medical treatment, after a vaginal delivery and with stable maternal hemodynamics, even if this indicates that a transfer is needed for embolization [4, 18].

15.4 Embolization

Transarterial embolization in PPH scenarios should be performed after failure of medical and conservative therapies.

An interventional radiologist should be involved, regardless of the severity and type of PPH: embolization, especially in the early phase of hemorrhage, is a useful treatment option for each type of bleeding.

Furthermore, if a first endovascular attempt failed, repeat embolization should be considered prior to performing a hysterectomy [19].

15.4.1 Preprocedural CT Evaluation

If the patient is hemodynamically stable and the clinical conditions allow, a pre-procedural CT should be acquired (Fig. 15.1); in these cases, the interventional radiologist carefully examines the arterial phase to individuate the source of bleeding and the type of lesion; imaging findings that represent acute bleeding foci are extravasation of the contrast agent (Fig. 15.2), pseudoaneurysms, and abruptly cutoff vessels [20]. Imaging exami-

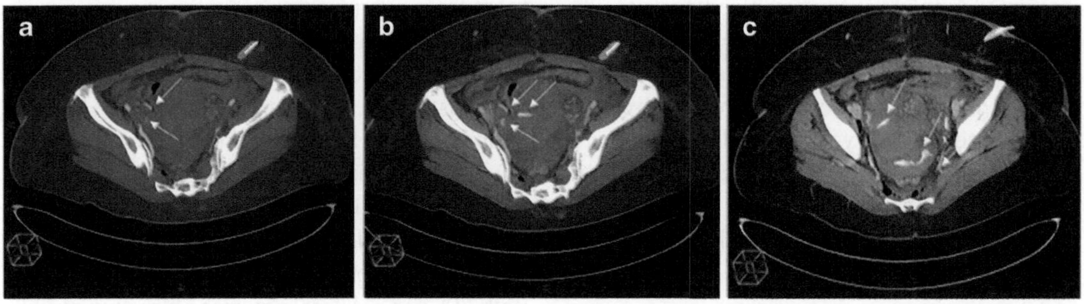

Fig. 15.1 A 28-year-old lady with severe and early PPH after cesarean delivery, one previous cesarean section; contrast-enhanced CT scan in axial plane with maximum intensity projections reconstruction, showing active hemorrhage with progressive increase of the extraluminal blush in arterial (**a**), venous (**b**), and delayed (**c**) phases. Dotted white arrows indicate the contrast agent extravasation, refurnished mainly from right uterine artery

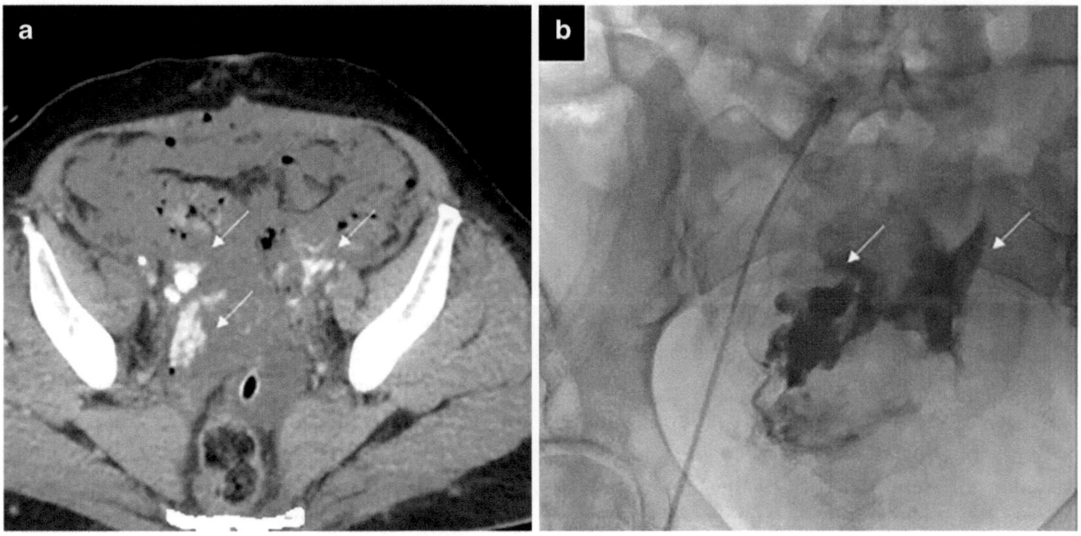

Fig. 15.2 A 44-year-old lady with severe and early PPH after cesarean delivery, two previous cesarean sections; (**a**) contrast-enhanced CT scan in axial plane showing active hemorrhage with extraluminal blushes (*white dotted arrows*) in pelvis; (**b**) fluoroscopy confirming massive contrast extravasation in pelvis (*white dotted arrows*) after injection from right uterine artery through a 2.7Fr microcatheter

nation algorithms, such as multiplanar reconstructions and maximum intensity projections, allow to plan a proper technical approach in terms of catheter curve, microcatheter size, and embolics selection.

15.4.2 Target Arteries

In the PPH scenario, the most involved artery is the uterine artery but bleeding refurnishments from other pelvic arteries can occur isolated or associated with uterine artery bleeding.

In the case of genital tract laceration, cervical arteries should be investigated: these might be involved in PPH in case of cesarean delivery in form of pseudoaneurysms [21]. Investigation of ovarian and round ligament arteries should be performed in case of persistent bleeding after uterine artery embolization (Fig. 15.3).

15.4.3 Technique

Pelvic embolization procedures in PPH emergent setting are usually performed through a 5Fr femoral access.

The artery can be punctured free-hand or under ultrasound guidance; when feasible, the latter approach should be preferred because of the lower incidence of complications (hematoma, arterio-venous fistula, pseudoaneurysm).

On a hydrophilic 0.035″ guidewire a 5Fr or 4Fr diagnostic catheter is advanced; an aorto-iliac arteriography through a pig-tail catheter can be acquired, according to operator preference, in case of unclear CT findings or when a CT has not been acquired before the intervention. It is also useful to individuate eventual bleeding refurnishment from ovarian arteries.

The left hypogastric artery is usually catheterized in cross with a Cobra catheter while the right hypogastric artery requires a reverse tip catheter (Simmons 1, RUC, or Shepherd tips, e.g.). Bilateral selective arteriography of the hypogastric artery and then of its anterior trunk are mandatory to depict the bleeding source. Antero-posterior projections must be integrated with 30° controlateral anterior oblique views [1].

Once the target artery is individuated and the proper projection is selected, digital roadmapping helps for subsequent coaxial microcatheterization. In these cases, attempts to catheterize the uterine artery directly with the diagnostic

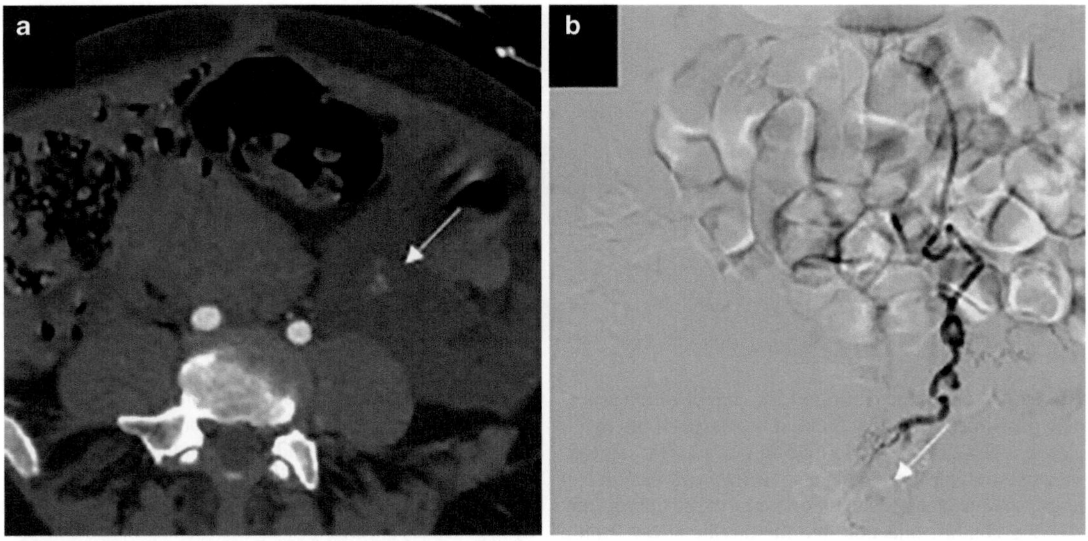

Fig. 15.3 A 41–year-old lady with severe PPH after cesarean delivery, one previous cesarean section. (**a**) Contrast-enhanced CT scan in axial plane showing active hemorrhage (*white dotted arrow*) in the left iliac region with hematoma; (**b**) left ovarian arteriography, performed through a 5Fr catheter, confirming distal extraluminal spots (*white dotted arrow*)

catheter should be avoided: indeed the microcatheter allows to distally reach the source of bleeding and also to reduce the risk of vascular spasm which occurs frequently in this category of patients (predisposing factors: young, female, bleeding). Once the embolization is accomplished, a final arteriography is acquired to exclude additional bleeding feeders.

15.4.4 Embolic Agents

Multiple embolics can be adopted to manage PPH: definitive (metallic, microparticles, and liquids) and temporary (gelatin sponge).

The choice depends on multiple factors and no standards of practice have been established. Operator preference and experience is certainly the main element influencing the choice; while metallic agents (coils and plugs), especially with controlled detachment technology, are easier to manipulate, particles and liquids (glue and DMSO-family agents) require longer training because of the higher risk of non-target embolization. Temporary sponge implies a lower risk of tissue necrosis (Fig. 15.4).

However, other factors must be taken into account (Table 15.2). First, not all the types of vascular lesions can be treated with all the embolics; for example, a pseudoaneurysm of the uterine artery cannot be embolized with spongel or microparticles, while a diffuse blush refurnished from multiple small vessels will require embolics that permeate into the tissues (gel sponge, particles, or liquids). A focal lesion, as a pseudoaneurysm or fistula, will be better treated with coils. In case of hemodynamic instability and large lesion where the whole vessel must be embolized, liquids are optimal agents allowing a fast and definitive embolization [21–25].

Another element to consider is the distalization of the microcatheter. When distal superselective microcatheterization is unfeasible and only proximal embolization is possible, definitive agents might induce non-target embolization with a risk of healthy tissues necrosis; in these cases, temporary spongel slurry should be preferred [1]. Instead, if distal microcatheterization is feasible, definitive agents such as coils or liquids allow to achieve a quick complete embolization.

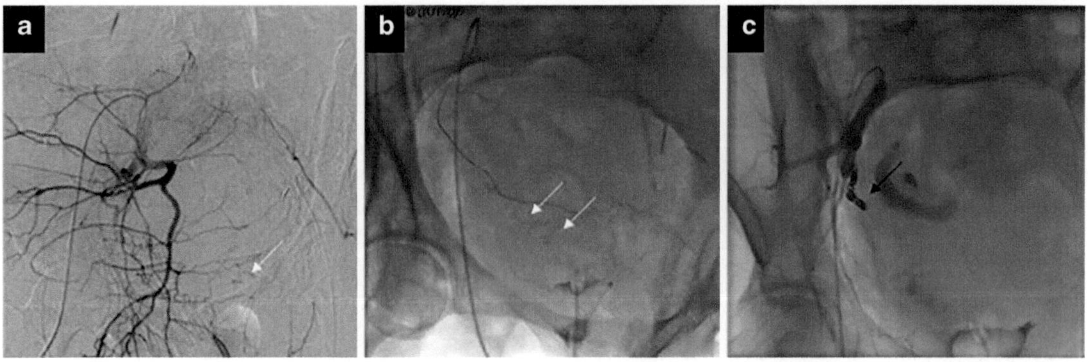

Fig. 15.4 Same patient of Fig. 15.1. Embolization procedure performed from right femoral access. (**a**) Right hypogastric arteriography, performed through a 5Fr catheter, showing multiple extraluminal spots (*white dotted arrow*) refurnished from a spastic uterine artery; (**b**) fluoroscopy showing contrast injection into the uterine artery from a 2.7Fr microcatheter; extraluminal blush is indicated by white dotted arrows; (**c**) embolization was performed by spongel slurry injection and sealing of the uterine artery at the origin with a microcoil (*black arrow*). Contralateral uterine artery embolization was performed with sole spongel slurry injection (images not shown)

Table 15.2 Embolic agents adopted for PPH and their indications according to the type of vascular lesion

Embolics	Duration	Vascular lesions
Coils	Permanent	Pseudoaneurysms, fistulas
Particles	Permanent	Multiple extraluminal spots
Spongel	Temporary	Multiple extraluminal spots, blind embolization
Glues	Permanent	Massive extraluminal blushes, large vessel lesions

The coagulation function must be investigated; in case of coagulopathies, metallic agents must be excluded because of lack of clot formation. In these cases, particulates and liquids must be adopted.

When choosing microparticles, since small particle size can induce definitive distal embolization of the capillary bed with ischemic complications, the use of particles >500 μm is preferred [21].

Overall the most common embolic material used in PPH treatment is gelatin sponge; this is mixed with saline and contrast agent to produce a slurry, which is injected into the arteries until stasis or occlusion of blood flow is evident during angiography. Its embolic power is temporary (recanalization happens in approximately 3–6 weeks) [1].

Furthermore, a temporary gelatin sponge is used in a specific PPH scenario: in case of clinical evidence of bleeding without angiographic direct signs of hemorrhage. In this case, blind embolization with sponge slurry injection into the anterior hypogastric trunk has proven to be effective [26].

15.4.5 Outcomes and Complications

Embolization for PPH is highly effective with clinical success rate ranging from 80% to near 90%; technical success rates, intended as bleeding control, are even higher approaching 98–100% [1].

Factors responsible for clinical failure of embolization are disseminated intravascular coagulation, hemodynamic instability, history of prior surgery, spasm of arteries, and unilateral and proximal embolization; interestingly, the success rate is not related to the mode of delivery, transfusion needs, time from delivery to embolization, or even hysterectomy before embolization [6].

In this category of patients, pregnancy rates following uterine artery embolization are comparable to age-adjusted rates in the general population [27, 28].

The complication rate [26] of embolization for PPH is 13%, and the most commonly reported complication is postembolization syndrome, including fever, nausea, and pelvic pain; other complications include menstrual abnormalities; more rare are neuropathy, organ ischemia, and hematomas.

Mortality of severe PPH after embolization is 0.9%.

Concerning uterine necrosis, this is a very rare but severe complication; in literature, it has been reported in the form of case reports, with approximately 19 cases up to date [29]; permanent embolics such as microcoils and microparticles have more chances to induce massive necrosis.

References

1. Corvino F, Giurazza F, Vallone M, et al. Postpartum hemorrhage: rescue. Semin Ultrasound CT MR. 2021;42(1):75–84.
2. Khan KS, Wojdyla D, Say L, et al. WHO analysis of causes of maternal death: a systematic review. Lancet. 2006;367:1066–74.
3. Sentilhes L, Merlot B, Madar H, et al. Postpartum haemorrhage: prevention and treatment. Expert Rev Hematol. 2016;9:1043–61.
4. Sentilhes L, Vayssière C, Deneux-Tharaux C, et al. Postpartum hemorrhage: guidelines for clinical practice from the French College of Gynaecologists and Obstetricians (CNGOF): in collaboration with the French Society of Anesthesiology and Intensive Care (SFAR). Eur J Obstet Gynecol Reprod Biol. 2016;198:12–21.
5. Abada HT, Golzarian J, Sun S. Interventional management of postpartum hemorrhage. In: Vascular embolotherapy: a comprehensive approach, vol. 1. Berlin: Springer, pp. 107–118; 2006.
6. Lindquist JD, Vogelzang RL. Pelvic artery embolization for treatment of postpartum hemorrhage. Semin Intervent Radiol. 2018;35:41–7.
7. Katz D, Beilin Y. Management of post-partum hemorrhage and the role of the obstetric anesthesiologist. J Matern Fetal Neonatal Med. 2021;34(9):1487–93.
8. Giurazza F, Angileri SA, Corvino F, et al. Postpartum hemorrhages: prevention. Semin Ultrasound CT MR. 2021;42(1):85–94.
9. Sentilhes L, Goffinet F, Vayssière C, et al. Comparison of postpartum haemorrhage guidelines: discrepancies underline our lack of knowledge. BJOG. 2017;124:718–22.
10. Donati S, Basevi V, et al. Emorragia post partum: come prevenirla, come curarla. Milano: Istituto Superiore di Sanità/Ministero della Salute Sistema Nazionale per le linee guida - Linee Guida; 2016.
11. American Society of Anesthesiologists Task Force on Perioperative Blood Management. Practice guidelines for perioperative blood management: an updated report by the American Society of Anesthesiologists Task Force on perioperative blood management*. Anesthesiology. 2015;122:241–75.
12. WOMAN Trial Collaborators. Effect of early tranexamic acid administration on mortality, hysterectomy, and other morbidities in women with postpartum haemorrhage (WOMAN): an international, randomised, double-blind, placebo-controlled trial. Lancet. 2017;389:2105–16.
13. Ferrazzani S, Iadarola R, Perrelli A, et al. Use of an intrauterine inflated catheter balloon in massive postpartum hemorrhage: a series of 52 cases. J Obstet Gynaecol Res. 2014;40:1603–10.
14. Laas E, Bui C, Popowski T, et al. Trends in the rate of invasive procedures after the addition of the intrauterine tamponade test to a protocol for management of severe postpartum hemorrhage. Am J Obstet Gynecol. 2012;207:281.e1–281.e2817.
15. Brotman S, Soderstrom CA, Oster-Granite M, et al. Management of severe bleeding in fractures of the pelvis. Surg Gynecol Obstet. 1981;153:823–6.
16. Gilmandyar D, Thornburg LL. Surgical management of postpartum hemorrhage. Semin Perinatol. 2019;43:27–34.
17. American College of Obstetricians and Gynecologists. ACOG practice bulletin: clinical management guidelines for obstetrician-gynecologists number 76, October 2006: postpartum hemorrhage. Obstet Gynecol. 2006;108:1039–47.
18. Wright JD, Devine P, Shah M, et al. Morbidity and mortality of peripartum hysterectomy. Obstet Gynecol. 2010;115:1187–93.
19. Niola R, Cavaliere C, Marcello L, et al. Role of interventional radiology in treating obstetric haemorrhages. Radiol Med. 2014;119:607–15.
20. Rebonato A, Mosca S, Fischer M, et al. Endovascular management of massive post-partum haemorrhage in abnormal placental implantation deliveries. Eur Radiol. 2016;26:1620–30.
21. Ganguli S, Stecker MS, Pyne D, et al. Uterine artery embolization in the treatment of postpartum uterine hemorrhage. J Vasc Interv Radiol. 2011;22:169–76.
22. Park KJ, Shin JH, Yoon HK, et al. Postpartum hemorrhage from extravasation or pseudoaneurysm: efficacy of transcatheter arterial embolization using N-butyl cyanoacrylate and comparison with gelatin sponge particle. J Vasc Interv Radiol. 2015;26:154–61.
23. Worthington-Kirsch RL. Uterine artery embolization: state of the art. Semin Intervent Radiol. 2004;21:37–42.
24. Naydich M, Friedman A, Aaron G, et al. Arterial embolization of vaginal arterial branches for severe postpartum hemorrhage despite hysterectomy. J Vasc Interv Radiol. 2007;18:1047–50.
25. Leleup G, Fohlen A, Dohan A, et al. Value of round ligament artery embolization in the management of postpartum hemorrhage. J Vasc Interv Radiol. 2017;28:696–701.

26. Zhang XQ, Chen XT, Zhang YT, Mai CX. The emergent pelvic artery embolization in the Management of Postpartum Hemorrhage: a systematic review and meta-analysis. Obstet Gynecol Surv. 2021;76(4):234–44.
27. Mohan PP, Hamblin MH, Vogelzang RL. Uterine artery embolization and its effect on fertility. J Vasc Interv Radiol. 2013;24:925–30.
28. Giurazza F, Corvino F, Silvestre M, et al. Role of interventional radiology in obstetric and gynecological diseases. J Radiol Rev. 2020;7:26–38.
29. Poujade O, Zappa M, Letendre I, et al. Predictive factors for failure of pelvic arterial embolization for postpartum hemorrhage. Int J Gynaecol Obstet. 2012;117:119–23.

16 Interventional Radiology in Postpartum Hemorrhage: Prevention Strategies

Francesco Giurazza, Fabio Corvino, and Raffaella Niola

16.1 Definitions

The standard definition of postpartum hemorrhage (PPH) is a blood loss >0.5 L within 24 h after vaginal delivery or >1 L after cesarean delivery [1].

PPH is considered primary if occurring during the first 24 h after delivery and secondary if occurring between 24 h and 12 weeks from delivery [2].

Severe PPH is a life-threatening hemorrhage associated with one or more of the following conditions: red blood cell units (RBCU) transfusion, transcatheter arterial embolization, conservative uterine surgery, hysterectomy, ICU admissions, peripartum hemoglobin reduction of 4 g/dL or more (considered equivalent to the loss of 1000 mL or more of blood), and maternal death [1].

16.2 Introduction

PPH is the leading cause of maternal death worldwide [3, 4], accounting for 25% approximately [5].

PPH diagnosis is furthermore underscored because the blood loss may not be properly calculated.

Literature data indicates that PPH and severe PPH occur, respectively, in 6% and 1.86% of all deliveries [5, 6]. Of note, up to 50% of cases [7] of PPH require intensive care unit admission.

Management of PPH includes conservative strategies, including uterotonics and embolization, and surgery; according to the local hospital facilities, endovascular embolization can be involved in different phases of patient care. Surgery includes postpartum hysterectomy, performed in life-threatening situations to prevent maternal death. Worldwide, the incidence of pregnancy-related hysterectomy is increasing over time (71.6–82.6 per 100.000 deliveries) [8]; the main indication for pregnancy-related hysterectomy is severe uterine bleeding that cannot be controlled by conservative measures [9].

The most common causes of postpartum hysterectomy for PPH are uterine atony (45.1%) and abnormally invasive placentation (AIP) (40.2%) [7] (Fig. 16.1). Nowadays risk factors for these anatomical pathological conditions have been clearly recognized [7, 10]:

- Previous cesarean sections
- Advanced maternal age (>35 years)
- Multiparity

In Western countries, the first two conditions are increasing in terms of occurrence due to social behaviors [11].

F. Giurazza (✉) · F. Corvino · R. Niola
Vascular and Interventional Radiology Department, Cardarelli Hospital, Naples, Italy

R. Niola et al. (eds.), *Diagnostic and Interventional Radiology in Gynecological and Obstetric Diseases*, https://doi.org/10.1007/978-3-031-11910-1_16

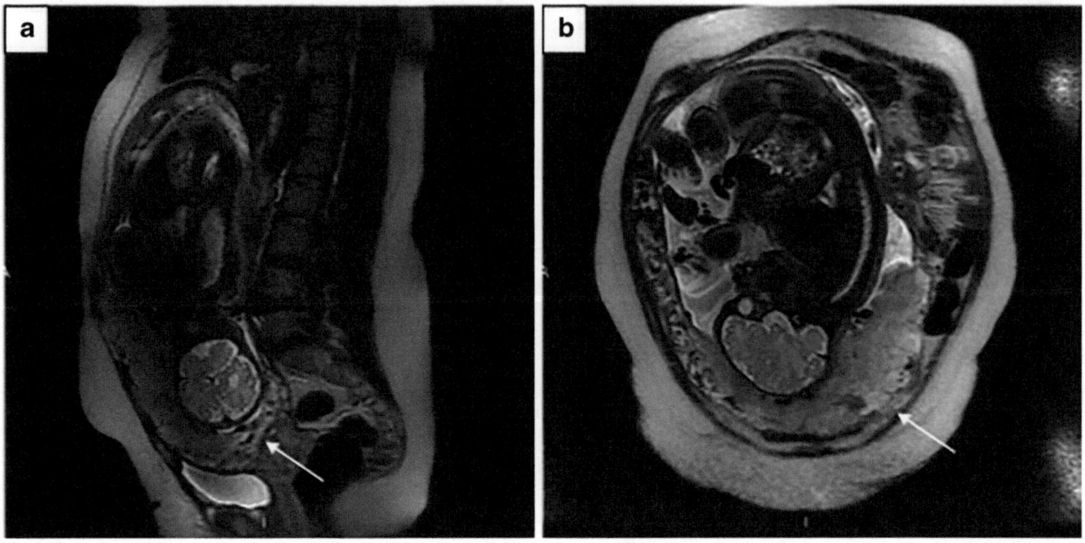

Fig. 16.1 Thirty-two-year-old lady at the 34th week of pregnancy, with placenta increta: magnetic resonance T2-weighted sequences in sagittal (**a**) and coronal (**b**) views showing placenta infiltration of the inferior margin of the uterus (*white arrows*) with the typical increta infiltration of the placenta into the myometrium wall

Patients with AIP require blood transfusions between 20% and 70% of the cases [12]. There is an increasing trend in the postpartum rate of massive transfusions (>10 RBCU), with women with AIP having the highest increased risk [10, 13]; patients undergoing massive transfusions are then at risk for developing disseminated intravascular coagulation, so there is a life-threatening events cascade that can develop from this scenario.

While it is obvious that, compared to uncomplicated deliveries, PPH patients require a challenging clinical management, the economic impact of PPH on the public health system with recognition of relevant cost increase been also evaluated [14].

Considering the increasing number of women affected by AIP [9] and being well-known the strict correlation between AIP and PPH, an antenatal diagnosis of AIP by ultrasound and/or magnetic resonance would certainly be advisable to improve their management: once the AIP is recognized, these patients should be directed to centers experienced in their management with high volumes; by scheduling the cesarean section, preventive strategies at the moment of delivery could be planned for avoiding hysterectomy and reducing the rate of massive transfusions.

Multiple studies [13, 15] have compared patients undergoing endovascular intervention with a control group without preventive endovascular support: all concluded that prophylactic endovascular procedures are effective for hemorrhage control during or after deliveries complicated by AIP, by significantly reducing blood loss volume.

All of these considerations have determined that nowadays endovascular interventional modalities for hemorrhage control during cesarean section for AIP are increasingly used [13] in experienced centers.

16.3 Preventive Strategies

The primary outcome of all the preventive strategies is to reduce the blood loss, while the secondary outcomes are to reduce hospital stay, minimize ICU admissions, and prevent hysterectomy.

The moment when the PPH is triggered is usually the surgical phase of the detachment of the placenta from the uterus wall; in case of uterine atony, the uterus does not contract strongly and placental blood vessels bleed freely; in case of

AIP condition with placental pathological infiltration into the muscular uterine wall, the placental detachment is incomplete and placental high-flow vessels are injured with consequent massive hemorrhage [9].

Multiple studies have described different approaches with encouraging experiences. However, a univoque standardized strategy still has to be recognized; there is indeed a lack of high-quality data because most published papers are retrospective case series or observational cohorts, large cohort trials missing; this may be due to the different instrumental facilities and local hospital settings that clinicians face in their daily medical practice. So, until now, there is no consensus regarding the best protocol.

It is sure that strict multidisciplinary cooperation between interventional radiologists, gynecologists, neonatologists, and anesthesiologists is mandatory to organize the best local protocol of shared management; finally this has to be functional for the gynecologist surgeon at the moment of delivery.

Altogether, two main different endovascular approaches can be recognized: embolization and balloon occlusion.

16.3.1 Embolization Approach

Embolization is the endovascular occlusion of a vessel; it is performed by releasing an embolic agent through a catheter. According to their physical status, the embolics can be mechanical, particulated, or liquid. While mechanical and liquid agents are permanent, particulated agents can be permanent or temporary, being reabsorbable as gelfoam, for example.

The embolization is performed by puncturing the common femoral artery and positioning a 4-French or a 5-French introducer; the access can be monolateral or bilateral; the monolateral technique presents the advantage of reducing the complications rate related to the vascular access; on the other hand, the bilateral technique reduces the procedural time and so the radiation dose. There is no clear consensus regarding which approach is to be performed; the choice mainly depends on the operator's preference.

In the PPH preventive setting, the embolization intervention has the goal of occluding the uterine artery bilaterally (UAs), the UA being the main placental feeders; the intervention can be performed immediately after or before the delivery (Table 16.1).

Table 16.1 Preventive embolization strategies, performed after or before cesarean section

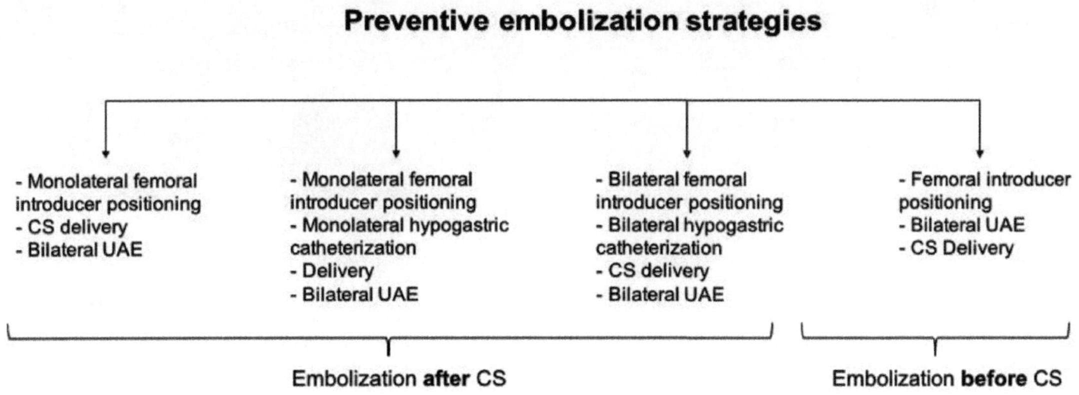

CS cesarean section, *UAE* uterine arteries embolization

16.3.1.1 Preventive Embolization After Cesarean Delivery

The rationale of conducting UAs embolization (UAE) immediately after cesarean delivery is to prevent a possible PPH, by occluding the target vessels just after an eventual arterial injury.

In order to reduce the delay between fetus extraction and embolization, the cesarean section can be performed in the angio-suite or the interventional radiologists can work with a mobile C-arm in the operating room; in both cases, these strategies allow to avoid patient transfer from the operating rooms to the angio-suites.

Literature data are varied, with different endovascular techniques. Results are not reported in a homogeneous fashion among the different papers; however, in all cases benefits from this kind of approach are reported compared to those patients managed without. Vascular access is usually obtained before surgery (Fig. 16.2).

Izbizky et al. [16] performed a ten-year retrospective analysis on 95 patients with suspected placenta accreta treated with prophylactic bilateral uterine artery catheterization before delivery and embolization after cesarean section; in that series, clinical success, defined as no maternal death or major blood loss, was achieved in 86% of patients; 14% of patients received large-volume blood transfusions, and 83% of patients underwent a hysterectomy.

Pan et al. [17] proposed to catheterize the left uterine artery before delivery and to embolize both uterine arteries with gelfoam pledgets immediately after cesarean delivery (Fig. 16.3). The mean fetal absorbed radiation and fluoroscopy time were 30.6 mGy and 158 s, respectively, while the mean maternal absorbed radiation and fluoroscopy time were 117.5 mGy and 612 s, respectively. Comparing two groups of patients (26 UAE vs. 19 control), they concluded that prophylactic intraoperative UAE was relatively safe and effective for reducing postpartum hemorrhage among patients with placenta accreta while the potential benefits could be lower among patients with placenta increta or percreta.

Li et al. [18] described more encouraging results on 12 patients (four previa, seven accreta, one percreta) managed with a procedural protocol similar to the one abovementioned by Pan et al. [17]; ten patients retained their uterus, the mean operative blood loss was 1391 mL, the

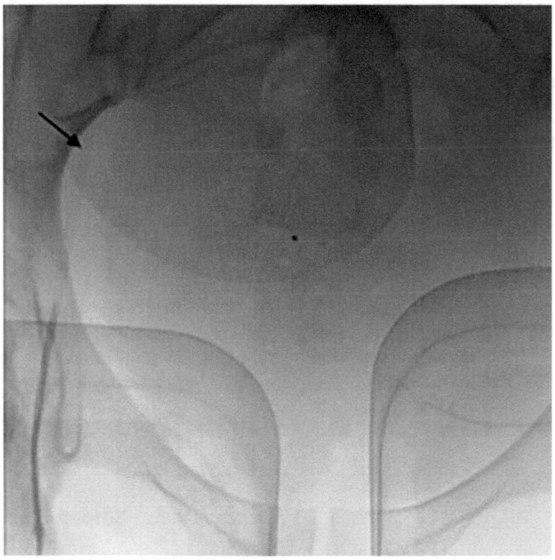

Fig. 16.2 Thirty-eight-year-old lady affected by placenta accreta. Right monolateral femoral 5French introducer positioned before cesarean section (*black arrow*); embolization was performed just after delivery. Fetus skull is evident (*black asterisk*)

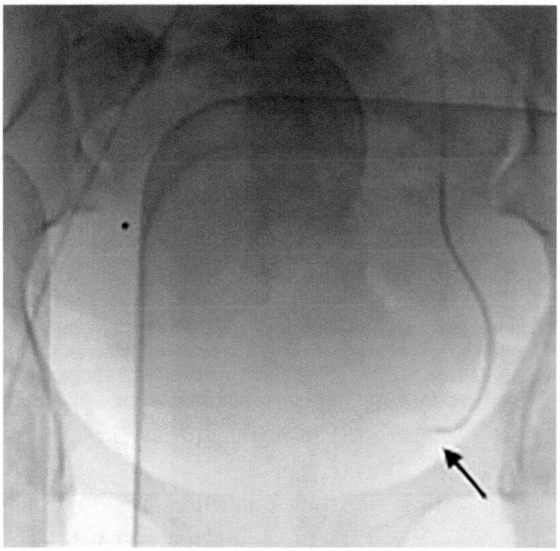

Fig. 16.3 Forty-year-old lady affected by placenta increta. By a right monolateral femoral access, the left uterine 5 French catheterization was performed before delivery (*black arrow*); after the cesarean section, embolization was performed with spongel pledgets. Fetus skull is evident (*black asterisk*)

average fetal X-ray dose was 17.66 mGy, and the average fluoroscopy time was 1 min 42 s.

Diop et al. [19] positioned bilateral femoral 4 French accesses in a group of six patients with placenta accreta. They transferred the patients from the operating room to the angio-suite immediately after delivery and they performed UAE with gelfoam or particles; comparing their data with a control group of 11 patients with accretism, they found a statistically significant difference in blood loss, favorable for the preventive group.

Bouvier et al. [20] reported their experience on 14 patients (ten accreta and four percreta) performing preventive hypogastric arteries embolization after cesarean delivery; in this study the authors described the feasibility of acting the cesarean delivery into the angio-suite in order to immediately proceed with embolization after newborn extraction. They positioned a 4 French introducer just before delivery and then embolized the vessels contributing to utero-placental perfusion with gelatin sponge or particles; 50% of the patients had PPH while in the other 50% blood loss was insignificant.

Lastly, in 2019, Yuan et al. [21] published their retrospective analysis on 54 patients with placenta accreta: in 28, a monolateral 5 Fr femoral access was positioned and after cesarean delivery in the angio-suite, preventive UAE was performed with gelfoam pledgets; compared to the control group of 26 patients, no differences in hysterectomy incidence or duration of ICU stay or postoperative hospitalization were appreciated; however, the incidence of disseminated intravascular coagulation (DIC), mean estimated blood loss, and blood transfusion ($P = 0.011$) were significantly lower in the UAE group.

16.3.1.2 Preventive Embolization Before Cesarean Delivery

The rationale of conducting UAE immediately before the cesarean delivery is to prevent a possible PPH, but in this case the procedural aim is to occlude the target vessels even before they might be injured, or else before placental detachment.

The whole procedure, intended from the vascular access to the embolics injection, is performed before cesarean surgery (Fig. 16.4).

An Italian group had proposed this strategy for the first time in 2016 [22] and then in 2018 [11]. The cesarean delivery was scheduled between the 35th week and the 36th week of gestation; the embolization was conducted in the gynecological operating room with a mobile C-arm. The procedure was performed just before the cesarean delivery through a monolateral femoral access. The embolizing agents adopted were gelfoam particles or calibrated microparticles 500–700 micron. Of 119 patients affected by placenta previa (55) and/or accretism (64) published in two studies [11, 22], the authors reported blood transfusion in 36%–47.8% with a mean of 0.7–1.2 blood units per patient. The hysterectomy rate ranged between 26% and 43.5%. Two patients were transferred to the ICU. The mean uterine dose, considered as the dose to the fetus, was in mean between 15.61 and 26.75 mGy. Concerning the newborn's conditions, no anomalies were reported considering the Apgar score at 5 min and the analysis of the neuro-developmental milestones in all children followed up at 6 months.

16.3.2 Balloon Occlusion Approach

Balloon occlusion is the temporary endovascular occlusion of a vessel, obtained by positioning a catheter presenting an inflatable balloon on its tip; the balloon is then inflated once in correspondence of the target arterial segment and finally deflated when required.

Firstly described by Dubois et al., the prophylactic iliac artery balloon occlusion technique reduces uterine perfusion to decrease the amount of bleeding especially in the area of surgery, improving visualization of the surgical field during cesarean delivery and reducing transfusion requirements [23].

In literature, three different balloon occlusion techniques are described based on different interpositions: prophylactic balloon occlusion (PBO) of the internal iliac arteries (IIA), of the common

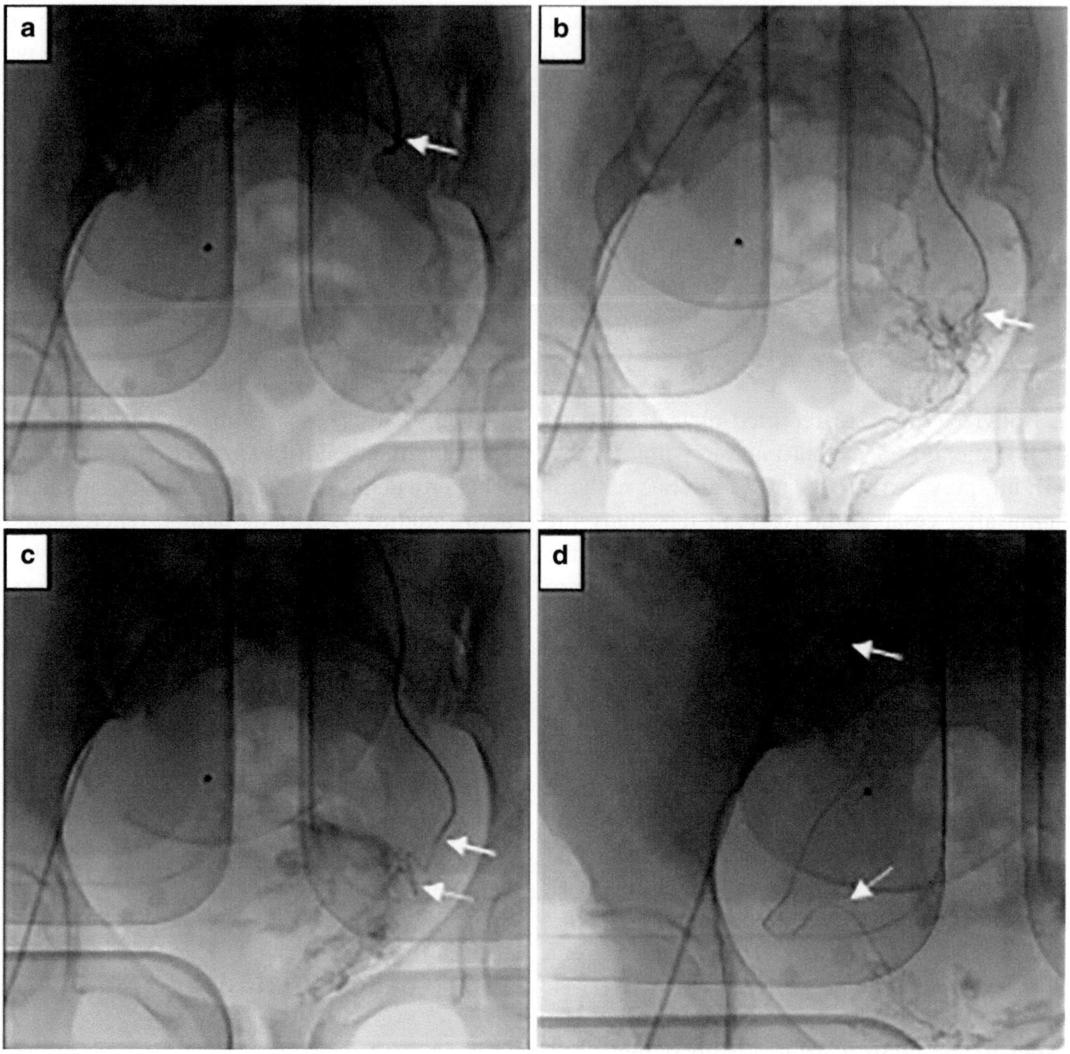

Fig. 16.4 Same patient of Fig. 16.1. Bilateral uterine artery embolization performed with a C-arm in the operating room immediately before delivery with right monolateral femoral access. (**a**) Left hypogastric 5 French catheterization (*white arrow*); (**b**) contrast injection into the hypogastric anterior trunk; (**c**) superselective 2.7 French microcatheterization (*white dotted arrow*) of the left uterine artery; (**d**) right 5 French hypogastric catheterization (*white arrow*) and 2.7 French uterine microcatheterization (*white dotted arrow*). Embolization was performed by injection of 500–700 micron microparticles. In all figures the fetus skull is appreciable (*black asterisk*)

iliac arteries (CIA), and of the infrarenal abdominal aorta (IAA). Figure 16.5 outlines the balloon position in these different techniques.

16.3.2.1 Iliac Artery Balloon Occlusion

Thirty-six publications [23–58] describe the use of the internal iliac artery balloon occlusion technique for PPH prevention in AIP patients.

These articles are divided into two Groups (A and B). Group A (Table 16.2) includes 32 studies [23–54] in which PPH prevention has been obtained by the use of prophylactic balloon occlusion of internal iliac arteries technique (Figs. 16.6 and 16.7). Group B (Table 16.3) includes five studies [52, 55–58] in which PPH prevention has been obtained by the use of prophylactic balloon occlusion of common iliac

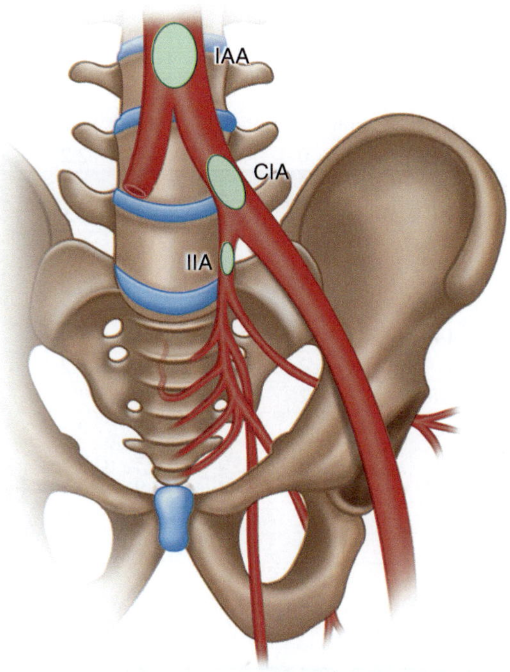

Fig. 16.5 Summary of different balloon-catheter positions into the arterious pelvic district

arteries technique. For each group, three main points are focused: estimated blood loss, number of red blood cell units (RBCU) transfusions, and incidence of hysterectomy.

In Group A, a total of 824 patients with AIP diagnosis at risk of PPH were identified. To evaluate the incidence of hysterectomy, eight articles were excluded describing hysterectomy as an elective procedure [23, 24, 29, 34, 35, 39, 46, 50].

The average incidence of hysterectomies performed in studies was from 0% to 83.3%. In Wang et al.'s [47] experience, hysterectomy had not been necessary in the 48 patients who underwent prophylactic balloon occlusion internal iliac artery technique to control PPH.

Minas et al. [57] showed three cases of hysterectomy: in two cases neither balloon inflation nor embolization can control bleeding and in one other case correlated to balloon rupture.

Fan et al. [42] reported a lower blood loss in patients who underwent balloon placement compared to the control group who were treated only surgically (1.2 L vs. 1.7 L; *p* value 0.01). The

Table 16.2 Group A, internal iliac artery balloon occlusion

Authors (year of publication)	No. of patients who underwent prophylactic balloon	Hysterectomy	Embolization	Complications	EBL (L)	RBC transfusion units
Dubois et al. (1997) [23]	2	2	2	0	1.7	0
Bodner et al. (2006) [24]	6	5	6	NR	2.8	6.5
Carnevale et al. (2011) [25]	21	21	NR	2	1.6	1.24
Nicholson et al. (2018) [26]	22	2	NR	0	1.4	2
Gulino et al. (2018) [27]	16	2	NR	1	1.1	2
Angileri et al. (2017) [28]	37	0	0	9	2	3.9
Shrivastava et al. (2007) [29]	19	19	0	3	2.7	10
Tan et al. (2007) [30]	11	5	5	3	2	3.4
Ojala et al. (2005) [31]	7	3	5	0	4.5	5.4
Sivan et al. (2010) [32]	30	2	23	5	2	4
Viñas et al. (2014) [33]	27	3	8	2	1	NR
Cali et al. (2014) [34]	30	30	NR	6	0.8	0.4
Picel et al. (2017) [35]	90	90	NR	21	2.3	3.5
Youwen et al. (2017) [36]	20	0	7	3	0.8	0.3
Zhou et al. (2019) [37]	58	4	0	8	1.2	1.4
Clausen et al. (2012) [38]	15	6	NR	5	4	5.8
Kidney et al. (2001) [39]	5	5	0	4	2.2	2
Feng et al. (2017) [40]	30	13	16	1	1	0

(continued)

Table 16.2 (continued)

Authors (year of publication)	No. of patients who underwent prophylactic balloon	Hysterectomy	Embolization	Complications	EBL (L)	RBC transfusion units
Tan et al. (2016) [41]	13	9	2	0	1	2.2
Fan et al. (2017) [42]	74	2	6	2	1.2	2.3
D'Souza et al. (2015) [43]	10	3	10	5	1.2	0.5
Broekman et al. (2015) [44]	42	NR	NR	0	0.8	0.2
Darwish et al. (2014) [45]	32	4	NR	21	1.9	2.9
Greenberg et al. (2007) [46]	1	1	0	2	2	9
Wang et al. (2017) [47]	48	NR	14	0	0.6	1.98
Salim et al. (2015) [48]	13	6	7	2	1.6	5.2
Krutman et al. (2013) [49]	15	8	NR	2	NR	2
Yi et al. (2010) [50]	1	1	0	0	0.8	0
Cho et al. (2017) [51]	18	3	8	0	1.9	6.4
Li et al. (2018) [52]	37	9	NR	1	2.9	3.9
Peng et al. (2020) [53]	48	14	NR	0	1.3	NR
Cho et al. (2020) [54]	17	2	8	0	2.3	NR

NR not reported, *EBL* estimated blood loss, *RBC* red blood cells

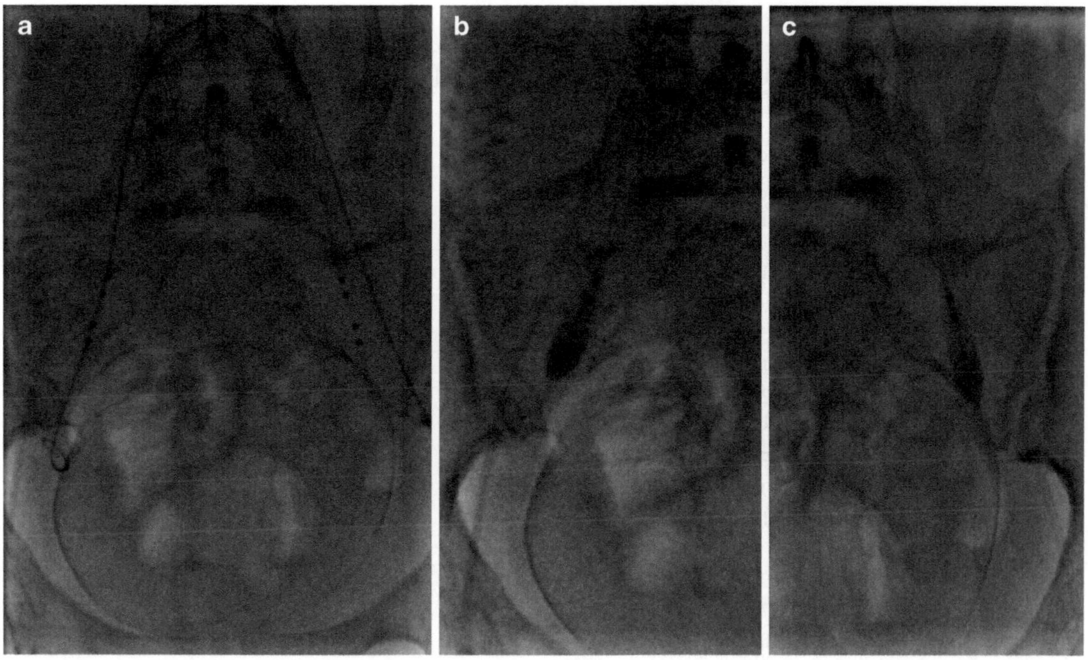

Fig. 16.6 Thirty-six-year-old lady affected by placenta accreta. Preventive IIA balloon placement before cesarean delivery. (**a**) Bilateral IIA catheterization and balloon placement were achieved with contralateral femoral approach (cross-over technique). Right (**b**) and left (**c**) IIA balloon inflated before delivery. *Courtesy of Angileri AS, IRCCS Hospital Maggiore Policlinico Milano, Italy*

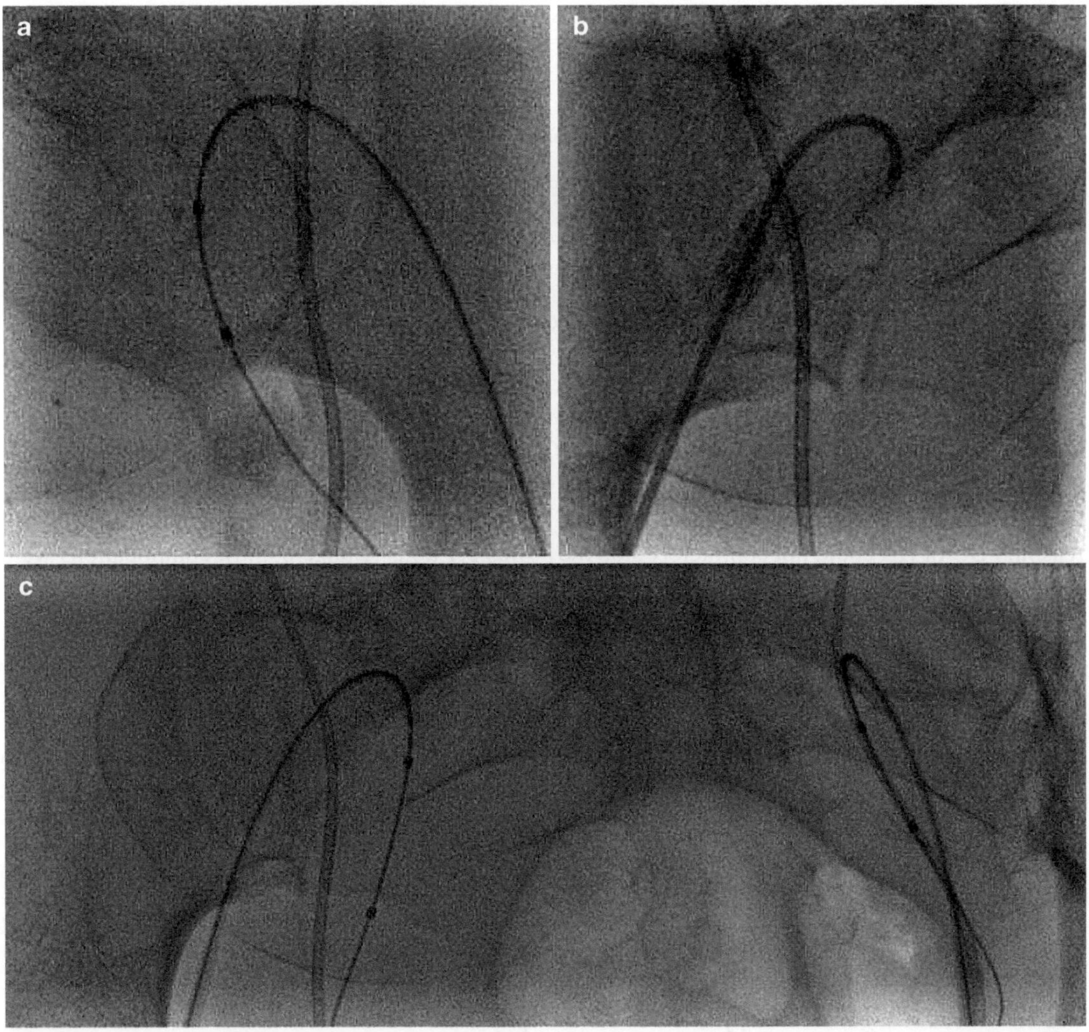

Fig. 16.7 Fluoroscopy images of left (**a**), right (**b**), and final bilateral balloon catheters placement (**c**), achieved with ipsilateral femoral approach, in both internal iliac arteries. *Courtesy of Vallone M, ARNAS Civic Hospital of Palermo, Italy*

average number of RBCU was 2.9 (range 0–10). The balloon placement group shows a lower blood transfusion number compared to control cases without balloon placement.

In the majority of cases, no complication was related to the interventional radiology procedure but to peripartum comorbidities or surgical maneuvers.

In Group B, 84 patients with AIP diagnosis at risk of PPH were identified. The average number of hysterectomies was between 7.1% and 84.6%.

Li et al. [52] reported 42 patients with AIP diagnosis treated preventively with common iliac artery balloon occlusion; only in three cases hysterectomies had been necessary due to uncontrollable bleeding. Moreover, a statistically significant lower blood loss rate had been demonstrated in subgroups where the balloon was positioned in the common iliac artery and infrarenal abdominal aorta group compared to the internal iliac artery (p value < 0.001). A possible explana-

Table 16.3 Group B, common iliac artery balloon occlusion

Authors (year of publication)	No. of patients who underwent prophylactic balloon	Hysterectomy	Embolization	Complications	EBL (L)	RBC transfusion units
Al-Hadethi et al. (2016) [55]	25	16	1	2	2.4	NR
Chou et al. (2015) [56]	13	11	1	3	1.9	NR
Minas et al. (2015) [57]	3	3	NR	0	3.2	4.6
Shish et al. (2005) [58]	1	1	0	1	0.8	1.06
Li et al. (2018) [64]	42	3	NR	1	1	0.06

NR not reported, *EBL* estimated blood loss, *RBC* red blood cells

tion is the existence of collateral circulation, that besides uterine arteries, support blood supply of the uterus through several arteries, including ovarian, femoral, and obturator arteries. For this reason, PBO of IIA could not completely stop the blood flow to the uterus.

The weighted average of blood loss was similar to group A, 1.6 L (range: 0.8–3.2 L). The average number of RBCU transfused was 0.88 (range: 0.6–4.6).

Chou et al. [56] in their experience with 13 patients reported a statistically significant decrease in blood loss for common iliac artery balloon occlusion group compared with controls of similar demographic groups previously published. However, two complications were correlated to the procedure: acute thrombosis of popliteal artery and of external iliac artery, both treated with anticoagulant therapy.

16.3.2.2 Aortic Balloon Occlusion

Sixteen articles [59–74] with aortic balloon placement in infrarenal aorta were considered for a total of 681 patients with AIP diagnosis (Table 16.4).

Hysterectomies incidence ranged from 0% to 22%. Inter-study range blood loss was between 0.6 and 4.5 L.

Xie et al. [62] reported a retrospective experience comparing two groups, with and without infrarenal aortic balloon placement. A significant lower blood loss and decrease in hemoglobin after surgery was found in aortic balloon group compared to the control one, treated only surgically. Moreover, the number of RBCU transfused was 2.1 units (Range 0–5.8); complications were mild and treated conservatively [74].

16.3.2.3 Balloons Technique Comparison

There is much debate in literature about which is the best vascular district for balloon placement to control blood loss and improves several perioperative outcomes in AIP patients. A univoque consensus is lacking.

Li et al. [52] showed a higher effectiveness in common iliac and aortic balloon placement group compared to the internal iliac artery group.

Shahin et al.'s [15] study concludes that prophylactic balloon occlusion of the abdominal aorta was associated with a lower rate of hysterectomy and less blood loss than other modalities.

Aortic occlusion may be a valid alternative compared to conventional treatment (i.e., surgery alone); this technique has considerable advantages in controlling intraoperative hemorrhage, shortening balloon occlusion time, and reducing radiation dose. However, this technique requires a larger introducer, in order to support the balloon against the aortic wall preventing its migration, and also a vascular closure device or surgical removal.

Table 16.4 Aortic balloon occlusion

Authors (year of publication)	No. of patients who underwent prophylactic balloon	Hysterectomy	Embolization	Complications	EBL (L)	RBC transfusion units
Cui et al. (2017) [59]	38	2	12	1	1.5	3.6
Liu et al. (2019) [60]	31	1	9	2	1.9	4
Wei et al. (2016) [61]	45	4	NR	2	0.8	1.7
Xie et al. (2017) [62]	30	5	NR	1	0.9	1.3
Wu et al. (2016) [63]	230	0	2	2	0.9	1.4
Li et al. (2018) [64]	24	2	NR	1	1.6	5.8
Peng et al. (2018) [65]	9	2	2	0	1.8	3.8
Zeng et al. (2017) [66]	48	2	0	5	1.4	5.4
Qiu et al. (2017) [67]	23	5	NR	1	1.7	2.3
Duan et al. (2015) [68]	42	1	42	0	0.6	1.04
Chen et al. (2016) [69]	20	0	1	0	1.1	0.5
Wang et al. (2017) [70]	57	2	16	0	0.4	1.4
Panici et al. (2012) [71]	15	2	NR	0	0.9	0
Masamoto et al. (2008) [72]	1	1	0	0	3.2	3.9
Sun et al. (2018) [73]	19	0	0	1	1.2	2.6
Blumenthal et al. (2018) [74]	16	15	0	7	2	2

NR not reported, *EBL* estimated blood loss, *RBC* red blood cells

16.4 Radiation Dose Reduction Protocols and Safety

In the preventive endovascular scenario, both with embolization and balloon occlusion approaches, it is of paramount importance to adopt all available strategies to keep the radiation dose as low as reasonably acceptable (ALARA protocol). During these procedures, X-ray exposure to the fetus and/or the mother are unavoidable.

The radiological technique must be standardized by applying several measures to achieve an appropriate balance between image quality and radiation dose. In accordance with the SIR and CIRSE guidelines for the use of radiation during pregnancy [75], these measures include:

- Low-dose rate pulsed fluoroscopy with the lowest pulse rate allowed by the equipment
- No angiography exposure
- Use of the "last image hold" to record the study and plan the procedure
- No enlargement of the field of view
- Use of a half-dose filter
- Postero-anterior beam projection
- X-ray tube at maximal distance from the patient
- Tube current as low as possible
- Tube potential as high as possible

Overall, the interventional radiologist should keep the beam-on time to an absolute minimum.

The lifetime cancer risk after a in utero radiation dose of 100 mGy during the third trimester would be the same as for children exposed to similar radiation levels up to the age of 10 years [76, 77]; furthermore, there is no evidence that a radiation dose in the diagnostic ranges (i.e., 100 mGy) is associated with an increased incidence of congenital malformation, stillbirth, miscarriage, or mental disability [78]. However, it should be considered that the risk of childhood cancer incrementally increases after the 10-mGy dose level [79].

The dose estimation should be performed in conjunction with a qualified medical physics expert [75], developing a conservative "worst-case" estimate of conceptus dose.

If the risk analysis of PPH is high, the optimized x-ray–based treatment is justified considering the 100-mGy threshold value [76].

Certainly, to minimize the radiation exposure and maximize the clinical outcome, these procedures should be always performed by experienced operators in the field of pelvic embolization.

References

1. Chen C, Lee SM, Kim JW, Shin JH. Recent update of embolization of postpartum hemorrhage. Korean J Radiol. 2018;19(4):585–96.
2. Delotte J, Novellas S, Koh C, Bongain A, Chevallier P. Obstetrical prognosis and pregnancy outcome following pelvic arterial embolisation for post-partum hemorrhage. Eur J Obstet Gynecol Reprod Biol. 2009;145:129–32.
3. Kassebaum NJ, Bertozzi-Villa A, Coggeshall MS, et al. Global, regional, and national levels and causes of maternal mortality during 1990-2013: a systematic analysis for the global burden of disease study 2013. Lancet. 2014;384:980–1004.
4. Donati S, Maraschini A, Lega I, D'Aloja P, Buoncristiano M, Manno V. Regional maternal mortality working group. Maternal mortality in Italy: results and perspectives of record-linkage analysis. Acta Obstet Gynecol Scand. 2018;97:1317–24.
5. Sheldon WR, Blum J, Vogel JP, Souza JP, Gülmezoglu AM, Winikoff B, WHO Multicountry Survey on Maternal and Newborn Health Research Network. Postpartum haemorrhage management, risks, and maternal outcomes: findings from the World Health Organization multicountry survey on maternal and newborn health. BJOG. 2014;121(Suppl 1):5–13.
6. Sentilhes L, Vayssire C, Deneux-Tharaux C, et al. Postpartum hemorrhage: guidelines for clinical practice from the French College of Gynaecologists and Obstetricians (CNGOF): in collaboration with the French Society of Anesthesiology and Intensive Care (SFAR). Eur J Obstet Gynecol Reprod Biol. 2016;198:12–21.
7. Maraschini A, Lega I, D'Aloja P, Buoncristiano M, Dell'Oro S, Donati S, Regional Obstetric Surveillance System Working Group. Women undergoing peripartum hysterectomy due to obstetric hemorrhage: a prospective population-based study. Acta Obstet Gynecol Scand. 2020 Feb;99(2):274–82.
8. Bateman BT, Mhyre JM, Callaghan WM, Kuklina EV. Peripartum hysterectomy in the United States: nationwide 14 year experience. Am J Obstet Gynecol. 2012;206(1):63.e1–8.
9. Tsolakidis D, Zouzoulas D, Pados G. Pregnancy-related hysterectomy for peripartum hemorrhage: a literature narrative review of the diagnosis, management, and techniques review. Biomed Res Int. 2021;2021:9958073.
10. Thurn L, Wikman A, Westgren M, Lindqvist PG. Massive blood transfusion in relation to delivery: incidence, trends and risk factors: a population-based cohort study. BJOG. 2019;126(13):1577–86.
11. Giurazza F, Albano G, Valentino L, et al. Predelivery uterine arteries embolization in patients affected by placental implant anomalies. Radiol Med. 2018;123(1):71–8.
12. Balayla J, Bondarenko HD. Placenta accrete and the risk of adverse maternal and neonatal outcomes. J Perinat Med. 2013;41:141–9.
13. Giurazza F, Angilleri SA, Corvino F, et al. Postpartum hemorrhages: prevention. Semin Ultrasound CT MR. 2021;42(1):85–94.
14. Niola R, Giurazza F, Torbica A, Schena E, Silvestre M, Maglione F. Predelivery uterine arteries embolization in patients with placental implant anomalies: a cost-effective procedure. Radiol Med. 2017;122(1):77–9.
15. Shahin Y, Pang CL. Endovascular interventional modalities for haemorrhage control in abnormal placental implantation deliveries: a systematic review and meta-analysis. Eur Radiol. 2018;28(7):2713–26.
16. Izbizky G, Meller C, Grasso M, et al. Feasibility and safety of prophylactic uterine artery catheterization and embolization in the management of placenta accreta. J Vasc Interv Radiol. 2015;26:162–9.
17. Pan Y, Zhou X, Yang Z, et al. Retrospective cohort study of prophylactic intraoperative uterine artery embolization for abnormally invasive placenta. Int J Gynaecol Obstet. 2017;137(1):45–50.
18. Li Q, Yang ZQ, Mohammed W, Feng YL, Shi HB, Zhou X. Prophylactic uterine artery embolization assisted cesarean section for the prevention of intrapartum hemorrhage in high-risk patients. Cardiovasc Intervent Radiol. 2014;37(6):1458–63.
19. Diop AN, Chabrot P, Bertrand A, et al. Placenta accreta: management with uterine artery embolization in 17 cases. J Vasc Interv Radiol. 2010;21:644–8.
20. Bouvier A, Sentilhes L, Thouveny F, et al. Planned caesarean in the interventional radiology cath lab to enable immediate uterine artery embolization for the conservative treatment of placenta accreta. Clin Radiol. 2012;67(11):1089–94.
21. Yuan Q, Jin Y, Chen L, Ling L, Bai XM. Prophylactic uterine artery embolization during cesarean delivery for placenta previa complicated by placenta accreta. Int J Gynaecol Obstet. 2020;149(1):43–7.
22. Niola R, Giurazza F, Nazzaro G, et al. Uterine artery embolization before delivery to prevent postpartum hemorrhage. J Vasc Interv Radiol. 2016;27(3):376–82.
23. Dubois J, Garel L, Grignon A, Lemay M, Leduc L. Placenta percreta: balloon occlusion and embolization of the internal iliac arteries to reduce intraoperative blood losses. Am J Obstet Gynecol. 1997;176(3):723–6.
24. Bodner LJ, Nosher JL, Gribbin C, et al. Balloon-assisted occlusion of the internal iliac arteries in

patients with placenta accreta/percreta. Cardiovasc Intervent Radiol. 2006;29:354–61.
25. Carnevale FC, Kondo MM, de Oliveira Sousa W Jr, et al. Perioperative temporary occlusion of the internal iliac arteries as prophylaxis in caesarean section at risk of hemorrhage in placenta accreta. Cardiovasc Intervent Radiol. 2011;34:758–64.
26. Nicholson PJ, O'Connor O, Buckley J, et al. Prophylactic placement of internal iliac balloons in patients with abnormal placental implantation: maternal and foetal outcomes. Cardiovasc Intervent Radiol. 2018;41:1488–93.
27. Gulino FA, Guardo FD, Zambrotta E, et al. Placenta accreta and balloon catheterization: the experience of a single center and an update of latest evidence of literature. Arch Gynecol Obstet. 2018;298:83–8.
28. Angileri SA, Mailli L, Raspanti C, et al. Prophylactic occlusion balloon placement in internal iliac arteries for the prevention of postpartum haemorrhage due to morbidly adherent placenta: short term outcomes. Radiol Med. 2017;122:798–806.
29. Shrivastava V, Nageotte M, Major C, et al. Case-control comparison of cesarean hysterectomy with and without prophylactic placement of intravascular balloon catheters for placenta accreta. Am J Obstet Gynecol. 2007;197:402.e1–402.e4025.
30. Tan CH, Tay KH, Sheah K, et al. Perioperative endovascular internal iliac artery occlusion balloon placement in management of placenta accreta. AJR Am J Roentgenol. 2007;189:1158–63.
31. Ojala K, Perala J, Kariniemi J, et al. Arterial embolization and prophylactic catheterization for the treatment for severe obstetric hemorrhage. Acta Obstet Gynecol Scand. 2005;84:1075–80.
32. Sivan E, Spira M, Achiron R, et al. Prophylactic pelvic artery catheterization and embolization in women with placenta accreta: can it prevent cesarean hysterectomy? Am J Perinatol. 2010;27:455–61.
33. Vinas MT, Chandraharan E, Moneta MV, et al. The role of interventional radiology in reducing haemorrhage and hysterectomy following caesarean section for morbidly adherent placenta. Clin Radiol. 2014;69:e345–51.
34. Cali G, Forlani F, Giambanco L, et al. Prophylactic use of intravascular balloon catheters in women with placenta accreta, increta and percreta. Eur J Obstet Gynecol Reprod Biol. 2014;179:36–41.
35. Picel AC, Wolford B, Cochran RL, et al. Prophylactic internal iliac artery occlusion balloon placement to reduce operative blood loss in patients with invasive placenta. J Vasc Interv Radiol. 2018;29:219–24.
36. Youwen M, Luo D, Lin Y. Clinical application of prophylactic internal iliac artery balloon occlusion combined with uterine artery embolization in patients with abnormally invasive placenta. J Matern Fetal Neonatal Med. 2018;31:3287–92.
37. Zhou X, Sun X, Wang M, et al. The effectiveness of prophylactic internal iliac artery balloon occlusion in the treatment of patients with pernicious placenta previa coexisting with placenta accreta. J Matern Fetal Neonatal Med. 2021;34(1):93–8.
38. Clausen C, Stensballe J, Albrechtsen CK, et al. Balloon occlusion of the internal iliac arteries in the multidisciplinary management of placenta percreta. Acta Obstet Gynecol Scand. 2013;92:386–91.
39. Kidney DD, Nguyen AM, Ahdoot D, et al. Prophylactic perioperative hypogastric artery balloon occlusion in abnormal placentation. AJR Am J Roentgenol. 2001;176:1521–4.
40. Feng S, Liao Z, Huang H. Effect of prophylactic placement of internal iliac artery balloon catheters on outcomes of women with placenta accreta: an impact study. Anaesthesia. 2017;72:853–8.
41. Tan YL, Suharjono H, Lau NL, et al. Prophylactic bilateral internal iliac artery balloon occlusion in the management of placenta accreta: a 36- month review. Med J Malaysia. 2016;71:111–6.
42. Fan Y, Gong X, Wang N, et al. A prospective observational study evaluating the efficacy of prophylactic internal iliac artery balloon catheterization in the management of placenta previa-accreta: a STROBE compliant article. Medicine (Baltimore). 2017;96:e8276.
43. D'Souza DL, Kingdom JC, Amsalem H, et al. Conservative management of invasive placenta using combined prophylactic internal iliac artery balloon occlusion and immediate postoperative uterine artery embolization. Can Assoc Radiol J. 2015;66:179–84.
44. Broekman EA, Versteeg H, Vos LD, et al. Temporary balloon occlusion of the internal iliac arteries to prevent massive hemorrhage during caesarean delivery among patients with placenta previa. Int J Gynaecol Obstet. 2015;128:118–21.
45. Darwish HS, Zaytoun HA, Kamel HA, et al. Prophylactic preoperative balloon occlusion of hypogastric arteries in abnormal placentation; 5 years experience. Egypt J Radiol Nucl Med. 2014;45:751–9.
46. Greenberg JI, Suliman A, Iranpour P, et al. Prophylactic balloon occlusion of the internal iliac arteries to treat abnormal placentation: a cautionary case. Am J Obstet Gynecol. 2007;197:470.e1–470.e4704.
47. Wang YL, Duan XH, Han XW, et al. Comparison of temporary abdominal aortic occlusion with internal iliac artery occlusion for patients with placenta accreta—a non-randomised prospective study. Vasa. 2017;46:53–7.
48. Salim R, Chulski A, Romano S, et al. Precesarean prophylactic balloon catheters for suspected placenta accreta: a randomized controlled trial. Obstet Gynecol. 2015;126:1022–8.
49. Krutman M, Galastri FL, Affonso BB, et al. Review of the cases of 15 patients at high risk of obstetric haemorrhage who underwent temporary bilateral occlusion of internal iliac arteries. J Vasc Bras. 2013;12:202–6.
50. Yi KW, Oh MJ, Seo TS, et al. Prophylactic hypogastric artery ballooning in a patient with complete placenta previa and increta. J Korean Med Sci. 2010;25:651–5.

51. Cho YJ, Oh YT, Kim SY, et al. The efficacy of pre-delivery prophylactic trans-catheter arterial balloon occlusion of bilateral internal iliac artery in patients with suspected placental adhesion. Obstet Gynecol Sci. 2017;60:18–25.
52. Li K, Zou Y, Sun J, et al. Prophylactic balloon occlusion of internal iliac arteries, common iliac arteries and infrarenal abdominal aorta in pregnancies complicated by placenta accreta: a retrospective cohort study. Eur Radiol. 2018;28:4959–67.
53. Peng Y, Jiang L, Peng C, et al. The application of prophylactic balloon occlusion of the internal iliac artery for the treatment of placenta accreta spectrum with placenta previa: a retrospective case-control study. BMC Pregnancy Childbirth. 2020;20:349.
54. Cho SB, Hong SJ, Lee S, Won JH, Choi HC, Ha JY, Moon JI, Park JK, Park JE, Park SE. Preoperative prophylactic balloon-assisted occlusion of the internal iliac arteries in the management of placenta increta/percreta. Medicina. 2020;56(8):368.
55. Al-Hadethi S, Fernando S, Hughes S, et al. Does temproray bilateral balloon occlusion of the common iliac arteries reduce the need for intraoperative blood transfusion in cases of placenta accretism? J Med Imaging Radiat Oncol. 2017;61:311–6.
56. Chou MM, Kung HF, Hwang JI, et al. Temporary prophylactic intravascular balloon occlusion of the common iliac arteries before caesarean hysterectomy for controlling operative blood loss in abnormal placentation. Taiwan J Obstet Gynecol. 2015;54:493–8.
57. Minas V, Gul N, Shaw E, et al. Prophylactic balloon occlusion of the common iliac arteries for the management of suspected placenta accreta/percreta: conclusions from a short case series. Arch Gynecol Obstet. 2015;291:461–5.
58. Shih JC, Liu KL, Shyu MK. Temporary balloon occlusion of the common iliac artery: new approach to bleeding control during caesarean hysterectomy for placenta percreta. Am J Obstet Gynecol. 2005;193:1756–8.
59. Cui S, Zhi Y, Cheng G, et al. Retrospective analysis of placenta previa with abnormal placentation with and without prophylactic use of abdominal aorta balloon occlusion. Int J Gynaecol Obstet. 2017;137:265–70.
60. Liu J, Wang Y, Jiao D, et al. Prophylactic occlusion balloon placement in the abdominal aorta combined with uterine or ovarian artery embolization for the prevention of cesarean hysterectomy due to placenta accreta: a retrospective study. Cardiovasc Intervent Radiol. 2019;42:829–34.
61. Wei X, Zhang J, Chu Q, et al. Prophylactic abdominal aorta balloon occlusion during caesarean section: a retrospective case series. Int J Obstet Anesth. 2016;27:3–8.
62. Xie L, Wang Y, Luo FY, et al. Prophylactic use of an infrarenal abdominal aorta balloon catheter in pregnancies complicated by placenta accreta. J Obstet Gynaecol. 2017;37:557–61.
63. Wu Q, Liu Z, Zhao X, et al. Outcome of pregnancies after balloon occlusion of the infrarenal abdominal aorta during caesarean in 230 patients with placenta praevia accreta. Cardiovasc Intervent Radiol. 2016;39:1573–9.
64. Li N, Yang T, Liu C, et al. Feasibility of infrarenal abdominal aorta balloon occlusion in pernicious placenta previa coexisting with placenta accrete. Biomed Res Int. 2018;6:4596189.
65. Peng ZH, Xiong Z, Zhao BS, et al. Prophylactic abdominal aortic balloon occlusion: an effective method of controlling hemorrhage in patients with placenta previa or accreta. Exp Ther Med. 2019;17:1492–6.
66. Zeng C, Yang M, Ding Y, et al. Preoperative infrarenal abdominal aorta balloon catheter occlusion combined with Bakri tamponade reduced maternal morbidity of placenta increta/percreta. Medicine (Baltimore). 2017;96:e8114.
67. Qiu Z, Hu J, Wu J, et al. Prophylactic temporary abdominal aorta balloon occlusion in women with placenta previa accretism during late gestation. Medicine (Baltimore). 2017;96:e8681.
68. Duan XH, Wang YL, Han XW, et al. Caesarean section combined with temporary aortic balloon occlusion followed by uterine artery embolization for the management of placenta accreta. Clin Radiol. 2015;70:932–7.
69. Chen M, Xie L. Clinical evaluation of balloon occlusion of the lower abdominal aorta in patients with placenta previa and previous caesarean section: a retrospective study on 43 cases. Int J Surg. 2016;34:6–9.
70. Wang YL, Su FM, Zhang HY, et al. Aortic balloon occlusion for controlling intraoperative hemorrhage in patients with placenta previa increta/percreta. J Matern Fetal Neonatal Med. 2017;30:2564–8.
71. Panici PB, Anceschi M, Borgia ML, et al. Intraoperative aorta balloon occlusion: fertility preservation in patients with placenta previa accreta/increta. J Matern Fetal Neonatal Med. 2012;25:2512–6.
72. Masamoto H, Uehara H, Gibo M, et al. Elective use of aortic balloon occlusion in cesarean hysterectomy for placenta previa percreta. Gynecol Obstet Investig. 2009;67:92–5.
73. Sun W, Duan S, Xin G, et al. Safety and efficacy of preoperative abdominal aortic balloon occlusion in placenta increta and/or percreta. J Surg Res. 2018;222:75–84.
74. Blumenthal E, Rao R, Murphy A, et al. Pilot study of intra-aortic balloon occlusion to limit morbidity in patients with adherent placentation undergoing cesarean hysterectomy. AJP Rep. 2018;8:e57–63.
75. Dauer LT, Thornton RH, Miller DL, et al. Radiation management for interventions using fluoroscopic or computed tomographic guidance during pregnancy: a joint guideline of the Society of Interventional Radiology and the cardiovascular and interventional

radiological Society of Europe with endorsement by the Canadian Interventional Radiology Association. J Vasc Interv Radiol. 2012;23:19–32.
76. Manninen AL, Ojala K, Nieminen MT, Perala J. Fetal radiation dose in prophylactic uterine arterial embolization. Cardiovasc Intervent Radiol. 2014;37:942–8.
77. International Commissionon Radiological Protection. Pregnancy and medical radiation. Ann ICRP. 2000;30:iii–viii, 1–43
78. Brent R. Saving lives and changing family histories: appropriate counselling of pregnant women and men and women of reproductive age, concerning the risk of diagnostic radiation exposures during and before pregnancy. Am J Obstet Gynecol. 2009;200:4–24.
79. Tapiovaara M, Siiskonen T. PCXMC: a Monte Carlo program for calculating patient doses in medical x-ray examinations. 2nd ed. https://www.julkari.fi/bitstream/handle/10024/124342/stuk-a231.pdf?sequence=1. Accessed 30 Aug 2021.

GPSR Compliance

The European Union's (EU) General Product Safety Regulation (GPSR) is a set of rules that requires consumer products to be safe and our obligations to ensure this.

If you have any concerns about our products, you can contact us on ProductSafety@springernature.com

In case Publisher is established outside the EU, the EU authorized representative is:

Springer Nature Customer Service Center GmbH
Europaplatz 3
69115 Heidelberg, Germany

Batch number: 10731385

Printed by Printforce, the Netherlands